PUBLIC HEALTH IN CHINA SERIES
Series Editor **Liming Li**

Tropical Diseases in China
Schistosomiasis

Editor Xiao-nong Zhou

People's Medical Publishing House

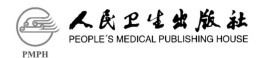

人民卫生出版社

PEOPLE'S MEDICAL PUBLISHING HOUSE

PMPH

Website: http://www.pmph.com/

Book Title: Tropical Diseases in China: Schistosomiasis

(Public Health in China Series)

中国公共卫生：热带病防治实践：血吸虫病（英文版）

Contact address: No. 19, Pan Jia Yuan Nan Li, Chaoyang District, Beijing 100021, P.R. China, phone/fax: 8610 5978 7584, E-mail: pmph@pmph.com

---

Disclaimer

This book is for educational and reference purposes only. In view of the possibility of human error or changes in medical science, the author, editor, publisher and any other party involved in the publication of this work do not guarantee that the information contained herein is in any respect accurate or complete. The medicinal therapies and treatment techniques presented in this book are provided for the purpose of reference only. If readers wish to attempt any of the techniques or utilize any of the medicinal therapies contained in this book, the publisher assumes no responsibility for any such actions. It is the responsibility of the readers to understand and adhere to local laws and regulations concerning the practice of these techniques and methods. The authors, editors and publishers disclaim all responsibility for any liability, loss, injury, or damage incurred as a consequence, directly or indirectly, of the use and application of any of the contents of this book.

First published: 2018
ISBN: 978-7-117-25999-6

Cataloguing in Publication Data:

A catalogue record for this book is available from the CIP-Database China.

Printed in The People's Republic of China

ISBN 978-7-117-25999-6

9 787117 259996 >

Contributors

Chunli Cao

National Institute of Parasitic Disease

Chinese Center for Diseases Control and Prevention

Shanghai, China

Lin Chen

Sichuan Institute of Parasitic Diseases, Sichuan Center for Disease

Control and Prevention

Chengdu, China

Jun Ge, MS

Jiangxi Provincial Institute of Parasitic Diseases

Nanchang, China

Wei Guan

National Institute of Parasitic Disease

Chinese Center for Disease Control and Prevention

Shanghai, China

Qingbiao Hong

Jiangsu Institute of Parasitic Diseases

Wuxi, China

Tiewu Jia, PhD

National Institute of Parasitic Diseases

Chinese Center for Disease Control and Prevention

Shanghai, China

Viktoria Khroundina

The Journal Infectious Diseases of Poverty

Melbourne, Australia

Kassegne Kokouvi, PhD

National Institute of Parasitic Diseases

Chinese Center for Disease Control and Prevention

Shanghai, China

Shi-zhu Li

National Institute of Parasitic Diseases

Chinese Center for Disease Control and Prevention

Shanghai, China

Yousheng Liang, PhD

Jiangsu Institute of Parasitic Diseases

Wuxi,China

Dandan Lin

Jiangxi Provincial Institute of Parasitic Diseases

Nanchang, China

Jiaojiao Lin

Shanghai Veterinary Research Institute,

Chinese Academy of Agricultural Sciences

Shanghai, China

Jianbing Liu

Institute of Schistosomiasis Control

Hubei Provincial Center for Disease Control and Prevention & Hubei Provincial Academy of Preventive Medicine

Wuhan, China

Jinming Liu, MM

Shanghai Veterinary Research Institute

Chinese Academy of Agricultural Sciences

Shanghai, China

Zhihong Luo, MPH
Hunan Institute of Parasitic Diseases
Yueyang, China

Yingjun Qian, MS
National Institute of Parasitic Diseases
Chinese Center for Disease Control and Prevention
Shanghai, China

Zhiqiang Qin, PhD
National Institute of Parasitic Diseases
Chinese Center for Disease Control and Prevention
Shanghai, China

Guanghui Ren
Hunan Institute of Parasitic Diseases
Yueyang, China

Leping Sun
Jiangsu Institute of Parasitic Diseases, China
Wuxi, China

Long Wan
Jianshui Research Station,Key Laboratory of State Forestry Administration on Soil and Water Conservation
School of Soil and Water Conservation, Beijing Forestry University
Beijing, China

Huilan Wang
Hunan Institute of Parasitic Diseases
Yueyang, China

Wei Wang
Jiangsu Institute of Parasitic Diseases
Wuxi, China

Liyong Wen
Institute of Parasitic Diseases, Zhejiang Academy of Medical Sciences
Hangzhou, China

Jing Xu

National Institute of Parasitic Diseases

Chinese Center for Disease control and Prevention

Shanghai, China

Guojing Yang

Jiangsu Institute of Parasitic Diseases

Wuxi, China

Kun Yang

Jiangsu Institute of Parasitic Diseses

Wuxi, China

Pin Yang, PhD

National Institute of Parasitic Diseases

Chinese Center for Disease Control and Prevention

Shanghai, China

Jianfeng Zhang

Institute of Parasitic Diseases

Zhejiang Academy of Medical Sciences

Hangzhou, China

Lijuan Zhang

National Institute of Parasitic Diseases

Chinese Center for Disease Control and Prevention

Shanghai, China

Shiqing Zhang

Anhui Provincial Institute of Schistosomiasis Control

Hefei, China

Yi Zhang

National Institute of Parasitic Diseases

Chinese Center for Disease Control and Prevention

Shanghai, China

Zhengyuan Zhao

Hunan Institute of Parasitic Diseases

Yueyang, China

Bo Zhong

Sichuan Institute of Parasitic Diseases, Sichuan Center for Disease Control and Prevention

Chengdu, China

Jie Zhou

Hunan Institute of Parasitic Diseases

Yueyang, China

Jinxing Zhou

Jianshui Research Station, Key Laboratory of State Forestry Administration on Soil and Water Conservation

School of Soil and Water Conservation, Beijing Forestry University

Beijing, China

Xiao-Nong Zhou, PhD

National Institute of Parasitic Diseases

Chinese Center for Disease Control and Prevention

Shanghai, China

Hong Zhu

Institute of Schistosomiasis Control

Hubei Provincial Center for Disease Control and Prevention & Hubei Provincial Academy of Preventive Medicine

Wuhan, China

Yonghui Zhu

Hunan Institute of Parasitic Diseases

Yueyang, China

Preface

The 60th anniversary of the poem titled "Farewell to the God of Plague" written by Mr. Mao Zedong, the first Chairman of the People's Republic of China, is marked in the year 2018. The major purpose of the poem was to call for the eradication of schistosomiasis in amenable endemic areas of China, after Mr. Mao read the news from People's Daily on 30th June, 2018, that schistosomiasis had been eliminated primarily in Yujiang county, Jiangxi province. The news boosted his confidence that the schistosomiasis eradication is achievable, and that the sufferings of the local people due to the disease in endemic areas will cease. Following Mr. Mao's call, arduous efforts have been made in the last 6 decades to control and eliminate schistosomiasis in China using various control strategies, such as snail control to reduce the intensity of the disease transmission, morbidity control to reduce disease prevalence, and integrated control strategies to block the disease transmission, supported by governments at different levels.

Although the first human case of schistosomiasis japonica was reported in 1905 in Changde, Hunan province, but schisotsomiasis has been epidemic in China for more than 2150 years as revealed through the schistosome eggs found from a corpse in Hunan province. However, the endemic areas of the disease was not clear until 1950 after careful national survey, it was found that more than 200 million people from 12 provinces in southern China, including Anhui, Fujian, Guangdong, Guangxi, Hubei, Hunan, Jiangsu, Jiangxi, Shanghai, Sichuan, Yunnan, and Zhejiang, were at risk of infection with *Schistosoma japonicum* based on the national survey results.

In spite of complexity in the nature of the zoonotic disease as well as social and environment factors, great achievements have been made with the reduction of schistosomiasis prevalence in endemic areas. Of the 12 endemic provinces, five provinces including Shanghai, Guangdong, Fujian, Guangxi and Zhejiang had achieved the criteria of schisotsomiasis elimination, Sichuan province achieved the criteria of transmission interruption, and four other provinces including Jiangsu, Anhui, Jiangxi, Hubei and Hunan achieved the criteria of transmission controlled by the end of 2017. Among 450 endemic counties in the country, schistosomiasis elimination and transmission interruption have been achieved in 229 and 139 counties, respectively. The remaining 82 counties have attained the status of transmission controlled with prevalence less than 1%. In 2014, State Council called for the elimination of schistosomiasis in China by 2030 to achieve the goal of Healthy China strategy.

As we all know that the life cycle of *Schistosoma japonicum* is very complicated, and its transmission was always influenced by various social and environmental factors. Its unique and serious morbidity of schistosomiasis japonica often occurred in human once no proper treatment is provided. However, only simple tools (not sophisticated) were available for use in the national schistosomiasis control programme at that time, which caused much more difficulties in the control programme. Lessons were learnt and experiences garnered while executing control programme from various stages, such as preparation stage, execution stage, elimination stage and consolidation stage. Altogether, these experiences enriched the outcome of the control efforts and more multi-sector resources were integrated into the programme, more innovative tools or approaches from various research projects were applied in the control programme, and more people from community level participated actively in the programme.

By consideration of the numerous combating activities with rich lessons contributed significantly to the successes of the programme, it is worthwhile to distill and synthesize the lessons learnt from the national schistosomiasis control programme in China, so that apply those successful working experiences and approaches into other LMICs. Therefore, this book is trying to i) analyze the changing patterns of schistosomiasis transmission in China at different stages, ii) review the scientific progress which technically support the control and surveillance of schistosomiasis in the field, and iii) summarize the working mechanism and control strategies of multi-sectoral collaboration to promote the national control programme leading to schistosomiasis elimination eventually. We expected that this book will provide adequate knowledge and working experience for infectious disease control and prevention as well as global health in other disease endemic countries to meet the challenges in achieving the United Nation's sustainable development goals by 2030.

Xiao-Nong Zhou

Contents

Chapter 1

History of Schistosomiasis Japonica in China

Ying-jun Qian, Chun-li Cao, Shi-qing Zhang, and Tie-wu Jia

1.1 Discovery of schistosomiasis in China

There is very little information on the discovery of *Schistosoma japonicum* in China. However, four facts as follows: i) the most ancient corpse with schistosome eggs discovered in 1972, ii) the first patient reported in international journal in 1905,[1] iii) the first books published in the field of schistosomiasis epidemiology in 1924, and iv) the first place of *Oncomalania hupensis* snails' habitat discovered in Hankou, Hubei province in 1881,[2] constitute the acquirable knowledge on the discovery of schistosomiasis in China.[3]

Although Chinese traditional medicine attempted to undertake schistosomiasis research described in the Chinese traditional medicine books, systematic studies on etiology, pathogenesis, treatment, and diseases identification were restricted by science and technology in the ancient time. Only clinical signs and symptoms of schistosomiasis were recorded in traditional Chinese medicine books. But, the history of schistosomiasis prevalence in China can be traced back to 2100 years ago on a female corpse. In 1972, during excavation of the Changsha Mawangdui tumulus, *S. japonicum* eggs were discovered in the liver and intestinal tissues of a female corpse (Figure 1.1), providing powerful evidence of over 2100 years of the schistosomiasis prevalence in China.[4]

The first patient was not discovered until 1905 that an American doctor, Logan, who was working in Guangde hospital in Changde, Hunan Province, detected *S. japonicum* eggs in feces of an 18-year-old farmer affected by diarrhea. He published his findings entitled 'A case of dysentery in Hunan Province caused by the trematode, *Schistosomum japonicum*' in the *Chinese Medical Missionary Journal*

1

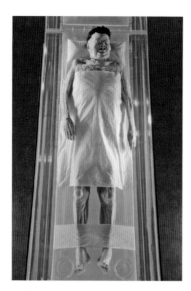

Figure 1.1 *Schistosoma japonicum* eggs discovered
in the liver and intestinal tissues of a female corpse in
Changsha Mawangdui tumulus.

(English version, 1905, 19: 243-245).[1] It was said that 'The patient was from Zhou-jiadian, Changde County. The case was 18 years old and started going fishing at 12. The feces were bloody. When he was 15, the patient was not able to work due to the development of the disease'. It was the first case reported in China. After that, schistosomiasis gradually came to be recognized by Chinese medical practitioners. In order to understand the status of schistosomiasis prevalence in China, early para-sitologists began to carry out many investigations since 1905. For example, Claude, an American doctor who was interested in schistosomiasis, found during his mis-sionary work in rural area of China in 1908 that half of his patients were infected with *S. japonicum*. With the aim to find the source of the infection, Barrow swal-lowed worms discharged from these patients. He found nothing in feces in the first instance, then he suggested that the digestive juice may have some negative effects on the experiment. Secondly, he took baking soda before swallowing and had dinner as usual. It was not until the third instance following this procedure that he excreted eggs. And thusly, he continued to repeat this experiment for one year, eventually taking medicine to kill the worms.[5]

In 1924, a monograph entitled 'Studies on schistosomiasis japonica' was authored by Faust *et al.* on the basis of schistosomiasis investigations in Suzhou, Jiangsu Province, and Jiaxing, Zhejiang Province, China.[2,6] This monograph was the first book published in the field of schistosomiasis prevalence in China, covering the morphology, biology, lifecycle, intermediate host, geographical distribution, pathological anatomy, clinical and laboratory detection, treatment, and the prophylactic aspects of schistosomiasis japonica. It was not until the publication of this book that the international academe started researches on the biology, epidemiology, diagnosis and treatment of schistosomiasis. Therefore, this research laid the foundations for a national public health campaign.

References

1. Logan OT. A case of dysentery in Hunan Province caused by the trematode, *Schistosomum japonicum*. Chin Med J, 1905, 19: 243- 245; 268- 269.

2. Wu ZD, Lv ZY, Zhang SM, et al. The 100th anniversary of the discovery of schistosomiasis in China -- research on schistosomiasis before 1949. J Trop Med, 2006, 6: 105-107 (in Chinese).

3. History of schistosomiasis in Hunan. Hunan Province People's Government counselor, Hunan Research Institute of Culture and History (http://www.hnscss.gov.cn/hxws/wssy/201502/wssw/201508/t20150805_1814931.html, excess on 5 Aug, 2015).

4. Wang LD. Memorizing the 100th anniversary of schistosomiasis discovery in China. People's Health Publish House, 2005. (in Chinese)

5. Zhuji. Crazy scientists. Qingnian Bolan, 2014, 23: 22-23 (in Chinese).

6. Faust EC, Meleney HE. Studies on schistosomasis japonica. Am J Hyg, Monographic Series, 1924, 3: 219.

1.2　History of the National Schistosomiasis Control Programme in China

The historical record for the schistosomiasis prevalence in China was back to 100 years ago. In 1905, Dr Logan, a medical doctor of the USA reported that he discovered *Schistosoma* spp. eggs in the feces of a dysentery patient from Changde City, Hunan Province of China. This was the first reported Chinese case of schistosomiasis in international journal. But, the first epidemiological study was not done until

1924 that Dr Faust conducted a survey on the *S. japonicum* infections in humans in Suzhou City of Jiangsu Province and Jiaxing City of Zhejiang Province.

The serious public health concern due to schistosomiasis was recognized by the government of the People's Republic of China since the beginning of 1950s. Very quickly, the national schistosomiasis control programme was initiated in the country in the 1950s. Up to now, the whole national schistosomiasis control programme can be divided into three stages: the first stage was from the beginning of 1949 to the 1980s, the second stage from the 1980s to the end of the 20th century (1999), and the third stage from the beginning of this century (2000) to the present.

In the first stage from the beginning of 1949 to the 1980s, the basic principle of schistosomiasis control in China was described as prevention by measures adapted to local conditions, with the primary measure being mollusciciding. Since *Oncomelania hupensis* is the sole intermediate snail host of *S. japonicum*, schistosome life cycle and transmission might be interrupted only by the killing of snails. At that time, several approaches, such as control of contamination with schistosome eggs and avoidance of water contact were not good ways for practice, and medicine for treatment of schistosomiasis patients was not so safe and effective. Thus, in an effort to reduce the risk of schistosome infections, an approach of snail killing was implemented. This strategy was performed by environmental modification based on the construction of basic irrigation through water conservation projects, and large-scale use of molluscicides. In addition, large-scale examination of patients and infected animals were also integrated into the programme. Other control measures were supplemented by water clearance of canals to reduce the snail habitats, manure management to reduce the contamination of the environment with parasitic eggs, personal protection by warring shoes, public health education to reduce water contact risks, etc.

In this stage, great achievements were made in schistosomiasis control programme in China, and the geographic range of the endemic areas was reduced significantly. Through the implementation of the national schistosomiasis control programme in the endemic areas, snail habitat area was limited along with the development of the economy in local settings. Consequently, schistosomiasis elimination was achieved in five provinces including Guangdong, Shanghai, Guangxi, Fujian and Zhejiang located in eastern China where there is a high population density. Control measures, such as snail control and chemotherapy in combination with other measures majorly contributed to the achievement of the programme. However, snail elimination was not only costly, but required long-term and repeated implementation. Moreover, molluscicding by using chemical compounds causes environmental pollution. Due to the wide distribution of *O. hupensis*, the breeding environment is too complex to control snail with the fluctuation of water level every year in the lake and mountainous regions, such as Hunan, Hubei, Jiangsu, Jiangxi, Anhui, Sichuan, and Yunnan provinces. Without a radical transformation involving the above measures it is hard to achieve the blocking of schistosomiasis transmission in the target.[1]

In the second stage, the foci of the control strategy were shifted to humans and human behavior, since the expert committee of World Health Organization (WHO) proposed a disease control strategy based on chemotherapy by using praziquantel in 1985, supported by a concept that schistosomiasis is transmitted by people not by snails. With the adjustment of the global schistosomiasis control strategy, the control measures for schistosomiasis in China were also changed significantly. The previous approach of "eliminating snails" was replaced by an approach of "synchronous chemotherapy for residents and livestock, supplemented by the elimination of snail intermediate host focused on areas where there are higher risks of infections, and strengthening activities on health education". The objectives of the national control programme also shifted from "interruption of transmission" to "disease control" through the introduction of World Bank loan project on schistosomiasis control, with an encouragement of active participation of the community.[2] This control strategy was effectively implemented across China with the following facts. First, between 1989 and 1995, the number of people infected with *S. japonicum* decreased from 1,638,103 to 865,084, in accordance to the estimated number of infected cases from two national sampling epidemiological surveys. However, although disease control measures based mostly on chemotherapy could quickly control the transmission of schistosomiasis, it was still difficult to reach the target rate of infection or re-infection. At the end of 2003, 17 counties had recorded the emergence of a transmission rebound. Infected snails with *S. japonicum* had occurred in 21 counties (cities, districts) out of 63 controlled counties (cities, districts).

Since 2004, the control strategy for the national schistosomiasis control programme has been changed to stop the risk of parasite contaminating the environment by eliminating infectious sources. This updated strategy is targeting to reduce human re-infection rate, based on transmission characteristics of schistosomiasis in the lake region of China. This strategic deployment in the national schistosomiasis control programme was supported by comprehensive measures, such as control of infected cattle by fencing water buffalos, building latrines, replacing water buffalos with machines, providing containers to boat-men, etc., supplemented by information, education and communications (IEC) and focal snail control through agricultural projects or water conservation projects. The programme was also supported by the new policy deployment from the central government, such as the State Council formulated the "Mid- and Long-term National Programme of Schistosomiasis Control from 2004 to 2015", and issued the "National Regulation for Schistosomiasis Control". All these policy documents adhered to the principle of "prevention priority, control with scientific measures, implementing by classified guideline in different settings", according to the different epidemic status and transmission characteristics.[3-10] After some years of efforts to effectively curb the epidemic trend, schistosomiasis was under controlled at national scale. This achievement provides more evidences that the control of infectious sources is able to reduce or even stop the disease transmission.

References

1. Wu ZD, Lv ZY, Zhang SM, et al. The 100th anniversary of the discovery of schistosomiasis in China -- research on schistosomiasis before 1949. J Trop Med, 2006, 6: 105-107. (in Chinese)

2. Chen MG, Feng Z. Schistosomiasis control in China. Parasitol Int, 1999, 48: 11-19.

3. Zhou XN, Jiang QW, Sun LP, et al. Schistosomiasis control and surveillance in China. Chin J Schisto Control, 2005, 17: 161-165. (in Chinese)

4. Xu J, Xu JF, Li SZ, et al. Integrated control programmes for schistosomiasis and other helminth infections in P.R. China. Acta Trop, 2015, 141: 332-341.

5. Wu XH, Xu J, Zheng J, et al. Challenges and control strategies in areas of schistosomiasis transmission controlled and interrupted in China. Chin J Schisto Control, 2004, 16: 1-3. (in Chinese)

6. Wang RB, Wang TP, Wang LY, et al. Study on the re-emerging situation of schistosomiasis epidemics in areas under control and interruption. Chin J Epidemiol, 2004, 25: 564-567. (in Chinese)

7. Wang LD, Zhou XN, Chen HG, et al. A new strategy to control transmission of *Schistosomiasis japonicum*. Eng Sci, 2009, 11: 37-43. (in Chinese)

8. Wang LD, Chen HG, Guo JG, et al. A strategy to control transmission of *Schistosoma japonicum* in China. N Engl J Med, 2009, 360: 121-128.

9. Wang LD, Guo JG, Wu XH, et al. China's new strategy to block *Schistosoma japonicum* transmission: experiences and impact beyond schistosomiasis [J]. Trop Med Int Health, 2009, 14: 1475-1483.

10. Yu Q, Zhao GM, Guo JG, et al. Evolvement of comprehensive strategy on schistosomiasis control in various control phases in China. Chin J Pathogen Biol, 2006, 1: 470-473. (in Chinese)

1.3 Epidemiological features of schistosomiasis in different endemic regions in China

Schistosomiasis japonica is distributed across the south of the Yangtze River basin and 12 provinces (municipalities, autonomous regions) in China. According to the geographical characteristics of snail habitats and epidemiological features, the endemic regions are divided into three types, namely: lake and marshland regions, plain regions with waterway networks, and hilly and mountainous regions. The control process is relatively slow and tortuous in lake and marshland regions, and faster in waterway network regions. Mainly endemic areas in plain regions with waterway networks, such as Guangdong, Guangxi, Shanghai, Zhejiang, and Fujian Provinces, achieved the criteria of transmission interruption in 1985, 1988, 1985, 1995, and 1987, respectively. Mainly endemic areas by lake and marshland areas such as Hunan, Hubei, Jiangxi, Anhui, and Jiangsu provinces, as well as hilly and mountainous areas such as Sichuan, Yunnan provinces, have not yet reached the criteria of transmission interruption by 2015. This part aims to introduce the epidemiological features of schistosomiasis in different endemic regions in China and provide a reference for schistosomiasis control.

1.3.1　Lake and marshland regions

Geographical features

Lake and marshland endemic regions are located in the middle and lower reaches of the Yangtze River and the adjacent areas of lakes interlinked with the Yangtze River. They are mainly distributed across Hunan, Hubei, Jiangxi, Anhui, and Jiangsu provinces. The marshland is exposed with large-scale lush vegetation after flooding subsides in fall. Lake and marshland endemic regions are divided into four sub-types comprising fork-beach, islet without embankment, islet with embankment, inner embankment, according to the variability of water levels, the type of snail habitat, geographic position of the residential districts, and epidemiological features (Figure 1.2).[1]

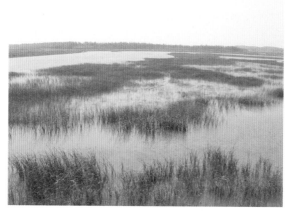

Figure 1.2   Geographical features of lake and marshland regions

Distribution of snails

The distribution of snails in lake and marshland regions is associated with the duration of annual flooding and vegetation. Snails often show a planar distribution with wide range and large scale in marshland areas. The areas "below water in summer and above water in winter" are potential snail habitats due to the uncontrollability of water levels, which results in specific snail distribution characteristics, namely, "two-lines and three-belts". The "two-lines" characteristic includes the lowest and highest snail hypsometric-curve, and the "three-belts" characteristic includes upper scarce snail distribution areas, middle dense snail distribution areas, and lower scarce snail distribution areas. Snails are generally distributed to a certain elevation in lake and marshland areas, while dense snail distribution areas are scattered across the bank and covered by floodwaters for 3 – 5 months of one year. Throughout the 60 years of progress in schistosomiasis control, the distribution of snails has changed greatly in China. The area inhabited by snails decreased from 1,421,000.00 hm^2 in 1950s to 364,324.38 hm^2 in 2014, i.e. a reduction of 74.42%. It is difficult to control snails by conventional means due to the complex environments in lake and marshland regions. The snail areas in lake and marshland regions comprise 96.62% of the total snail areas in China in 2014 (Table 1.1).

Table 1.1   Changes in snail distribution in different types of endemic regions in China.

Year	Water-network regions		Lake and marshland regions		Hilly and mountainous regions	
	Area (hm^2)	Constituent ratio (%)	Area (hm^2)	Constituent ratio (%)	Area (hm^2)	Constituent ratio (%)
1950s	112,000.00	7.89	1,130,000.00	79.52	179,000.00	12.59
2014	147.28	0.04	352,003.76	96.62	12,173.38	3.34

Sources of infection

Livestock is the main source of infection in lake and marshland endemic regions. At the advent of schistosomiasis control, more than 50% of bovines were detected to be schistosome positive.[2] The type of source of infection and its implications for schistosomiasis transmission varied in different regions. Some studies on the contamination index of wild stool in marshland areas have revealed that bovine feces account for more than 90% of infections and domestic pigs account for 6–8% of infections, while other livestock account for smaller proportions. Infected bovines are the primary source of infection in the marshlands of Poyang Lake.[3] A survey conducted in Hanbei River revealed that bovine feces were highly positive with schistosome eggs, which accounted for 97.5% of wild stool and 89.5% of eggs per day (EPD) excreted by the hosts.[4] There are large-scale marshlands along the Yangtze River in Anhui and Jiangsu Provinces, and cattle graze freely by the banks. The infection rate of bovines is generally very high, and reaches as much as 77.3% in some places. The mean infection rate of bovines was 45.42% and the rate of contamination was 99.8% in river beach areas in Anhui Province.[5] A five-year prospective study reported a mean infection rate of 8.23% in cattle, and bovine feces accounted for 85.15% of wild stool in marshland areas in Jiangsu Province.[6]

With developments in livestock husbandry, the sheep population is on the rise. Sheep are a susceptible host for schistosomiasis with higher infection rates, and generally grazing in the habitats of snails. During the period in which waters are rising, fishermen may act as an important source of infection as they live on fishing boats and contaminate the water easily. Thus, the infection rate among snails is generally higher in the moorings. Across different seasons, there are some differences in the types and effects of the main sources of infection in lake and marshland endemic areas: free-ranging cattle and pig are the main source of infection during drought period, while fishermen are the main source of infection during periods of flooding in which water levels raise.[7]

Water contact and infection of residents

There are significant variations in the mode and frequency of contact with contaminated water in lake and marshland areas with variations in geographical environments and living habits. The frequency of contact with infested water of residents in islet without marshland areas is 10 times higher than that of fork-beach areas and embankment areas. There is remarkable seasonal variation in the frequency of contact with infested water in fork-beach and islet with embankment areas, where higher frequencies are usually observed in April, May, October and November. The modes of contact with contaminated water comprised fishing, laundry and dallying in marshlands, and wading, grazing and fishing in fork-beach and islet with embankment areas.[8] Adult males become exposed to infested water primarily through work on paddy fields in the inner embankment areas. Besides this, adult females might be exposed to contaminated water via other means, for example, washing clothes and dishes, while the primary manners of contact with infested water among teenagers include washing clothes and dishes, catching fish, and playing in the water.[9] Generally, the seasons with the highest frequency of contact with infested water are in the spring and summer times, followed by the fall and winter times in lake and marshland areas. The manner of contact with contaminated water primarily includes mowing grass in the spring, washing clothes, swimming, catching fish/shrimp in the summer, and catching fish/shrimp in the fall. Infection can occur throughout the year, except in the winter. Infection rates vary across different types of endemic area, and people living in island and inner embankment areas have the highest infection rate.

At the beginning of the national schistosomiasis control programme, the mean infection rate was above 20% in marshland and embankment endemic areas in the 1950s. The infection rate was positively correlated with the distance from resident housing where local residents live to marshlands. The infection rate among people in marshland regions was 15–30% when the distance was less than 500 m, and 5% when the distance was from 500 m to 1,000 m, and less than 3% when the distance was more than 1,000 m.[10] The infection rate among people in island endemic areas was significantly higher than that in other types of endemic area, and the infection rate could be as high as 50–80% among people living in a distance less than 500 m from living houses to marshlands, while the infection rate was about 30% when the distance was from 500 to 1,000 m. Fishermen were very easily infected with schistosome due to their long periods living on the water and frequent contact with infested water. Acute infection was hard to avoid in lake and marshland endemic regions due to frequent exposure to contaminated water. The outbreak of acute schistosomiasis might take place when a large number of people made contact with infested water due to flooding, harvesting, and swimming. Studies revealed that acute infection was positively correlated with water level of floods, and that the outbreak of acute schistosomiasis might take place in flood years.

1.3.2 Plain regions with waterway networks

Geographical features

Plain regions with waterway networks are primarily distributed across the broad plains between the Yangtze River and the Qiantang River or the plains in the Yangtze River delta region (Figure 1.3). Such regions have convenient traffic condition and

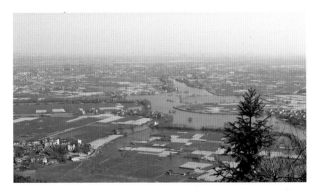

Figure 1.3   Geographical features of plain regions with waterway networks.

are densely populated that people move frequently. The terrain is relatively flat, and waterway networks are arranged in a crisscross pattern. The water level in the river changes marginally in any given year. Waterway network regions are mainly located in Shanghai, and Jiangsu, Zhejiang, Anhui, and Guangdong provinces (Table 1.2).

Table 1.2 Constituent ratio of different types of the endemic regions in China in 1950s.

Municipality/ Province	Water-network regions Constituent ratio (%)	Marshlands and lakes regions Constituent ratio (%)	Hilly and mountainous regions Constituent ratio (%)
Shanghai	14.84	0	0
Jiangsu	59.06	5.91	3.51
Zhejiang	20.32	0.09	22.57
Anhui	5.44	7.9	16.66
Fujian	0	17.7	1.52
Jiangxi	0	36.46	20.5
Hubei	0	31.16	6.83
Hunan	0	0.77	0.73
Guangdong	0.35	0	0.32
Guangxi	0	0	1.46
Sichuan	0	0	14.03
Yunnan	0	0	11.88

Distribution of snails

Oncomelania hupensis snails show a linear distribution along irrigation water systems in plain regions with waterway networks. Snails are generally found within the irrigation ditches through which water flows slowly and in which water levels change marginally, ponds which interlink with rivers and ditches, and the location of import and export of ridges. Rivers, ditches, paddy fields, and beaches are the main breeding habitats for snails in water-network regions. Crisscrossing canals and gullies, field ditches, and sub-lateral canals are the most suitable environments for the breeding of snails in flatland areas. Snails in the paddy fields are generally located along the ridge within 5 m of the inlet or along the ridge near ditches that contain snails. Snails can also be discovered within smaller environments of graveyards, water pools, springs, ponds, dry land, bamboo forests, etc. Snails have been controlled effectively in the past 60 years in plain regions with waterway networks, such that there were only snail infected area of 147.28 hm^2 by the end of 2014 in China (see Table 1.1).

Sources of infection

Sources of infection in water-network regions are mainly patients and animals (cattle, dogs, rats). In water-network areas, livestock are often housed near the houses of local residents. Wild animals have less direct impact due to their distance from residential areas. Adjacent to residential areas, rats are also an important infectious source in water-network regions.

Water contact and infection of residents

Residents in water-network regions live near snail habitats and contact contaminated water frequently in the course of daily life and production. The most significant means of exposure are swimming in rivers, work on farmlands, fishing, washing, etc. The infection rate among people was much higher in the early stages of schis-tosomiasis control programme as higher as over 90% in local residents, of which 34.3% of the total number of patients came from water-network areas. The highest infection rate among people was in the 15–24 year old group. Fisherman, sailors, and farmers had the highest infection rate, followed by rural students and children. The infection rate among males was usually higher than that among females. Acute schistosomiasis usually occurred in summer and fall due to swimming and fishing in rivers.

1.3.3 Hilly and mountainous regions

Geographical feature

In addition to Shanghai, hilly and mountainous regions are distributed across the other eleven endemic provinces in China (see Table 1.2). These regions are charac-terized by sparse population density, large landmasses, and complex topology. The environment is complex, comprising lofty mountain ranges, intermountain basins, and rolling hills (Figure 1.4). Such environments are typically divided into three subtypes, mainly: flat highlands, hills, and high mountain endemic regions.[11] The flat highland subtype areas are mainly located in the basin area of Sichuan and Yunnan provinces, with subtropical climate and developed water systems incorporating rivers and canals. About 50.23% of the endemic villages in Sichuan Province belong to the flatland subtype.[12] In the hill subtype regions, most cultivated hills have terrace style farming of rice and upland crops due to large differences in altitude, and rugged and scattered terrain. The high mountain subtype regions are mainly distributed in the lofty mountains and steep hills of Sichuan and Yunnan provinces. These areas are characterized by complex geographic environments, relatively isolated water system, opening up of hillside terraces, and grassy slopes overgrown with weeds.[13]

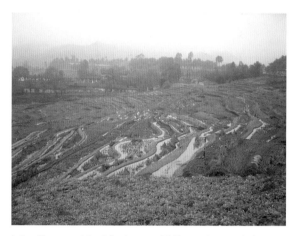

Figure 1.4   Geographical features of hilly and mountainous regions.

Distribution of snails

Snails usually show linear or dot distribution in hilly and mountainous regions. Snails are widely distributed across the edge of flat highland areas or in the central basin in hilly subtype areas, and scattered in various environments, such as terraced fields, ditches, dry land, ponds, wooded land, etc.[14] In high mountain areas, snails take on clustered or dotted distributions. The primary environment for the breeding of snails comprises terrace ridges, small transverse furrows, waste lands, mud fields, permeable rocks, water seepage slopes, seepage lands, valleys, graveyards, etc.[13] Snails on the top of mountains could also spread downhill with rainstorms. In mountain areas, wild lands and drainage ditches are the primary environment for snails. Flatland areas are similar to plain regions with waterway networks of some extent, and snails are mainly distributed in ditches and are easily controlled.

Sources of infection

In hilly and mountainous endemic regions, the major sources of infection are people and domestic animals, such as cattle, horses, sheep, etc. In flat highland areas, the number of eggs per gram (EPG) of people, cattle and dogs take up 87.44%, 12.32% and 0.23% respectively, and humans play a dominant role in sources of infection, followed by cattle.[15] However, there are a large number of domestic animals such as cattle, horses, etc., in the hilly areas. Cattle and human being are the primary sources of infection, followed by pigs and dogs.[16] Pastoral agriculture is the major economic activity due to limited arable land in high mountain endemic areas. The numbers of such domestic animals as cattle, sheep, horses, etc., are enormous, and the numbers of domestic animals exceed even that of the local residents in some regions. The frequent trade of livestock and other domestic animals promotes the flow of infected animals throughout the endemic regions.

Water contact and infection of residents

The infection of residents is influenced by the terrain and the activities that vary in different subtype regions. In hilly subtype endemic areas, people generally have contact with contaminated water by way of farming and daily living, such as washing in the ditches near houses, swimming and fishing in ponds around villages, harvesting, irrigating, etc. The infection rate among people gradually decreases with rising altitude. The infection rate of schistosomiasis shows two temporal peaks, namely, in June and September. A historical review shows that residents living in hilly regions have a higher schistosome infection rate than those living in flatland areas. In high mountain areas, the human infection rate shows strong seasonal trends. Local residents are infected mainly by way of production, while children and teenagers get infected mostly by playing in water. Infection sites are mainly terraced fields and ditches. In flat highland areas, both daily living and production are the most important means of contact with contaminated water. Infection sites are mostly in ditches. The infection rate among males is higher than that among females. Due to the different proportions of paddy fields and dry lands, risks for residents to be contaminated with infested water in production and living also differ, and, even in neighboring villages of the same countryside, the infection rates of residents also differ to some extent. Schistosome infection is closely linked to Personal characteristics, suchas educational attainment, family income, water contact, and ethnicity. The infection rate of residents who are engaged in crop cultivation is significantly higher than that of other workers.

References

1. Chen KX. Sub-type of habitats of *Oncomelania hupensis* in marshland endemic regions. Acta Hunan Med Coll, 1980, 5: 129-130. (in Chinese)

2. Shen W. Review and suggestion on animal schistosomiasis control. Chin J Schisto Control, 1992, 4: 82-85. (in Chinese)

3. Lin DD, Liu YM, Hu F, et al. Animal host of *Schistosoma japonicum* and transmission of schistosomiasis in Poyang Lake regions. J Trop Med, 2003, 3: 383-387. (in Chinese)

4. Huang YJ. Characteristic of wild feces contamination in the river beach. J Prac Parasit Dis, 1998, 6: 86. (in Chinese)

5. He JC, Wang EM, Wang TP, et al. The prevalence situation of schistosomiasis of cattle and transmission role in river beach region in Anhui Province. Chin J Schisto Control, 1995, 7: 288-289. (in Chinese)

6. Sun LP, Zhang YP, Cao Q, et al. Schistosomiasis transmission role of farm cattle in marshland region in Jiangsu Province. J Prac Parasit Dis, 1997, 5: 66-68. (in Chinese)

7. Wu ZW, Xie MS, Zhuo SJ, et al. The relevance of human behavior to the endemicity and control of schistosomiasis japonica in Dongting Lake region. Chin J Schisto Control, 1991, 3: 7-11. (in Chinese)

8. He N, Yuan HC, Zhang SJ, et al. Quantitative research on human water contact after reclamation in an Islet region of *Schistosoma japonicum*. Chin J Parasitol Parasit Dis, 1997, 5: 410-414. (in Chinese)

9. Guan WH, Yuan HC, Zhao GM, et al. A quantitative study on human water contact in dam circled marsh region of *Schistosoma japonicum*. Chin J Schisto Control, 1999, 11: 211-214. (in Chinese)

10. Lin DD, Zhang SJ. Geographical environment and schistosomiasis transmission in Poyang Lake regions. Chin J Epidemiol, 2002, 23: 90-93. (in Chinese)

11. Mao SB. Schistosomiasis biology and schistosomiasis control. Beijing: People's Health Publishing House, 1991. (in Chinese)

12. Yin ZC, Gu XG, Qiu DC, et al. Schistosomiasis situation in Sichuan Province - report of sampling survey in 2001. J Prac Parasit Dis, 2002, 10: 97-103. (in Chinese)

13. Dong XQ, Feng XG, Dong Y, et al. Epidemiological characteristics and control strategies of schistosomiasis in mountainous areas of Yunnan Province. Chin J Schisto Control, 2008, 2: 135-137. (in Chinese)

14. Gu JG. Prevalence and control of schistosomiasis in hilly endemic regions in China. Chin J Prev Med, 2008, 42: 547-548. (in Chinese)

15. Xu FS, Gu XG, Zhao WX, et al. The role on the transmission of schistosomiasis by different sources of infection in hilly endemic regions. J Prac Parasit Dis, 1995, 3: 129. (in Chinese)

16. Yin ZC, Qian XH, Wu ZS, et al. Analysis on schistosomiasis infection among farm cattle in Sichuan during 2001. Parasit Infect Dis, 2003, 1: 104-107. (in Chinese)

1.4 Burden and impact of schistosomiasis

Schistosoma japonicum infection remains one of the most important public health concerns in China, because the disease causes great loss of human health and socioeconomic development. In the 1950s, schistosomiasis was endemic in 433 counties and cities of china, affecting 12 provinces along the Yangtze River and in the south area of the Yangtze River. When the Chinese population was approximately 600 million (United Nations, 2002), an estimated 100 million were at risk of schistosomiasis and about 11.6 million people were infected with *S. japonicum*. The numbers of advanced cases and those with acute schistosomiasis were estimated at around 600,000 and more than 10,000, respectively. Mortality due to advanced schistosomiasis was high, with an estimated case fatality rate of 1%. There were 1.2 million infected cattle and an area of 14,300 km^2 was infested by the intermediate host snail, *Oncomelania hupensis*.

Since the mid 1950s, great achievements have been made in the control of schistosomiasis in China after initiation of the national schistosomiasis control programme. In both humans and livestock, *S. japonicum* infections and snail-infested areas have decreased dramatically. In 2000, the number of infected people had been reduced to an estimated 694,788, snail-infested areas had been decreased by more than 75%, and the disease had been eliminated in five of the 12 previously endemic provinces. Between the mid 1980s and 2003, the criteria of transmission interruption had been reached in 260 counties (60%) and transmission control had been achieved in 63 counties (14.5%). By the end of 2013, there were 184,943 schistosomiasis cases in China, including a total of 29,796 advanced cases. Nationally, there were around 365,467.99 hm^2 of *Oncomelania* snail infested areas in total, with 9.25 hm^2 inhabited by *S. japonicum*-infected snails in 2013. Moreover, 962,065 cattle were estimated to be raised in endemic regions, with 633 determined as positive for schistosomiasis based on stool examinations in 2013. Generally, all data from surveillance show that the endemicity of schistosomiasis in China has decreased in recent 10 years.

1.4.1　Individual impact

The impact of schistosome infections to individuals can be seen in six specific domains, including ordinary life, growth, fertility, production, livelihood and happiness. There is universal consensus that morbidity represents the largest share of schistosomiasis burden, but its true extent is debated. Compared with *S. mansoni* or *S. haematobium* infections, the clinical symptoms of schistosomiasis japonica are more severe than other forms of schistosomiasis. These include fever, headache and lethargy to serious fibro-obstructive pathology, leading to portal hypertension, ascites, and hepatosplenomegaly, and can finally cause death if treatment is not properly provided (Figure 1.5). With the same intensity of infection, the morbidity of the infected persons varies due to the localities of egg deposit. Eggs deposited in the intestine

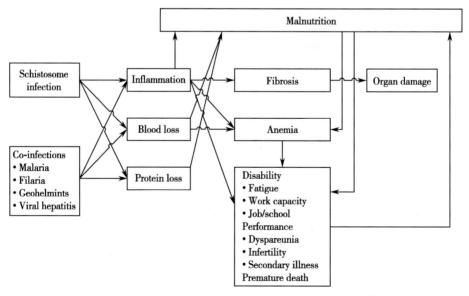

Figure 1.5　Sequelae resulting from schistosomiasis.[1]

usually cause lighter morbidity, compared with those deposited in the brain and spinal cord, as well as in the lungs. A great number of eggs deposited in the lungs could induce pulmonary hypertension, and even cardio-pulmonale. Eggs deposited in the central nerve system could cause severe cerebral or spinal cord schistosomiasis, as demonstrated by surgery or autopsy results.

Based on the duration of the infection and its main clinical manifestations, the disease is divided into three categories in China: i) acute schistosomiasis; ii) chronic schistosomiasis; and iii) advanced schistosomiasis.

Acute cases

Infected persons may or may not have a clear history of infested water contact. Acute infections tend to occur in late spring through to fall. Appearances of acute cases are usually seen in summer and fall, peaking from June to October. People usually get acute infections by swimming, playing, fishing, mowing in marshlands, harvesting crops, combating floods, and so on. Acute clinical disease, or Katayama fever, is usually observed either in persons living in the endemic area at the time of their first exposure or in uninfected persons who reside elsewhere and enter the endemic area for the first time. Fever is the main symptom of an acute infection. Most individuals present with intermittent or remittent fever that peaks in the early morning. Rigor, sweating, headache, general muscular pain, and gastrointestinal disturbances are usually associated with the fever.

Clinically, symptoms in acute *S. japonicum* infection are more severe than those in other forms of schistosome infection. Before praziquantel (PZQ) was available, mortality varied between 2.2% and 20.7% according to reports from different hospitals in China. A historical record of high mortality occurred in 1950 in Xinmin, Gaoyou County, Jiangsu Province. During a flood season, 4,019 out of approximately 7,000 villagers acquired acute *S. japonicum* infection after being contaminated with infested water, and 1,335 patients died. In one village, among 72 residents in 18 families, 46 (63.8%) died of acute *S. japonicum* infection, and seven of the 18 families disappeared. The fatality rate of acute schistosomiasis has significantly decreased since PZQ has been made available. However, without specific treatment, a portion of acute cases may progress to the chronic disease phase, with automatic subsidence of fever and other clinical symptoms, possibly due to a mechanism of endogenous desensitization.

Chronic cases

Usually, more than half of the chronic cases of schistosomiasis are asymptomatic although stool sample examinations may reveal ova of *S. japonicum*.[2] The severity of the disease may be related to the intensity and duration of the infection, location of the egg deposition, immune status of the host, and concomitant diseases. Many of the individuals who have clinical symptoms present with intermittent chronic diarrhea or dysentery. Abdominal pain, diarrhea, or diarrheas with mucus are significant after an individual has been tired or caught a cold. These symptoms lighten or disappear after a period of rest. Hepatomegaly and splenomegaly are common. Infected individuals usually have normal appetites and their working capacities are not, or are only slightly hindered. The consequences of chronic schistosomiasis are manifold, but there are two major aspects: direct morbidity and indirect morbidity. Direct morbidity refers to pathological changes and clinical manifestations induced by the deposition of schistosome eggs in tissues, and subsequent inflammatory immune reactions and calcification of dead eggs. This causes hepatomegaly, splenomegaly, hepatic fibrosis, and various other symptoms; for example, abdominal pain, diarrhea, and mucous bloody stool. Indirect morbidity is not specific. It is often difficult to distinguish this status from the consequences of other infectious diseases, especially soil-transmitted helminth (STH) infections. Indirect morbidity includes nutritional consequences of schistosome infections, such as anemia and growth retardation, and functional consequences, such as cognition impairment and loss of productivity. In addition, the symptoms and signs of chronic cases may become aggravated, resulting in advanced schistosomiasis without timely treatment.

Advanced cases

Advanced or late-stage schistosomiasis japonica can be regarded as an extreme phase of chronic Asian schistosomiasis. It is similar to the advanced hepatosplenic disease caused by *S. mansoni*, which is an infection found in Africa and South

America. In China, advanced schistosomiasis is a chronic disabling condition associated with portal hypertension, splenomegaly, ascites, and gastro-oesophageal variceal bleeding. It can also be linked to severe growth retardation or granuloma-tous disease of the large intestine. In china, advanced cases are registered and man-aged independently from patients with general chronic schistosomiasis. Advanced schistosomiasis is much more common in highly endemic areas because repeated, and heavy exposure to cercariae means that early-stage chronic cases may not be effectively treated in routine control programmes. After two to five years or more, parasite-induced periportal fibrosis may progress to cause obstruction of the portal vessels and damage to the liver parenchyma, leading to the development of advanced schistosomiasis. Mortality eventually results from bleeding of the upper gastrointestinal tract, spontaneous bacterial peritonitis, hepatic failure, and so on. Based on its major symptoms, advanced schistosomiasis japonica in China repre-sents a common, serious health burden. It is classified according to four clinical sub-types: i) ascites; ii) megalosplenia; iii) colonic tumoroid proliferation; and iv) dwarfism.

In the 1950s, it was estimated that 5–10% of the *S. japonicum*-infected indi-viduals in areas highly endemic for schistosomiasis would develop to the advanced stages of disease. At that time, there were approximately 500,000 advanced cases in China. Terms such as "villages of widows" and "villages where all are dead" were used to describe the devastating impact of schistosomiasis across southern China. Over the last 50 years, the implementation of integrated control approaches has suc-ceeded in greatly reducing the health burden due to schistosomiasis in China. At present, dwarfism and colonic tumoroid proliferation are rarely found. However, ascites and megalosplenia are still common, typically in foci of high transmission intensity. These two clinical sub-types can also be found in areas where the transmis-sion of schistosomiasis has been controlled and interrupted for several decades; for example, in Zhejiang Province where schistosomiasis transmision has been inter-rupted since 1995.

By the end of 2008, a total of 412,927 cases of schistosomiasis were found in China. Among these, 30,030 (7.3%) suffered from the advanced form of chronic schistosomiasis japonica. Schistosome infection may play a predisposing role in the causation of colorectal cancer and may have a high relation with viral hepatitis. Several studies have shown that there is a higher prevalence rate of cancers in the large intestine in endemic areas than in non-endemic areas. For example, 44.19 per 100,000 people had cancers in the large intestine in schistosomiasis endemic areas of Jiashan County, whereas only 2.87 per 100,000 people had these types of cancer in non-endemic areas. The incidence rate of hepatitis B in *S. japonicum*-infected persons has also been shown to be four times higher than that of non-endemic populations.

Socioeconomic impact

Schistosomiasis is a drain to social and economic development, especially in the remote and impoverished countryside. Before the P.R. China was founded, a large number of people died from the disease. As a result, a number of families, even entire villages disappeared. In Lantianban Village, Yujiang County, for example, over the course of 50 years before the founding of the P.R. China, the disease had killed over 3,000 people, 20 villages were in ruins, and 14,000 *mou* (over 2,000 acres) of agrarian lands were laid to waste. People who did not die from the disease were emaciated with distended abdomens and unable to hold heavy farm implements. Poor harvests led to famine, and 10% of the peasant population depended on aid from the local government. During a 40-year period between 1909 and 1949 in 34 counties of Jiangxi Province, data from studies have shown that approximately 310,000 people in 1,362 villages died and 26,000 families were affected as a result of schistosomiasis infections. In 1953, in two counties in Anhui Province, Ningguo and Xixian, 132 hectares of cultivated land were unplanted because of a lack of labor and 1,948 houses collapsed because almost all of the residents had died of schistosomiasis.

Schistosomiasis has also greatly impaired the labor power of agricultural populations. About 40% of individuals infected with *S. japonicum* had various degrees of symptoms, resulting in the loss of labor power, with 5 – 10% of those persons suffering from advanced cases unable to do any physical work whatsoever. Schistosomiasis has hindered the growth and development of infected children to such an extent that they may become dwarfs. Endemic populations not only suffer

in terms of their health, but they are also affiliated with poverty. Agricultural production and economic development in rural communities have been significantly
impaired. The disease could also have a negative impact on military defense
capacities. In the summer of 1949, for example, tens of thousands of soldiers and
cadres in the army, who came from northern parts of China (non-endemic areas),
contracted S. japonicum infections during their military training and recreation
activities in the Yangtze River delta areas. This weakened their health and diminished their fighting capacities. At the same time, few young people in endemic
areas were unable to join the army due to schistosome infections. For example, in
1963, a total of 559 young people in Diadong, Kunshan County, Jiangsu Province
had enlisted to join the military, but none of them passed the physical examination—mainly because of schistosomiasis infections. During the 1950s, no young
men were permitted to join the military in schistosomiasis endemic areas of Chili
County, Hubei Province.

1.4.2 Burden of disease

The DALY (disability-adjusted life year) is the metric developed to quantify the
global burden of disease (GBD) in the early 1990s. It is a summary measure of the
health of a population, which combines in a single indicator consisting of years
lost from premature death (YLL) and years of life lived with disability (YLD). One
DALY can be regarded as one lost year of "healthy life". According to the GBD
2013 report, the global DALY for schistosomiasis is 3.06 million health years. This
indicates a burden of disease that is ranked nearly first among neglected tropical
diseases, just after the burden of leishmaniasis (4.28 million DALYs). Community-
based studies on chronic and advanced cases of schistosomiasis in China have
shown that the age-specific disability weights of chronic schistosomiasis ranged
from 0.095 (5 – 14 years) to 0.246 ($\geqslant$60) and those of advanced cases ranged from
0.378 (30 – 44 years) to 0.510 ($\geqslant$60). This data has contributed to the revision and
update of the disability weight of schistosomiasis in the GBD study. Before this, the
GBD programme input "asymptomatic infection" as the majority (approximately
50%) of chronic schistosome infections, which would lead to an underestimation of
the YLD related to schistosomiasis.

References

1. Ross AG, Sleigh AC, Li Y, et al. Schistosomiasis in the People's Republic of China: prospects and challenges for the 21st century. Clin Microbiol Rev, 2001, 14: 270-295.

2. King CH, Dickman K, Tisch DJ. Reassessment of the cost of chronic helmintic infection: a meta-analysis of disability-related outcomes in endemic schistosomiasis. Lancet, 2005, 365: 1561-1569.

Chapter 2

Schistosomiasis Endemic, Diagnosis and Treatment in China

Jing Xu, Zhi-qiang Qin, Zheng-yuan Zhao, Yong-hui Zhu, Jie Zhou, and Zhi-hong Luo

2.1 Diagnosis and treatment of acute schistosomiasis

Within endemic populations, schistosomiasis is a chronic helminthic infection that establishes a long-term, multi-year association with its human host. Acute schistosomiasis can occur from 14 to 84 days after non-immune individuals are exposed to a primary infection or heavy reinfection, especially in high transmission areas. It has an average incubation period of 41.5 days. The acute form of the disease was first described in Japan more than 100 years ago as Katayama fever. More recently, it is referred to as Katayama syndrome. The outbreak of acute schistosomiasis has a serious impact on an individual's health and hinders the development of social economics in endemic areas. Effective prevention, early diagnosis, and treatment will significantly decrease the burdens associated with acute schistosomiasis.

2.1.1 Epidemic features of acute schistosomiasis

Population distribution

The infection of acute schistosomiasis normally occurs in immunologically naïve populations, such as students from primary and junior high schools or migrant workers who are accidentally exposed to infested water containing cercaria. Because of the nature of their work, individuals from endemic areas (for example, fishermen or boatmen) can also be contaminated by large amounts of cercaria and develop acute schistosomiasis syndromes. Recent statistics have shown that more than 40%

of acute cases were school children in the 7 – 18-year age group; the second largest group with acute schistosomiasis was the 31 – 40-year-old population.[1-3]

Seasonal characteristics

Infections with acute schistosomiasis normally occur from May to October in China. The infection season in hilly and mountainous regions tends to be one to two months earlier than that of lake and marshland regions. In hilly and mountainous regions, the number of acute schistosomiasis cases usually reaches a peak during May and June. In lake and marshland regions, the number of acute schistosomiasis cases has two peaks: the first occurs during June and July, and the second during September and October. In recent years, the tendency of the peak value has become weak due to the significant reduction in acute schistosomiasis cases as a result of effective control activities.

Spatial distribution

When acute schistosomiasis occurs, interviews with affected individuals can be helpful to determine the location of the suspected waterbody with which they came in contact. Infected snails and/or livestock are normally found in the foci after con-ducting a survey around the suspected waterbody. Most contaminated waterbodies are located near the residence of infected individuals; for example, around their vil-lages, especially in hilly and mountainous regions, or in cattle grazing areas. Cur-rently, more than 90% of acute cases have been reported in the lake and marshland regions of Hunan, Hubei, Jiangxi, Anhui, and Jiangsu Provinces, with concentration along the Yangtze River and nearby Poyang/Dongting Lake.[1,2,4] Over the last 10 years, there has been an increased pattern in the percentage of imported acute cases reported from non-endemic areas or interrupted areas due to population movements.[5]

2.1.2 Symptomatology

In many cases, acute infections are asymptomatic. The onset of acute schistosomia-sis is related to migrating schistosomula larvae and egg deposition by adult female worms. High-grade nocturnal fever and eosinophilia are generally reported to occur and should alert the clinician to the parasitic nature of the illness, once other potential causes of fever and eosinophilia have been ruled out. Although most patients recover spontaneously after two to 10 weeks, some develop persistent and more serious symptoms, including weight loss, dyspnea, diarrhea, diffuse abdominal pain, hepatomegaly, and generalized rash.

Cercariae dermatitis

After exposure to water containing schistosome cercaria, patients present symptoms such as pruritus erythema or papules. These are caused by the penetration of the skin by cercaria. There are two kinds of cercariae dermatitis. One type is caused by the cercaria of *S. japonicum*, which leads to pimples about the same size as a soybean. Individuals feel itching and numbness. These symptoms disappear after several hours or in two to three days. The second type of cercaria dermatitis is caused by bird or non-human schistosome cercaria. The parasites are trapped in the skin and fail to complete their migration, thus causing an allergic reaction. This is manifest as severe dermatitis, the symptoms of which may take four to seven days to resolve. Sometimes the skin becomes blistered, following by a bacterial infection.

Sensitized individuals who have a history of contact with cercaria often break out in a rash. Those who are infected by cercaria for the first time normally present no or only light symptoms. It may be impossible to determine which type of cercaria has caused the dermatitis. It is also possible that individuals are sometimes co-infested by two kinds of cercaria simultaneously. It has been reported that 12 – 90% of acute schistosomiasis infections have presented with cercaria dermatitis.[6]

Fever

Fever is the primary symptom of an acute infection. It is also an important indicator for assessing the morbidity caused by schistosomiasis. Fever can persist for two weeks and up to one month. Body temperature and the duration of the fever are related to the intensity of the infection and the immune status of infected individuals. There are three types of fever caused by *S. japonicum*: i) Mild fever: 25% of cases present light fever, with body temperature less than 38℃. The systematic symptoms are normally slight and the fever disappears automatically. ii) Intermittent or remittent fever: The majority of cases (70%) present with intermittent or remittent fever, which reaches a peak of 40℃ in the late evening. The temperature returns to normal or below 38℃ after midnight or in the early morning. Patients often have other symptoms at the same time, such as chills, sweating, dizziness, and headache. iii) Relapsing fever: Approximately 5% of acute cases present this kind of fever. The body temperature remains around 40℃. Toxemia syndrome, such as diminished mental capacities, rigor, and dizziness also occur.

Gastrointestinal symptoms

Abdominal symptoms may develop within a few weeks because of the migration of juvenile worms and egg deposition of mature female worms. Gastrointestinal disturbances are prominent. These consist of loss of appetite, nausea, abdominal pain and distension, diarrhea with mucus, and bloody stools. In some cases, individuals present with significant constipation. In a few cases, individuals present with ascites. This may be caused by the widespread formation of acute egg granulomas in the liver and intestines, leading to lymph leaking into the stomach.

Respiratory symptoms

Clinical pulmonary schistosomiasis is frequently seen in the acute phase of the infection. Approximately half of acute patients complain about coughing, with some sputum and occasionally bloody sputum. Coughing is a predominant symptom associated with fever and other acute symptoms. On auscultation, dry or moist rales can be heard. Radiological appearances of the chest have been well documented in previous Chinese literature. There are mainly diffuse, mottled opacities or miliary shadows, poorly or well defined, according to the stage of the acute infection. Hazy shadows also occur, with symmetrical distribution in the mid and lower lung field. The pulmonary hilus is usually enlarged and vascular markings are increased.

Abnormal lung roentgenograms and pulmonary symptoms have been variously reported to occur. Within three to six months after chemotherapy, the abnormal radiological signs disappear. The clinical respiratory symptoms regress within one to four weeks. These symptoms and signs in the lung are considered to be related to hypersensitivity, an inflammatory reaction induced by newly deposited eggs.

Hepatosplenomegaly

Hepatomegaly is common in most cases. Usually, the left lobe of the liver is significantly more enlarged than the right lobe. Individuals may consciously feel pain in liver region. They also experience obvious tenderness when receiving a physical examination. Hepatomegaly may occur 5 cm below the xiphoid, and even more than 6 cm in some cases. A slightly enlarged spleen can be palpated in approximately half of the patients. The spleen may feel soft, with no tenderness.

Other symptoms

Other common symptoms include maransis, weakness, dizziness, arthralgia, hives, and so on. Symptoms of meningoencephalitis, with or without epilepsy, may also appear in the acute phase. The symptoms of meningoencephalitis are suspected to be caused by biochemical or immunological effects of the eggs, with or without cerebral egg deposition.

2.1.3　Detection of acute schistosomiasis

Acute schistosomiasis may be difficult to diagnose in individuals with light infections, since they are likely to possess low worm burden, with low egg production and excretion. The delay in symptom manifestation by weeks to months after exposure adds to diagnostic difficulties.

Laboratory-based examination
Regular blood test

The blood leucocytes and eosinophil count are usually above normal limits during acute schistosomiasis. The peripheral leucocyte count is usually within $(10 - 30) \times 10^9$/L, but may be as high as 50×10^9/L. Eosinophils generally account for $15 - 50\%$ of the total blood leucocytes, but occasionally $> 90\%$.

Liver function test

On electrophoresis, the γ-globulin fraction is usually elevated. Levels of serum alanine aminotransferase (ALT) are increased in partial acute schistosomiasis cases. The concentration of IgM, IgG and IgE increases, while the lymphocyte transformation rate is markedly depressed in acute schistosomiasis.

Immunological test

The cercarien hullen reaction (CHR) is the earliest immunological test that can be given to detect acute schistosomiasis two weeks after infection (exposure to infested water), with positive rates of 95–100%. The circumoval precipitin test, the enzyme-linked immunosorbent assay (ELISA), the indirect hemagglutination test, and recently developed rapid diagnostic kits, such as the dot immunogold filtration assay (DIGFA) and the dipstick dye immunoassay (DDIA) can detect acute schistosomiasis with a sensitivity of nearly 100%. The positive rate of circulating antigen detection can be attained at a rate of 90 – 100%. Nonetheless, there are issues that need to be mentioned. First, serological findings are usually negative at the onset of clinical signs. Consequently, serological investigations must be repeated to identify seroconversion, which may appear up to three weeks after the onset of symptoms and six weeks after being exposed to contaminated water. Upon primary investigation by a physician, serological findings are positive in no more than 65% of the cases. Second, the sensitivity and specificity of serological tests vary with the antigens used. The tests are not uniform throughout the world and most can only be performed in research laboratories.

Parasitological test

Microscopy

Acute schistosomiasis is determined by parasitological tests by finding typical eggs or miracidia in feces under microscopy. The eggs of *S. japonicum* are generally 51 – 73 mm. When the eggs are excreted in the stool, they contain a mature miracidia. Kato–Katz and miracidial hatching techniques are the methods that are normally used, and final check performs under microscopy.

Ova production begins at the end of adult maturation and migration to the mesenteric veins, with at least 30 – 50 days from skin penetration to egg laying. Moreover, early treatment with PZQ can delay egg laying. In the early stages of acute schistosomiasis, a search for ova in stools is typically negative and will remain so until the end of the entire life cycle. Increasing the number of test slides prepared from the same fecal specimen or multiple stool samples tested five weeks after infection would increase the detection rate.

Sigmoidoscopy

Congestion and edema are the main lesions that are manifest in the rectum and sigmoid colon as a result of an acute schistosomiasis infection. The rate of detecting living eggs of schistosome in mucosa of these parts of the body is 50%, which is lower than that of chronic schistosomiasis. This may be due to the short time frame in which adult worms have laid their eggs.

B-ultrasonography

Enlargement of the liver and spleen can be detected through the use of B-ultrasonography. The echo of the liver parenchyma is enhanced and spots on the liver are thicker. The inside diameter is not enlarged and the echoes of partial vein walls are enhanced.

X-ray examination

Two months after infection, flocculent, irregular, massive, and miliary shadows in the middle and lower part of the lungs are present on X-ray films. The increase and thickness of lung texture and the enlargement of pulmonary hilus usually disappear three to six months after infection. Pathogenic treatment could accelerate the disappearance of these symptoms.

2.1.4   Diagnostic criteria

Criteria

Acute schistosomiasis cases are classified into three different categories: suspected cases, clinical cases, and confirmed cases, based on the criteria of schistosomiasis diagnosis issued by Chinese Ministry of Health. A case falls into one of these categories according to epidemiological history, clinical symptoms, and laboratory-based examinations. Specific indicators to help with classification of a case include:

i) A recent history (two weeks and up to one month ago) of water contact in endemic regions before the onset of schistosomiasis.

ii) Clinically presents for fever, hepatomegaly, and increased peripheral eosinophils percentages, accompanied by tenderness in the liver region, splenomegaly, cough, abdominal pain, and abdominal distension.

iii) Presents a positive reaction to immunological tests.

iv) Eggs or miracidia of schistosomes are found as a result of parasitological tests or a sigmoidoscopy.

v) PZQ treatment has been effective.

Suspected cases: Must meet the criteria in i) and ii)

Clinical cases: Must meet the criteria in i), ii), and iii), or i), ii), and v)

Confirmed cases: Must meet the criteria in i), ii), and iv)

Differential diagnosis

Differential diagnosis should be conducted to distinguish acute schistosomiasis from other diseases, such as typhoid, paratyphoid, amebic abscess, miliaris phthisis, and bacillary dysentery. These diseases present clinical symptoms that are similar to acute schistosomiasis, such as fever, hepatosplenomegaly, respiratory symptoms, etc.

2.1.5　Treatment

In contrast to acute *S. haematobium* and *S. mansoni* infections, which are usually self-limited, acute *S. japonicum* infections cause severe morbidity. If untreated, Katayama syndrome infrequently causes death. It is also generally self-limited and simply progresses to the chronic phase. For acute cases with light symptoms and a body temperature lower than 39℃, pathogenic treatment can be given as soon as possible. If cases present serious morbidity, symptomatic treatment should be given first to treat combined infections to improve the condition of the body, then followed by pathogenic treatment at the right time.

Pathogenic treatment

Preziquantel (PZQ) is the best choice for treating acute schistosomiasis. Before PZQ was available in China, the mortality rates among patients in hospital with the severe form of acute infection ranged between 2.2% of 138, 2.8% of 629 and 20.7% of 87, according to different studies. The dose of PZQ for treating acute schistosomiasis for adults and children in China is 120 mg/kg and 140 mg/kg of body weight respectively, over a six-day period. Half of the total dose of the medication is administered in the first two days, while the other half is taken over the remaining four days of the treatment period. PZQ is administrated three times a day. If the body weight of the patient is over 60 kg, the dose of PZQ is equal to that of a patient with a body weight of 60 kg.

　Because PZQ is a fast-acting medicine, the body temperature of patients with light symptoms should return to normal within two to four days after a course of treatment. In patients with medium or severe symptoms, the fever should disappear one week or more after the medication has been administered. Half of acute cases will present Herxheimer Reaction, such as chills or high fever. Body temperature will also increase by 1°C or more than that before treatment. The rebound of body temperature may be caused by the body reacting to the heterologous proteins that are released when a large number of worms die. Great attention should be paid to those patients who experience the Herxheimer Reaction because it may lead to serious morbidity and even death. To prevent or decrease the Herxheimer Reaction, adrenocortical hormones could be administrated simultaneously with PZQ. In order to avoid the inhibition of normal immune response and the occurrence of other side effects, the principle of short-term and appropriate dosage should be applied.

The rebound of body temperature can happen in approximately 20 – 30% of acute schistosomiasis cases. In these instances, patients are suspected to have been infected by schistosomes several times as a result of repeated exposure to infested water. For these cases, a total dose of PZQ at 60mg/kg of body weight over two days or 120 mg/kg of body weight over three or four days should be administered. Positive stool samples obtained as a result of the hatching technique should become negative 18 to 20 days after treatment. Six to 12 months after treatment, the cure rate should be higher than 90%. In a patient whose fever persists for two weeks after one course of treatment, treatment can be repeated once eggs are found in a stool sample 20 days after the first round of treatment. In a patient whose body temperature was normal before treatment, the dose of PZQ that should be given is the same as that for chronic schistosomiasis cases.

PZQ is only effective on two stages of schistosome, including adult worms and early (3 – 8 hour) skin-stage schistosomula. The co-existence of mature and immature worms in infected subjects may prolong fever after PZQ treatment, necessitating additional chemotherapy. Furthermore, some individuals do not respond well to PZQ, especially if they have had repeated exposure to infested water before the onset of the disease. Artemether (AM), used for the treatment of malaria, is also effective against juvenile schistosomes in animals and humans. It has been developed as a prophylactic for the prevention of schistosome infections. In animals, combination therapy with PZQ plus AM is safe and results in higher worm reduction rates than PZQ alone. However, a randomized, double-blind, placebo-controlled trial for the treatment of acute schistosomiasis in China has shown that the combination of AM and PZQ chemotherapy did not improve treatment efficacy compared with PZQ alone.[7]

Adjuvant treatment

Given the symptoms that are presented in acute schistosomiasis cases, symptomatic treatment could be given to balance water and electrolytes. This includes supplements of vitamins, liquids, potassium, etc. For patients with high fever or symptoms of poisoning, corticosteroids could be added to the treatment regime in order to increase the effectiveness of fever reduction and to improve the condition of the body. When concurrent infection occurs, antibiotics should be used in a timely manner.

Corticosteroids (for example, prednisone at 1.5 – 2.0 mg/kg per day for three weeks) are used to treat Katayama syndrome within two months of exposure to infested water. They are also used for the treatment of schistosomal encephalopathy during the oviposition (egg laying) stage. Corticosteroids and anticonvulsants may be needed as adjuvants to PZQ in neuroschistosomiasis, which requires specialized care. Corticosteroids help to alleviate acute allergic reactions and prevent the mass effects caused by excessive granulomatous inflammation in the central nervous system. Anticonvulsants are used to treat seizures associated with cerebral schistosomiasis, but lifelong use is rarely indicated. Surgery should be reserved for particular patients, such as those with evidence of medullary compression and for those who deteriorate despite clinical treatment.

Liver protection

When the liver is damaged due to an acute schistosome infection, treatment for protecting the liver should be administrated simultaneously with pathogenic treatment. These drugs for protection of liver include: i) unspecific hepatinica (antioxidant drugs; for example, vitamins, reduced glutathione, taurine, N-acetyl cysteine); ii) enzyme lowering medicines, such as diammonium glycyrrhizinate, glycyrrhizinic acid, biphenyl dimethyl ester, radix sophorae subprostrata; and iii) xanthate retreating drugs (ademetionine, yinzihuang, corydalis saxicola bunting, and anethol trithione).

2.1.6　Case study

Case 1: The outbreak of acute schistosomiasis in Yangyuan Community in 1989

Yangyuan is located in the south of Wuhan City in China, administering 30 administrative villages with 55,000 people. During the flood season in 1989, a large number of people visited Yujiatou beach, along the Yangtze River. An outbreak of acute schistosomiasis occurred. Based on in-depth analysis of 732 acute schistosomiasis cases with complete data, the transmission pattern of acute schistosomiasis was identified, as follows:[8]

i) Males accounted for 62.70% of acute cases, while the number of acute cases peaked in two age groups of 6 – 14 years old and 20 – 39 years old.

ii) The majority of acute cases were workers (42.08%) and students (38.39%). All of them had a history of swimming at Yujiatou Beach.

iii) Those who contracted acute schistosomiasis had a history of water contact from late June to the middle of August, with peaks in mid and late July. Symptoms were presented from early August to late September.

Case 2: The outbreak of acute schistosomiasis in Hukou County in 2013

On 31 August 2013, an outbreak of acute schistosomiasis was reported through the disease reporting system established in China. Eight cases were from Hukou, where schistosomiasis had reached the stage of transmission controlled. According to the criteria of schistosomiasis diagnosis issued by the Chinese Ministry of Health, there were five comfirmed cases (eggs were found in stool specimens) and three clinical cases (history of water contact, serological positive results, and related clinical symptoms). The eight individuals who contracted the infection were aged from 16 – 49 years old. Five of them were students, one was a teacher, one a worker and one unemployed. Detail information linked to these cases is listed in Table 2.1.

The first case, as indicating patient, presented clinical symptoms on 20 June 2013 and the final case presented on 17 August 2013. The remaining cases presented symptoms from 15 July to 20 July 2013. The typical symptoms of these cases included fever, increased eosinophilic granulocyte, with or without itchy skin. According to the epidemiological survey, all of the patients were infected at the marshland in Helongyan, near Pingfeng Village, Shunde Township, Hukou County during May and June. After diagnosis, all of the patients were administrated a dosage of PZQ over a six-day period. The patients were cured and discharged from the hospital.

Table 2.1   Information of 8 reported acute schistosomiasis cases
in Hukou County in 2013.

No. of cases	Gender	Age	Occupation	Date presented symptoms	Date received diagnosis	Date reported	Category of infection
1	M	28	worker	20/6/2013	31/7/2013	31/8/2013	confirmed case
2	M	17	student	15/7/2013	20/8/2013	31/8/2013	clinical case
3	M	16	unemployed	16/7/2013	15/8/2013	31/8/2013	confirmed case
4	M	20	student	18/7/2013	20/8/2013	31/8/2013	confirmed case
5	M	49	teacher	18/7/2013	24/8/2013	31/8/2013	confirmed case
6	M	17	student	19/7/2013	21/8/2013	31/8/2013	confirmed case
7	M	17	student	20/7/2013	20/8/2013	31/8/2013	clinical case
8	M	16	student	17/8/2013	18/8/2013	31/8/2013	clinical case

References

1. Li SZ, Luz A, Wang XH, et al. Schistosomiasis in China: acute infections during 2005-2008. Chin Med J (Engl), 2009, 122: 1009-1014.

2. Lin CW, Li XR, Guo YH, et al. Simultaneous giant mucinous cystadenoma of the appendix and intestinal schistosomiasis: 'case report and brief review'. World J Surg Oncol. 2014, 12: 385.

3. Li SZ, Zheng H, Abe EM, et al. Reduction patterns of acute schistosomiasis in the People's Republic of China. PLoS Negl Trop Dis. 2014, 8: e2849.

4. Zhang LJ, Gao FH, Xu ZM, et al. A cluster analysis of cases of schistosomiasis japonica using retrospective space-time permutation scan statistics. J Pathogen Biol, 2014, 9: 109-112.

5. Wang Q, Xu J, Zhang L, et al. Analysis of endemic changes of schistosomiasis in China from 2002 to 2010. Chin J Schisto Control, 2015, 27: 229-234. (in Chinese)

6. Zhao WX, Gao SF. Practical schistosomiasis. Beijing: Renwei Publishing House; 1996. (in Chinese)

7. Hou XY, MaManus DP, Gray DJ, et al. A randomized, double-blind, placebo-controlled trial of safety and efficacy of combined praziquantel and artemether treatment for acute schistsomiasis japonica in China. Bull World Health Organ, 2008, 86: 788-795.

8. Zhan ZW, Chen F, Mao CX, et al. Survey on 732 acute schistosomiasis cases in Yanguan District in Wuchang. Chin J Schisto Control, 1991, 3: 60. (in Chinese)

2.2 Diagnosis and treatment of chronic schistosomiasis

Schistosomiasis is a chronic disease caused by parasitic worms called trematodes or blood flukes. It is transmitted through contact with fresh water infested with the cercarial schistosome of a parasite that penetrates human skin. Three species of the genus *Schistosoma* are of major medical importance: *Schistosoma japonicum, S. mansoni, and S. haematobium. S. japonicum* is the most pathogenic schistosome of medical importance Occoured only in southeast Asia including china. The complications of zoonotic transmission for *S. japonicum* increase the difficulty of control, which can only be achieved by integrated interventions.

Chronic schistosomiasis will occur when people are exposed to infested water with schistosome cercaria repeatedly or are infected by small dose of cercaria several times or frequently in daily life. Acute schistosomiasis can evolve into chronic schistosomiasis if patients are not cured timely.[1] The clinical manifestation of chronic schistosomiasis is light, normally with no symptoms or signs of the infection. A few infected individuals develop periportal fibrosis of the liver, which may result in the hepatosplenic form of the disease.

2.2.1 Symptomatology

Chronic schistosomal patients may complain of recurrent vague abdominal symptoms, or disturbances to their bowel habits. Chronic diarrhea or rectal bleeding may mimic ulcerative colitis. Chronic hepatic schistosomiasis is far more serious. It affects immunogenetically predisposed young and middle-aged adults.[2] Its severity correlates with the intensity of infection. The fibrotic, thickened portal tracts appear as "pipe stems", which confer a histopathological characteristic and ultra-sonographic appearance. Most of the accompanying liver enlargement occurs in the left lobe. Eventually the liver shrinks, with typical pre-sinusoidal portal hypertension, which manifests by splenomegaly, portosystemic collaterals, and ascites. The spleen may feel soft, with no tenderness.

2.2.2   Detection of chronic schistosomiasis

Laboratory-based tests

Routine blood examination

Blood leucocytes and eosinophil count usually maintain normal levels in individuals with chronic schistosomiasis. The peripheral leucocyte count is usually within $(10-30) \times 10^9/L$. Some patients occasionally manifest clinical symptoms of anemia, particularly occurred in children.

Parasitological tests

Detection of parasite eggs or miracidia in the stool, or finding eggs through rectal biopsy is the parasitological method to determine the infection of *S. japonicum*.

Immunological tests

With the decrease of prevalence and infection intensity of schistosomiasis, immunological methods were developed to detect antibody or circulating schistosome antigens based on various labelling techniques. Antibody detection-based assays such as indirect hamagglutination test (IHA), enzyme-linked immunosorbent assay (ELISA), rapid diagnostic assays, etc., are widely used for screening of chronic schistosomiasis with relative high sensitivity, easy use and rapidity.[3] The detection of circulating antigens (CAg) is the most direct method as the amount of released antigens from the adult worms in the host varies in direct relation to a change in the worm burden. However, currently they are not widely used due to unsatisfactory sensitivity in patients infected with *S. japonicum*, especially with light infections.

Physical examinations

B-ultrasonography

Enlargement of the liver and spleen can be detected through the use of B-ultrasonography. The echo of the liver parenchyma is enhanced and spots on the liver are thicker. The stages of chronic schistosomiasis always showed clear, smooth or not slippery liver contour, and liver enlargement especially in left lobe. A light spot or band type change, and the echoes of partial vein walls are enhanced. The length and diameter of the spleen in some patients were increased. Particularly the thickness of periportal fibrosis as determined by ultrasound echogenicity is an important indicator, which correlates with liver biopsies in pathological studies. Therefore, in addition to the clinical examination, ultrasound measurements—such as liver size, portal-vein diameter, thickness of the walls of central and peripheral portal branches, spleen size, and splenic vein diameters—improve efforts to determine the stage of the chronic schistosomiasis.

Colonoscopy examination

Adult worms live in the portal vein and its tributaries, notably the inferior mesenteric vein. Although all segments of the colon may be affected, the rectum, sigmoid and descending colon, and the domain of the inferior mesenteric vein are the main sites of pathology in more than 90% of cases. Egg deposition in the submucosa leads to granuloma formation, congestion, edema and polyp formation, and ulceration. Procto-colonoscopy examination helps to establish the diagnosis of *S. japonicum* infections, exclude similar lesions such as ulcerative and amebic colitis, and categorize the histopathological patterns.[4]

2.2.3　Diagnositic criteria

Criteria

The diagnosis criteria for the clinical and confirmed chronic case of schistosomiasisi japonica has been documented as follows:

Clinical chronic case

- Lived in endemic areas or had multiple contamination of water with cercaria of schistosome
- Without symptoms, or presenting abdominal pain, diarrhea, bloody stool occasionally. Most cases have liver enlargement mainly in left lobe while a few patients present symptoms of splenomegaly
- At least one of immunological tests performed positive result

Confirmed chronic case

- Lived in endemic areas or had multiple contamination of water with cercaria of schistosome
- Without symptoms, or presenting abdominal pain, diarrhea, bloody stool occasionally. Most cases have liver enlargement mainly in left lobe while a few patients present symptoms of splenomegaly
- At least one of immunological tests performed positive result
- Found eggs or miracidium of schistosome by parasitological examination or biopsy.

Differential diagnosis

From chronic dysentery, chronic colitis, intestinal tuberculosis

Chronic diarrhea or colitis can be confirmed by detecting *Bacillus dysenteriae*, *Shigella*, amoeba, and other pathogenic bacteria in stool cultures. Chronic dysentery, also called chronic colitis or intestinal tuberculosis, is accompanied by fever and other toxic symptoms. A gastrointestinal barium meal or an endoscopic examination is helpful to obtain an accurate diagnosis.

From chronic viral hepatitis

Most of chronic viral hepatitis patients present with loss of appetite, pain in their liver region, obvious lack of energy and other symptoms, and increased levels of aminotransferase. However, there were no obvious symptoms or signs of viral hepatitis in most of the chronic schistosomiasis patients. Hepatitis B antigen, anti- hepatitis B antibody, especially anti-Hbe IgM (HBeAb), can help to diagnosis hepatitis B virus (HBV) infection.

2.2.4   Treatment

Pathogenic treatment

At present, the drug of choice for anti-schistosomal chemotherapy is PZQ, which is a pyrazinoisoquinoline derivative.[5] The recommended therapeutic dose for adults with chronic schistosomiasis is 60 mg/kg of body weight, administered in two or three equal doses per day in two consecutive days. The recommended therapeutic dose for children with chronic schistosomiasis is 70 mg/kg PZQ in children weighing less than 30 kg. It could be recommended a single oral dose of 40 mg/kg PZQ (once to two times in one day treatment) while in mass treatment programmes.

Adjuvant treatment for liver protection

When the liver is damaged or has lost function due to chronic schistosomiasis, it may be necessary to administer liver-protection medicine simultaneous to the pathogenic treatment. Liver-protection drugs include vitamins, diammonium, glycyrrhizinate, colchicine, ademetionine, radix sophorae subprostrata, and N-acetyl cysteine. Adjuvant treatment with some liver-protection medicine has been successful in reducing fibrosis in clinical patients.

Adverse reactions and contraindications

PZQ is safe, but a few side effects have been reported. These include abdominal pain, headaches, dizziness, and skin rash. Adverse reactions to orally administered PZQ generally occur within a few hours after taking the drug. The duration of these adverse reactions is short.

Symptomatic treatment should deal with patients who show a severe reaction to PZQ treatment. The main adverse reactions are summarized as follows.

Nervous system

The most common symptoms are dizziness and headache. A second set of symptoms for some patients included: insomnia, dizziness, sweating, and muscle twitches. Individual patients also experienced epilepsy and other symptoms. The use of PZQ for psychiatric patients should be prohibited.

Digestive system

The primary symptoms are abdominal pain and abdominal distension. A second set of symptoms for some patients included nausea, vomiting, and diarrhea.

Circulatory system

Many research results indicated that PZQ treatment is safe for the heart. However, if patients show severe heart rate turbulence and/or heart failure, PZQ is not recommended. It is also not advocated in patients with very poor liver compensatory function or renal function with severe disabilities.

References

1. Caldas IR, Campi-Azevedo AC, Oliveira LF, et al. Human schistosomiasis mansoni: immune responses during acute and chronic phases of the infection. Acta Trop, 2008, 108: 109-117.

2. Maizels RM, Pearce EJ, Artis D, et al. Regulation of pathogenesis and immunity in helminth infections. J Exp Med, 2009, 206: 2059-2066.

3. Xu J, Peeling RW, Chen JX, et al. Evaluation of immunoassays for the diagnosis of *Schistosoma japonicum* infection using archived sera. PLoS Negl Trop Dis, 2011,5: e949.

4. Hosho K, Ikebuchi Y, Ueki M, et al. Schistosomiasis japonica identified by laparoscopic and colonoscopic examination. 2010, 22: 133-136.

5. Mahmoud AA. Praziquantel for the treatment of helminthic infections. Adv Int Med, 1987,32: 193-206.

2.3 Diagnosis and treatment of advanced schistosomiasis

Advanced schistosomiasis is one form of chronic schistosomiasis japonica, resulting from one infection with a large quantity of schistosome cercariae or repeated exposure to smaller quantities of cercariae infections, and lack of timely and effectively schistosomicidal treatment. Advanced schistosomiasis mainly manifests as portal hypertension, gastrointestinal bleeding and hepatosplenomegaly. In the 1950s, there were about 600,000 advanced schistosomiasis patients reported in China, accounting for 5 – 10% of total cases.[1] Without good medical conditions and efficacious drugs at that time, the final outcome of advanced schistosomiasis patients tended to be death gradually. In the 1950s, Chairman Mao wrote in a poem entitled "Farewell to the God of Plague" about "hundreds of villages choked with weeds, men wasted away; thousands of homes deserted, ghosts chanted mournfully". This poem vividly reflects the actual horrors of advanced schistosomiasis at that time.

Since the founding of the P.R. China, the Chinese government has paid great attention on medical care and welfare of patients of advanced schistosomiasis. In the era of the Chinese planned economy before 1980s, advanced schistosomiasis case was treated as a work injury and medical care to patients was freely provided by hospitals at all levels, subsidized by local government. Since 1980s, those with advanced cases also had to seek medical services at their own expense partially. After 2004, a large-scale and long-term project titled "Treatment Project on Advanced Schistosomiasis in China" was initiated. Under this treatment project, a certain amount of medical expenses would be subsided by the government if patients reached the standard of hospitalization assessed by "Technical Committee for Treatment Project on Advanced Schistosomiasis in China" and went to the designated hospitals for their treatment.[2] Although at present the endemic situation of schistosomiasis in China has entered the stage of transmission control or elimination, the number of advanced schistosomiasis cases still remains at 29,000 patients.[3]

2.3.1　Clinical subtypes

Owing to the complexity of symptoms, Chinese scientists classified advanced schistosomiasis japonica into four clinical subtypes: i) ascites; ii) megalosplenia; iii) colonic tumoroid proliferation; and iv) dwarfism (Figure 2.1). Other four and raw subtypes are noticed as i) universal; ii) bleeding; iii) hepatic coma; and iv) miscellaneous.[4]

2.3.2   Clinical features

At the advanced stage of schistosomiasis, a variety of clinical manifestations can be observed. These may range from mild to severe, with several gradations in between. Clinically, the most severe manifestations of advanced schistosomiasis are characterized by splenomegaly, portal hypertension, esophageal varices, gastrointestinal hemorrhage, hepatomegaly (typically on the left lobe of the liver), and so on.

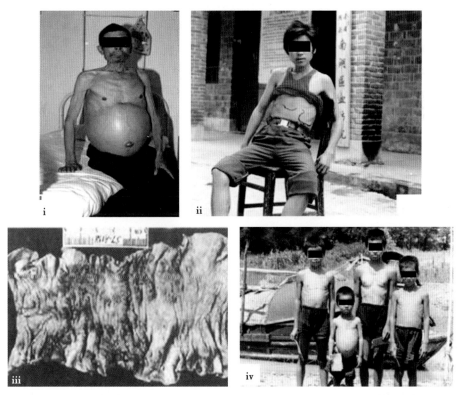

Figure 2.1   Four subtypes of advanced schistosomiasis in China: i) ascites; ii) megalosplenia; iii) colonic tumoroid proliferation; and iv) dwarfism.

General appearance

In the compensated state of advanced schistosomiasis, the stigmata of chronic liver disease are generally absent and the liver function tests are usually within normal limits. Occasionally, an elevation of the r-globulins and moderate elevation of the alkaline phosphatase exist. Sometimes, the large spleen and the prominent, hard left lobe of the liver are the only clinical clues hinting at the existence of the disease.

In the decompensated state of advanced schistosomiasis, patients will present with some degree of portal hypertension, ascites, and a few or all of the clinical stigmata of chronic liver disease. The laboratory tests in these patients often show hypoalbuminemia and variable degrees of derangement of all other tests of liver function.[5]

In most conditions, advanced schistosomiasis occurs in all gradations of inter-mediate forms between the well-compensated and the severely decompensated cases.

Esophageal varices and hemorrhage

Esophageal varices of advanced schistosomiasis occur more frequently than they do in Laennec's cirrhosis. Because of their extensive deep portal collateral circulation and high incidence of esophageal varices, gastrointestinal hemorrhage is a common event. It is often the only reason for which compensated cases seek medical care. Generally, tolerance to hemorrhage in advanced schistosomiasis is good. The mortal-ity rate from bleeding varices is far below that observed in cirrhotic patients. In cir-rhosis, the mortality rate varies from 30 – 80%, yet in advanced schistosomiasis the mortality rate is only 8%.[5] Because of their good tolerance to hemorrhage, the medi-cal management of ruptured esophageal varices in advanced schistosomiasis seems to be very effective. Spontaneous cessation of the hemorrhage starts to occur before any treatment in about one third of the cases. Even so, acute upper gastrointestinal hemorrhage is still a major cause of death in patients with advanced schistosomiasis in China.

Hepatic coma and ammonia tolerance

Hepatic encephalopathy is a severe complication of advanced schistosomiasis. The factors that cause this complication in advanced schistosomiasis can be roughly divided into the following four aspects: i) the increase in nitrogen substance (ammo-nia) and other poisons in the blood; ii) the hypokalemic alkalosis that results from extensive use of diuresis or a large volume of ascites tapping; iii) certain factors that seriously affect the portal system shunt and further deteriorate the damaged liver; and iv) misuse of sedatives and narcotics. The mortality rate of hemorrhage in advanced schistosomiasis is low, which reflects the rarity with which advanced patients develop hepatic coma. The majority of these patients, who belong in the compensated category, are well able to tolerate the overload of ammonia in blood brought about by the hemorrhage into the gut. Only patients with decompensated advanced schistosomiasis show a rise in their arterial blood ammonia. The elevated blood ammonia of decompensated advanced schistosomiasis may mainly be caused by the severely damaged liver. Damage decreases the ability of the liver to metabolize ammonia and makes ammonia directly into the blood circulation without liver metabolism under the condition of portosystemic shunt. The increase in blood ammonia concentration is the most important cause of hepatic encephalopathy. Its clinical symptoms are manifested in changes to intellectual functions and personality, behavior disturbances, disorder of consciousness, and coma.[6]

Ascites

Ascites is clinically graded as mild, moderate, and severe. It is the major clinical sign of the decompensation state of advanced schistosomiasis. It is absent in all compensated cases and is independent of the severity of portal hypertension. Occasionally, severe hemorrhage induces the development of transient ascites and becomes a temporary decompensation in a borderline case. In such cases, there is usually a prompt response to salt restriction and to diuretics. After the bleeding episode, patients may go back to a normal diet. Usually, advanced schistosomiasis patients with pure ascites have a normal appetite and good mental capacities, with frequent diarrhea and emaciation. In severe cases, cachexia, countenance of liver disease, liver palm, and spider telangiectasia are presented, but rarely with jaundice. Glutamic-pyruvic transaminase is usually confirmed in the normal range, or it is slightly elevated. Patients with severe ascites usually manifest as hydrothorax, umbilical hernia or femoral hernia, periumbilical varices, and positive Cruveilh-Baumgerten syndrome.[7]

Jaundice

For decompensated advanced schistosomiasis, mild to moderate hyperbilirubinemia only occurs in a few cases. In these patients, schistosomal cor pulmonale, passive congestion of the liver, and deep jaundice may ensue. After portacaval shunts are done, jaundice may also appear due to hepatic failure, hemolysis, and other factors.[5]

Abdominal wall collaterals

In view of the extensive deep portal collateral circulation, as shown by esophagoscopy or splenoportography, superficial collaterals such as dilated veins on the abdominal wall are uncommon. Hence, venous collaterals on the abdominal wall are clearly not a sensitive clinical index of portal hypertension in advanced schistosomiasis.

Growth retardation and cognitive defects

Fifty years ago, dwarfism affected up to 5% of the population in areas of hyperendemicity. It has now virtually disappeared. The pathogenesis is unknown, but the clinical presentation indicated pituitary growth failure. Schistosomiasis dwarfs had normal mental abilities, but remained sexually immature, with atrophy of the pituitary and gonads. This dwarfism is thought to have been caused by heavy infection of schistosomiasis in early childhood. Cure of schistosomiasis and early hormonal treatment could substantially improve the condition.[8]

Schistosome infection in childhood also causes substantial wasting and growth retardation without pituitary dwarfism.[9] Recent research in Sichuan province in China also indicates that infected children suffer cognitive impairment, with significant adverse effects on memory.[10]

For dwarfism in adolescents with advanced schistosomiasis, protein undernutrition may be responsible for the lack of normal growth. Another possible reason is a peripheral blockade to the action of growth hormone and gonadotrophins, although the production of hypophyseal hormones has been shown to be normal in such patients.[5,11]

2.3.3 Diagnostic approach

Medical history

A history of exposure to infested water is very important, particularly when such exposure took place in a group of individuals who develop a similar clinical course. The clinical findings of outstanding significance are fever, diarrhea, abdominal pain, intermittent blood in the stool, and later, palpable liver and spleen. The diagnosis should be confirmed by positive laboratory results.

Parasitological examination

Schistosome eggs are easy to detect and identify on microscopy, owing to their characteristic size and shape, with a lateral or terminal spine. Currently, the Kato-Katz thick-smear technique is widely used, as it is cost effective, easy to learn, and not technically difficult, and requires limited special resources. This rapid, simple and inexpensive method requires 40–50mg of feces. Generally, as the numbers of stool samples collected and slides prepared increase per patient, so does the sensitivity. Another method is the miracidial hatching test, which has been widely used in China. The test is initiated by the concentration of ova from saline, using fresh feces in a nylon tissue bag and suspension in distilled water.[12] Miracidia that hatch from ova are visualized macroscopically and their presence is diagnostic of infection. This method for detecting a *S. japonicum* infection is easily influenced by environmental factors, such as air temperature, water temperature, light, water pH, etc. It is important to note that both the Kato-Katz technique and the miracidial hatching methods are not suitable for etiologic diagnosis of those advanced cases that have repeatedly received schistosomacidal treatment or have serious granuloma fibrosis of intestinal tract.

For patients with a typical clinical presentation, but negative for fecal eggs, especially in advanced schistosomiasis, a biopsy of the rectal mucosa should be considered for diagnosis. The eggs in the tissues are revealed by pressing the tissue between the slides and examining the tissue under microscopy or by the usual pathological technique of preparing slides from a block of suspected tissues (Figure 2.2).

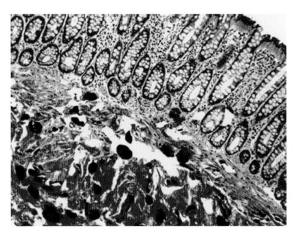

Figure 2.2 Calcified schistosomal ova in a rectal biopsy. Normal mucosa overlying submucosal layer containing numerous calcified *S. japonicum* eggs.[13]

Biochemical markers

Generally, biochemical markers are not very specific given the generalized presentation of the disease. Up to now, biochemical markers of liver fibrosis, such as procollagen peptide types III and IV, the Pl fragment of laminin, hyaluronic acid, fibrosin, tumor necrosis factor, alpha receptor II, and soluble inter-cellular adhesion molecule-1 (sICAM-1), could be measured in serum. These biochemical markers have the potential to provide a highly sensitive and cost-effective method for the assessment of schistosome-induced fibrosis, but are still under investigation.[14]

Scan image examination

Ultrasound

Imaging techniques to diagnose advanced schistosomiasis have mostly focused on ultrasonography. Early use of grayscale ultrasound in the diagnosis of S. mansoni demonstrated lesions on the liver typical of schistosome-induced fibrosis such as periportal fibrosis. These appeared as echogenic tubular shadows with anechoic lumen that radiated from the portahepatis. When viewed crosswise, these tubular structures appeared as bull's eye lesions due to the appearance of the concentric ring of fibrosis surrounding portal venous vasculature.[15] Other ultrasonographic signs of schistosomiasis include hypertrophy of the left hepatic lobe, atrophy of the right hepatic lobe, gallbladder wall thickening, granulomas, and splenic nodules. Stigmata of portal venous hypertension are also demonstrated. In the diagnosis of schistosomiasis liver pathology, in addition to lesions similar to S. mansoni, ultrasonography recorded a mosaic or network pattern typical only for a S. japonicum infection (Figure 2.3).[15,16]

Doppler ultrasound now offers a better future in the detection and diagnosis of advanced schistosomiasis. The fibrotic, thickened portal tracts appear as pipe stems that confer a characteristic histopathological and ultrasonographic appearance. Evidence to date indicated that the trunk of the portal vein, portal vein blood flow, thickness of spleen, width of splenic vein, and the maximum oblique diameter of the hepatic right lobe have correlated well with the degree of liver fibrosis. Doppler sonographic measurements of portal perfusion have been correlated with the presence and degree of esophageal varices, probability of gastrointestinal bleed-

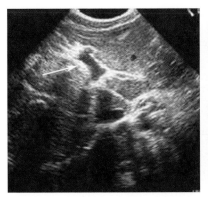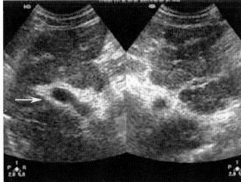

Figure 2.3   Ultrasonographic images in hepatic schistosomiasis. Note the central peripor-tal fibrosis (white arrow) and fibrosis on the periphery of the liver (red arrows) in a patient with advanced schistosomiasis.[17]

ing, and survival in patients with cirrhosis.[18] The limitations of Doppler ultrasound in the diagnosis of advanced schistosomiasis include the following three aspects: i) it is more expensive than the ultrasound model with basic function; ii) it has not been extensively used in the field settings; and iii) personnel who use this technique require additional training.[19]

Computed Tomography (CT) ultrasound

Compared to grayscale and Doppler ultrasonography, the disadvantages of CT ultra-sound are higher equipment and procedure costs, as well as the use of ionizing radia-tion. Like ultrasound, CT can show schistosomiasis-induced changes in liver mor-phology, including atrophy of the right lobe and hypertrophy of the left lobe. CT depicts periportal fibrosis as a band of low attenuation around portal vein branches throughout the liver, which is enhanced following intravenous administration of a contrast media. Similar to ultrasonographic findings, these enhancing periportal regions can be seen as both rounded foci and linear branching patterns, depending on the cross-sectional orientation.[20] The bull's eye lesion on the liver that is demon-strated by ultrasound is seen as concentric layers of periportal enhancement in CT. Some authors regard this as a more specific indicator of schistosomiasis than peri-portal enhancement. Compared with ultrasound, the CT scan can provide accurate diagnosis of ectopic forms of schistosomiasis involving the central nervous system, pulmonary, and other organ sites (Figure 2.4).

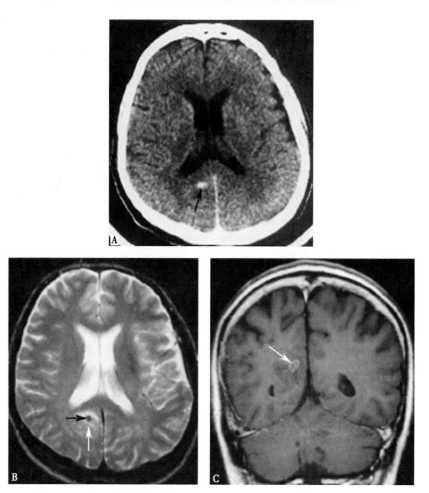

Figure 2.4 Cerebral schistosomiasis. A, an unenhanced axial computed tomography (CT) scan shows a small, oval, hyperdense lesion (black arrow) in the paraventricular zone, dorsal of the right posterior horn; B, an axial T2-weighted magnetic resonance imaging (MRI) shows a hypointense lesion (white arrow) with a small, centrally located area with an intermediate signal (black arrow); C, a coronal contrast-enhanced T1-weighted MR image shows an oval lesion with an intermediate signal (white arrow), with ring-like and septum-like contrast enhancement.[21]

CT can also show splenomegaly, ascites, and prominent collateral circulation, including the formation of varicose veins in the gastric fundus and the distal oesophagus.[22]

MRI

Compared to both ultrasound and CT, MRI is a more expensive imaging modality.

It is similar to CT in its capacity to detect ectopic forms of schistosomiasis, such as schistosomal myeloradiculopathy (SMR) and cerebral schistosomiasis. Its main advantage over CT is its lack of ionizing radiation. The contrast media used for MRI is gadolinium based, rather than the iodine-based contrast media for CT. The hyperechoic periportal is seen on MRI as an accentuation of the periportal signal on T2-weighted images, and of the hypointense signal in relation to the normal liver parenchyma in T1-weighted sequences. The periportal signal becomes accentuated on contrast enhanced T1-weighted images. It has been suggested that the hyperintense signal observed in T2-weighted sequences may differentiate periportal inflammation from fibrosis, which may not be achievable by ultrasound examination.[23] Portal vein thrombosis (PVT), which can occur in patients with advanced schistosomiasis, is best diagnosed by MRI. However, cavernous transformation of the portal vein (CTPV) due to PVT can be detected by Doppler ultrasound, CT, and MRI.

Immunological methods

Immunodiagnostic techniques have a long history to be used in diagnosis of schistosomiasis in China. New ones have been developed and have superseded older ones. In China, there are currently five immunological assays that can serve as an auxiliary diagnosis of advanced schistosomiasis. It is important to note that at present, the primary and common defects of the serologic tests applied in the detection of schistosomiasis make it difficult to distinguish between a recent infection and the history of an infection.

IHA

The assays have shown a high sensitivity (93 – 100%). The false positive rate in healthy people has declined to 1.7 – 3.0%. However, the cross reaction of these assays with *Paragonimus westermani infection* reaches 64 – 84% with the soluble egg antigen (SEA) and 31.3% with a purified egg antigen.[24] IHA is a simple and rapid test,so that it continues to be widely applied for case screening in China.

ELISA

This approach has a higher efficacy on evaluation of cure after treatment. The negative conversion rate one year after effective treatment can be arrived at 42.5 – 100% of cases.[25] When a 107 – 121 kDa fraction of SEA is used as the detecting antigen, the results are further improved. There is no cross reaction with other parasites.[26]

DDIA

The assay is basically a chromatography technique using SEA, labeled with a dye as the indicator system. The test shows a high sensitivity and adequate specificity in healthy people. Aside from *Paragonimus westermani*, cross-reactions with other common parasitic diseases are low.[27]

Polymerase chain reaction (PCR)

Researchers have developed specific and highly sensitive PCR-based assays for the detection of *S. japonicum* DNA in feces or serum/plasma specimens of infected hosts. This potentially provides a test for early diagnosis and therapy evaluation in humans.[28] Recently, a PCR test for the detection of cell-free parasite DNA (CFPD) in human plasma has been devised. This test is showing good prospects for providing a new laboratory tool in the diagnosis of schistosomiasis in all clinical phases of the disease.[29]

2.3.4　Diagnostic criteria

Criteria

Based on the Chinese National Criteria on Diagnosis of Schistosomiasis Japonica, the advanced stage of schistosomiasis japonica is divided into three types of cases: i) suspected; ii) clinically diagnosed; and iii) confirmed. For the suspected case, patients need to match the following conditions: i) have a long-term or repeated history of contact with infested water; or have a definite history of schistosomiasis treatment; and ii) clinically, have symptoms or signs regarding portal hypertension, or show indications of dwarfism or colon granuloma.

For the clinically diagnosed case, patients need supportive data from serum examination—in addition to manifesting the conditions of the suspected phase. That is, for cases without a history of schistosomiasis treatment, or with a treatment history that is more than three years ago, IHA and/or ELISA should be positive. For untreated cases or cases that have been treated at least one year ago, the serum circulating antigen should be positive.

For the confirmed case, in addition to fulfilling the conditions of the clinically diagnosed phase, patients need to manifest with eggs or miracidia detected in their feces or, in untreated cases, living eggs are found in fecal examination; in treated cases, recently modified eggs are found by rectal biopsy.[30]

Differential diagnosis

The disease spectrum in the endemic areas for schistosomiasis and the cumulative experiences in the diagnosis and treatment of advanced schistosomiasis indicate a need to differentiate advanced schistosomiasis from the following diseases, with which it shares similar clinical symptoms: nodular liver cirrhosis; primary liver cancer; malaria; tuberculous peritonitis; chronic myelogenous leukemia; and so on.[31]

Nodular liver cirrhosis

Nodular liver cirrhosis is generally caused by viral hepatitis. Liver cells are seriously damaged and, clinically, the disease is often accompanied by malaise, loss of appetite, distension, jaundice, spider angioma, liver palm, and gynecomastia. The nodules on the surface of the liver are often palpable. In the late stage of the disease, the liver frequently atrophies and becomes difficult to palpate. The spleen is obviously enlarged. This is generally a result of liver dysfunction, in particular elevated levels of alanine aminotransferase in the blood. The hepatitis B surface antigen (HBsAg) and core antibody (HBc) can be detected. The disease progresses quickly and has a poor prognosis. It is notable that advanced schistosomiasis often coexists with an infection of HBV, and manifests as mixed liver cirrhosis dominated by hepatitis.[31,32]

Primary liver cancer

Primary liver cancer progresses quickly. It is often accompanied by fever, significant weight loss, and persistent liver pain. The liver is progressively enlarged and shows a hardening texture and an uneven surface. Serious jaundice and ascites can rapidly appear. Ascites can be a light yellowish or hemorrhagic liquid. Serum alkaline phosphatase is increased and AFP is positive. Space-occupying lesions are present in ultrasound, radionuclide scans, CT, etc.[32]

Malaria

Malaria patients have a history of repeated fever episodes. The main clinical manifestations of malaria include periodic fever, chills and sweating. After long-term repeated attacks, malaria can lead to anemia and splenomegaly. *Plasmodium* parasites can be found in blood smears. Anti-malaria treatments are effective.[31,32]

Tuberculous peritonitis

Patients with tuberculous peritonitis lack portal hypertension and often have fever.

Primary tuberculosis lesions in the lungs can be found. Ascites is a small or medium volume, exudate in nature, and occasionally bloody. Diagnosis should be made on the basis of clinical characteristics, auxiliary examinations, and the efficacy of anti-tuberculous therapy. Laparoscopy is an effective method of diagnosis for tuberculous peritonitis.[31,32]

Chronic myelogenous leukemia

In patients with chronic myelogenous leukemia, the spleen is obviously enlarged and can even manifest megalosplenia. The disease if often accompanied by mild fever. Leukocyte levels are significantly increased in the peripheral blood and korocytes appear. Bone marrow puncture helps with diagnosis.[31,32]

HBV

There are indications that the more heavily a patient is infected with *S. japonicum*, the more susceptible he or she is to a HBV infection. This is especially noticeable among patients with signs of advanced schistosomiasis.[33] Lyra also finds that decompensated cases show a higher proportion of positive HBsAg (12%) than compensated cases (7.7%).[34] It seems possible that patients with advanced schistosomiasis may be especially susceptible to the development of HBV-induced chronic active hepatitis. The presumably reason is that schistosomes (worms and eggs) may impair cell-mediated immunity, which makes hosts more susceptible to HBV.

2.3.5　Treatment

Advanced schistosomiasis has complex symptoms and signs, and often accompanied by complications and comorbidities. It is difficult to apply a fixed treatment mode that can be used in all subtypes of advanced schistosomiasis. Treatment procedures must be individually based.

Parasitological therapy

Praziquantel (PZQ) has been used for more than 30 years. It is considered to be a safe anti-schistosome drug. It has been observed that PZQ may not only eliminate the parasites, but also influence the immune responses of the host.[35] This means that PZQ has the potential to be used for the treatment of liver fibrosis in advanced schistosomiasis, consequently exerting dual effects on schistosome infections.

Treatment of variceal bleeding

Variceal bleeding in the esophagogastric region is the most frequent cause of death in advanced schistosomiasis japonica. It is often cause by portal hypertension. Treatment for this complication of advanced schistosomiasis involves a complex process.

Pharmacologic therapy

At present, there are three types of drugs used in portal hypertension and upper gastrointestinal bleeding that result from advanced schistosomiasis. These are vasopresssors, β-blockers, and somatostatin analogs.

All vasopressor infusions were titrated and tapered to maintain a target blood pressure. Terlipressin, a vasopressin analogue, can reduce the hepatic venous pressure gradient, variceal pressure, and azygos blood flow. Terlipressin has been found to decrease renal vasoconstrictor system activity and improve renal function in patients with hepatorenal syndrome. However, terlipressin can induce ischemic complications, particularly in cases of severe hypovolemic shock.[36] It is contraindicated in patients with cardiovascular disease: arterial disease with severe obstruction, cardiac insufficiency, arrhythmias, and hypertension. Terlipressin is a good choice to combine with the use of vasodilators that contain nitroglycerin or regitine so as to increase curative effect, reduce portal vein pressure, improve hemostasis rate, and decrease adverse drug reactions.

β-blockers can effectively reduce portal pressure and varicose vein internal pressure, as well as reduce varicose vein blood flow.[37] The hepatic venous pressure gradient could be measured to evaluate the efficiency of β-blocker treatment.[38] Studies have shown that variceal bleeding does not occur if the gradient is reduced to below 12 mmHg, or that bleeding occurs at a low rate if the gradient is reduced by at least 20% of the basal value, thereby reducing fatal hemorrhages and the case fatality rate. β-blockers are appropriate in patients with moderate to severe varicose veins or with red sign (hemorrhage). They are not appropriate for patients with advanced liver cirrhosis or a heart rate that is less than 60 beats per minute. During administration, the dose of β-blockers should be decreased gradually in order to avoid a rebound of the reduced portal pressure.[39]

Somatostatin and its analogues octreotide and vapreotide can significantly reduce the hepatic venous pressure gradient, variceal pressure, and azygos blood flow. However, because its hemodynamic effect is transient, continuous infusion is required.[40] Octreotide and vapreotide have a longer half-life than somatostatin and are useful in the treatment of portal hypertension. Octreotide decreases the hepatic venous pressure gradient and azygos blood flow, but it does not reduce variceal pressure.[41,42] Vapreotide, a long-acting analogue of somatostatin, was administered before endoscopic treatment. It was found to result in fewer blood transfusions and better control of bleeding than endoscopic treatment alone. No major toxic effects and practically no complications are associated with the use of somatostatin and its analogues.[43]

Endoscopic treatment

Endoscopy is presently a priority in the treatment of acute varices bleeding because it has definite effects in the control of acute bleeding. It is also effective in the prevention of early rebleeding. Three endoscopic techniques are currently used: endoscopic band ligation, endoscopic sclerotherapy, and variceal obturation with glue.

Endoscopic band ligation is the first choice for currently endoscopic treatment of esophagogastric varices. The evidence that endoscopic band ligation (EBL) has greater efficacy and fewer side effects than endoscopic injection sclerotherapy has renewed interest in endoscopic treatments for portal hypertension. The introduction of multishot band devices, which allow the placement of 5 – 10 bands at a time, has made the technique much easier to perform, avoiding the use of overtubes and their related complications. EBL sessions are usually repeated at 2 week intervals until varices are obliterated, which is achieved in about 90% of patients after 2 – 4 sessions. Variceal recurrence is frequent, with 20 – 75% of patients requiring repeated EBL sessions.[44]

Endoscopic sclerotherapy: There are several sclerosant agents, including polidocanol, ethanolamine, ethanol, tetradecyl sulfate, and sodium morrhuate, all of which provide similar results. The treatment involves intravariceal or paravariceal injections of the sclerosant agent every one to three weeks until obliteration of the varices. Frequent complications of endoscopic sclerotherapy include retrosternal pain, dysphagia, and post-sclerotherapy bleeding ulcers.[45]

Variceal occlusion with glue: This technique is especially useful in patients who have had gastric or gastroesophageal variceal bleeding. It consists of embolization of the varices by injecting them with the tissue adhesive N-butyl-2-cyanoacrylate. The adhesive polymerizes in contact with blood. The most serious risk associated with this procedure is embolization of the lung, spleen, or brain.[46]

Transjugular intrahepatic portosystemic shunt (TIPS)

Percutaneous creation of a TIPS through a jugular route connects the hepatic and portal veins in the liver. The goal of TIPS is to reduce portal pressure and thus prevent variceal bleeding. TIPS diverts portal blood flow from the liver, but it increases the risk of encephalopathy.[47] In most cases, encephalopathy responds to standard therapy. Thrombosis and stenosis are the complications that can cause TIPS dysfunction.[48] It has been reported that the morbidity of hepatic encephalopathy induced by TIPS is 30%. The contraindications of TIPS are hepatic encephalopathy, cardiac insufficiency, and patients who are more than 70 years old and/or have a Child-Pugh score that is more than 12 points.[49]

Balloon tamponade

In case of massive or uncontrolled bleeding, balloon tamponade provides a bridge to definitive treatment with TIPS, a portosystemic surgical shunt, or further endoscopic therapy. The continuous use of balloon tamponade should not exceed 24 hours. Otherwise, esophageal mucosal erosion in the segment that is pressed by balloon tamponade is much more likely to happen. The most frequently used balloon is the four-lumen modification of the Sengstaken-Blakemore tube, which employs a gastric and esophageal balloon. In cases of bleeding gastric varices, use of the Linton-Nachlas tube with a large gastric balloon is recommended. Currently, balloon tamponade is not used much anymore, except as an emergency hemostatic measure. Decreased use of balloon tamponade is due to improvements in and the increasing efficacy of hemostasis drugs. However, balloon tamponade is still used in approximately 5 – 10% of patients who have intractable hemorrhage (persistent bleeding or rebleeding in the short-term) and present with drug resistance.[50,51]

General treatment

General treatment aims to correct hypovolemia and to prevent complications. Blood volume replacement should be done cautiously using concentrated erythrocytes to obtain a hemoglobin level of about 70 – 80 g/L. Overtransfusion should be avoided given the risk of increased portal pressure and continued or recurrent bleeding.

Plasma expanders are used to maintain hemodynamic stability and renal perfusion pressure. Either a crystalloid (isotonic saline solution) or colloid solution can be used, but a crystalloid solution is preferred because it is harmless.

Bacterial infection occurs in 25 – 50% of patients with cirrhosis and gastrointestinal bleeding. Failure to control bleeding and rates of death are increased in patients with infections. The early administration of antibiotic prophylaxis benefits all patients with variceal bleeding and improves survival rates. One recommended protocol is oral administration of norfloxacin.[52]

Surgical procedures

Many kinds of surgical methods have been developed to treat the portal hypertension that is caused by advanced schistosomiasis. Surgical procedures can be divided into the following 10 subtypes. These are grouped into three major categories, or general types of surgery (Table 2.2). Each surgical subtype has its own indications and contraindications.[53]

Table 2.2　Surgical procedures used to treat portal hypertension
caused by advanced schistosomiasis.

Types of surgery in portal hypertension	Subtypes of surgery in portal hypertension
Esophagogastric devascularization, with or without splenectomy, and with or without direct ligation of varices or esophageal transection	i) Sugiura procedure
	ii) Modified Hassab's procedure (splenectomy with esophagogastric devascularization)
	iii) Johnston's stapled esophageal transection and reanastomosis
	iv) Transabdominal esophagogastric devascularization with gastroesophageal stapling, with or without splenectomy
Nonselective portosystemic shunts	i) Side-to-side portocaval shunts (s-s PCS)
	ii) Proximal splenorenal shunt (PSRS) with splenectomy
	iii) S-side splenorenal shunt without splenectomy
Selective or partial portosystemic shunts	i) Distal splenorenal shunt (DSRS)
	ii) Sarfeh's small diameter (8mm) interposition (H graft) PCS
	iii) Inokuchi's coronary caval shunt

In other words, these surgical approaches can be divided into two kinds. The first is devascularization surgery, which blocks the abnormal blood flow between portal vein and azygos vein to achieve the goal of hemostasis. The second is shunt surgery, including selective and non-selective portosystemic shunts, to reduce portal vein hypertension.

In addition, liver transplantation—as a new treatment for terminal-stage liver diseases—has made remarkable strides in the past decades.

It is important to select the corresponding surgical method based on the specific condition of the patient. Overall, periesophagogastric devascularization is the most commonly used surgical approach because it is considered to have the most efficacy in controlling portal hypertension. This operation can also be performed completely with laparoscopy. Most specialists give preference to a combination of splenectomy plus either transesophageal ligation of the varices or another type of azygoportal disconnection. It should be emphasized, however, that there is no well-controlled study to justify these surgical preferences.

Thrombosis of the splenic vein may result in bleeding from gastric varices arising from short gastric veins. In these uncommon cases, splenectomy is the definitive treatment. Portal hypertension-associated hypersplenism with thrombocytopenia is not an indication for splenectomy.[54]

Treatment of ascites

For subclinical ascites that is detectable only by ultrasonography, no specific treatment is necessary. However, a reduction in daily sodium intake is recommended. In cases of moderate ascites, renal function is usually preserved and treatment can be administered on an outpatient basis. Moderate dietary sodium restrictions should be imposed. Spironolactone, an anti-mineralocorticoid, is the drug of choice at the onset of treatment because it promotes better natriuresis more often than do loop diuretics. Spironolactone blocks the aldosterone-dependent exchange of sodium in the distal and collecting renal tubules, thus increasing the excretion of sodium and water.[55]

In the presence of edema, treatment with furosemide may be added for a few days to increase natriuresis. In cirrhosis, the effect of loop diuretic monotherapy is limited. It is therefore more commonly used as an adjunct to spironolactone therapy. Amiloride may be used when spironolactone is contraindicated or if side effects, such as gynecomastia, occur. Amiloride also acts in the distal tubule. Diuretic therapy should be monitored by daily measurements of patient weight and levels of serum electrolytes, urea, and creatinine. Maximum weight loss should not exceed 500 g/d in patients without peripheral edema and 1,000 g/d in those with it. If the therapeutic effect is insufficient, urinary sodium excretion should be determined to identify nonresponsive patients.[56]

Patients with severe ascites have marked abdominal discomfort. In such cases, higher diuretic doses are needed. However, in some patients, free-water excretion is impaired and severe hyponatremia may develop. Frequently, large-volume paracentesis should be done. Paracentesis should be routinely combined with plasma volume expansion. If the volume of ascites removed is less than 5 L, a synthetic plasma substitute may be used. If more than 5 L of ascitic fluid is removed, albumin should be given at a dose of 8 g per liter of fluid removed.[56]

A relatively efficient method for the treatment of severe ascites consists in concentrating self-ascites and reinfusion. However, some side effects can occur during treatment, such as fever, hypotension, and so on. By means of dialyzer or artificial kidney, a volume of 5,000 – 10,000 ml ascites can be tapped within two to three hours, which is further ultrafiltrated and concentrated to a volume of 500 – 1,000 ml, and then retransfused into the body. This method can create favorable conditions for surgery.

Refractory ascites develops in about 10% of patients. In such cases, liver transplantation should be considered. In the meantime, therapeutic strategies can involve repeated large-volume paracentesis and plasma volume expansion with albumin or TIPS. TIPS improves renal function and sodium excretion by suppressing the natriuresis resistance system. It is more effective than paracentesis in removing ascites. Four weeks after TIPS, renal function should change for the better and renal natriuresis should be increased (Figure 2.5).

Treatment of dwarfism

Due to the large-scale schistosomiasis control campaign, advanced schistosomiasis with dwarfism is now rarely seen. In most cases of dwarfism patients, symptoms and signs are generally improved by the timely administration of schistosomacide treatment and a splenotomy. For patients with treatment failure, the use of growth hormones is recommended. In male patients, it is recommended to add a gonadal hormone, such as styrene acrylic acid nandrolone or testosterone propionate. In female patients, diethylstilbestrol should be supplemented.[57]

Treatment of colon proliferative

Generally, the treatment for this subtype of advanced schistosomiasis needs to be combined with internal medicine and surgery. If granuloma is light, and colon polyps and narrow lesions in the tract are not visible on X-rays and in endoscopy, internal therapy supplemented by symptomatic management (including support therapy, liver-protecting treatment, schistosomacide, gastrointestinal treatment, etc.) is adequate. If colon proliferative leads to intestinal obstruction, or creates broad and

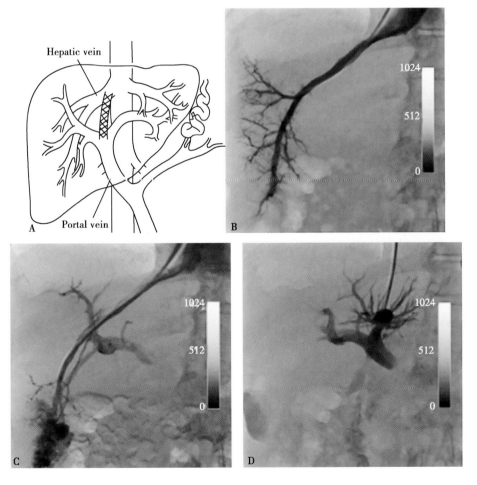

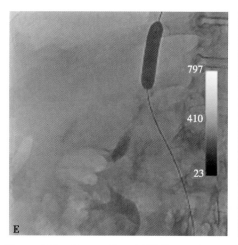
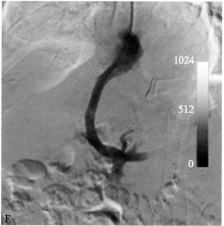

Figure 2.5 Conventional TIPS creation technique. A, Schematic diagram shows TIPS connecting the right hepatic vein to the right portal vein. The shunt extends from the main portal vein to the confluence of the right hepatic vein and inferior vena cava; B, right hepatic venogram shows the path of the hepatic vein; C, transhepatic portogram using iodinated contrast material shows the course of the portal veins; D, injection of contrast medium through a Colapinto needle confirms needle position within the portal vein before passage of a guidewire; E, dilatation of a tract through the hepatic parenchyma that is interposed between the hepatic and portal veins; F, portal venogram obtained after TIPS insertion shows flow through the FLUENCY polytetrafluoroethylene-covered stent. Peripheral portal vein branches are no longer opacified because of reversal of flow.

multiple polyps, and/or a malignant tendency in the mucosa is prompted in biopsy, surgery should be performed as soon as possible.[58]

2.3.6 Case study

Typical treatment course

A 52-year-old Chinese-born woman was admitted to the affiliated Xiangyue Hospital of Hunan Institute of Parasitic Diseases in March 2016, with a six-month history of abdominal distension and indigestion. She had a history of contact with infested water in areas endemic for schistosomiasis several years prior to her admission to hospital and had recently suffered from hypertension and hysterectomy. The only abnormal findings revealed by physical examination were splenomegaly and caput medusae. Findings from abdominal ultrasonography and gastroscope were abnormal, but findings from ELISA and liver function were normal. After the consent of family members, the victim underwent periesoph-agogastric devascularization and splenectomy, accompanied by open liver biopsy. The pathological evidence from the liver tissue indicated a hyperplasia of the hepatic fibrous tissue, and the helminthic ova were circumscribed and infiltrated by chronic inflammatory cells (Figure 2.6).

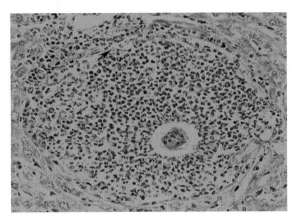

Figure 2.6　Characteristic perioval granuloma formed around *S. japonicum* egg in liver tissue.

The patient was discharged without complications eight days after surgery. She was followed up with three months later. Her symptoms had been completely resolved.

Introduction of "Treatment Project on Advanced Schistosomiasis in China"

With the termination of the "World Bank Loan Project on Schistosomiasis" in 2001, the prevalence of schistosomiasis began to rise in China. A considerable number of advanced schistosomiasis patients were sustained. Given the severity of the disease, its prolonged course, the poor effect of treatment, and the high cost of treatment, advanced schistosomiasis resulted in patients with a huge disease burden, a poor quality of life, and a worsening economic status. It is a common situation in China that advanced schistosomiasis creates a downward spiral defined in terms of "circulating from disease to poverty, and from poverty to more serious state of the disease". This is a sharp contrast to the goal of a harmonious society and sustainable development that the Chinese government has recently been pursuing.

Hence, in 2003, the Chinese government identified schistosomiasis as one of the country's major public health concerns. To address this, from 2004 onward, a special fund was created to carry out a nationwide treatment project for advanced schistosomiasis. The objective of this project is to reduce the economic burdens of this disease, alleviate the pain and suffering of the disease, and prolong the life span and improve the quality of life of patients. Technical groups consisting of experts and administrative committees were set up at all levels to carry out the work. Treatment standards were formulated and then subjects who reached the standard were screened from China's advanced schistosomiasis pools. For patients who were treated by internal medicine, the medical fees of RMB 3,000 – 6,000 were subsidized based on the degree of hepatic lesions. Patients treated by surgical management received an amount of RMB 7,500 as government assistance.

At present, China's advanced schistosomiasis treatment project has lasted more than 10 years. During this time, the treatment concept has been improved— changing from individuated treatment to a comprehensive method based on a multidisciplinary approach. Data management of the treatment project has also been modernized, from the traditional manual processing to the use of modern electronic information technology for handling. A recent survey has shown that the average cure rate of advanced schistosomiasis patients increased by 13.08% from 2004 to 2015. More than 60% of patients experienced improvements in their health condition, nearly 70% had better psychological conditions, and more than 70% experienced improved self-help abilities and social contact. Family happiness also increased. In addition, the annual average cost of caretakers decreased by RMB 2,000.

Although the endemic situation of schistosomiasis in China has attained the criteria of transmission control, a considerable number of advanced schistosomiasis patients still exist throughout the country. This is despite the implementation of a dedicated treatment programme for more than 10 years. Given the serious and persistent nature of this public health problem in China, it is clear that this large-scale public health project is still necessary and must continue into the foreseeable future.

References

1. Zhou XN, Wang LY, Chen MG, et al. The public health significance and control of schistosomiasis in China—then and now. Acta Trop, 2005, 96: 97-105.

2. Li SM, Zhao ZY, Peng ZZ, et al. Evaluation on effect of treatment and assistance to advanced schistosomiasis patients in Hunan Province from 2004 to 2013. Zhongguo Xue Xi Chong Bing Fang Zhi Za Zhi, 2014, 26: 362-366. (in Chinese)

3. Zhang LJ, Xu ZM, Qian YJ, et al. Endemic status of schistosomiasis in People's Republic of China in 2015. Zhongguo Xue Xi Chong Bing Fang Zhi Za Zhi, 2016, 28: 611-617. (in Chinese)

4. Ministry of Health, P.R. China. Manual of Schistosomiasis Prevention and Control. 3rd edition. Shanghai Science and Technology Press, Shanghai, 2000, pp.63-64. (in Chinese)

5. Reboucas G. Clinical aspects of hepatosplenic schistosomiasis: a contrast with cirrhosis. Yale J Bio Med, 1975, 48: 369-376.

6. Warren KS, Reboucas G. Blood ammonia during bleeding from esophageal varices in patients with hepatosplenic schistosomiasis. N Eng J Med, 1964, 271: 921-926.

7. Bisseru B, Patel JS. Cruveilhier-Baumgarten (C-B) disease. Gut, 1989, 30: 36-137.

8. Ross AG, Sleigh AC, Li Y, et al. Schistosomiasis in the People's Republic of China: Prospects and challenges for the 21st Century. Clin Microbiol Rev, 2001, 14: 270-295.

9. McGarvey ST, Wu GL, Zhang S, et al. Child growth, nutritional status and schistosomiasis japonica in Jiangxi, People's Republic of China. Am J Trop Med Hyg, 1993, 48: 547-553.

10. Nokes C, McGarvey ST, Shiue L, et al. Evidence for an improvement in cognitive function following treatment of *Schistosoma japonicum* infection in Chinese primary schoolchildren. Am J Trop Med Hyg, 1999, 60: 556-565.

11. Carvalho ACM, Horwith M. Hepatosplenic schistosomiasis mansoni associated with retarded growth and sexual development: Endocrine evaluation. Gas Med Bahia, 1972, 72: 69-84.

12. Ross AGP, Li YS, Sleigh AS, et al. Epidemiologic features of *Schistosoma japonicum* among fishermen and other occupational groups in the Dongting Lake region (Hunan Province) of China. Am J Trop Med Hyg, 1997, 57: 302-308.

13. Bharti AR, Weidner N, Ramamoorthy S. Chronic schistosomiasis in a patient with rectal

cancer. Am J Trop Med Hyg, 2009, 80: 1-2.

14. Ellis MK, Li Y, Hou X, et al. sTNFR-II and sICAM-1 are associated with acute disease and hepatic inflammation in schistosomiasis japonica. Int J Parasitol, 2008, 38: 717-723.

15. Hussain S, Hawass ND, Zaidi AJ. Ultrasonographic diagnosis of schistosomal periportal fibrosis. J Ultrasound Med, 1984, 3: 449-452.

16. Pereira LM, Domingues AL, Spinelli V, et al. Ultrasonography of the liver and spleen in Brazilian patients with hepatosplenic schistosomiasis and cirrhosis. Trans R Soc Trop Med Hyg, 1998, 92: 639-642.

17. Lambertucci JR, dos Santos Silva LC, Andrade LM, et al. Imaging techniques in the evaluation of morbidity in schistosomiasis mansoni. Acta Trop, 2008, 108:209-217.

18. Kardorff R, Olveda RM, Acosta LP, et al. Hepatosplenic morbidity in schistosomiasis japonica: evaluation with Doppler sonography. Am J Trop Med Hyg, 1999, 60: 954-959.

19. Olveda DU, Olveda RM, Lam AK, et al. Utility of diagnostic imaging in the diagnosis and management of schistosomiasis. Clin Microbial, 2014, 3: 142.

20. Fataar S, Bassiony H, Satyanath S, et al. CT of hepatic schistosomiasis mansoni. Am J Roentgenol, 1985, 145: 63-66.

21. Preidler K, Riepl T, Szolar D, et al. Cerebral Schistosomiasis: MR and CT Appearance. Am J Neuroradiol, 1996, 17: 1598-1600.

22. Passos MC, Silva LC, Ferrari TC, et al. Ultrasound and CT findings in hepatic and pancreatic parenchyma in acute schistosomiasis. Br J Radiol, 2009, 82: e145-147.

23. Silva LCS, Maciel PE, Ribas JGR, et al. Treatment of schistosomal myeloradiculopathy with praziquantel and corticosteroids and evaluation by magnetic resonance imaging: A longitudinal study. Clin Infec Dis, 2004, 39: 1618-1624.

24. Wu F, Xie Z, Yuan S, et al. Studies on the diagnosis of schistosomiasis with IHA. Zhongguo Xue Xi Chong Bing Fang Zhi Za Zhi, 1991, 3: 138-140. (in Chinese)

25. Hua W, Zhu Y, He W, et al. Analysis of fraction antigens of soluble egg antigen (SEA) of *Schistosoma japonicum.* Zhongguo Xue Xi Chong Bing Fang Zhi Za Zhi, 1996, 8: 274-276. (in Chinese)

26. Zhu Y, Hua W, Liu Y, et al. A study on evaluation of efficacy of chemotherapy for schistosomiasis with fraction antigen of soluble egg antigen of *Schistosoma japonicum.* Zhongguo Xue Xi Chong Bing Fang Zhi Za Zhi, 1996, 8: 321-324. (in Chinese)

27. Zhu Y, Socheat D, Bounlu K, et al. Application of dipstick bye immunoassay (DDIA) kit for

the diagnosis of schistosomiasis mekongi. Acta Trop, 2005, 96: 137-141.

28. Xia CM, Rong R, Lu ZX, et al. *Schistosoma japonicum*: a PCR assay for the early detection and evaluation of treatment in a rabbit model. Exp Parasitol, 2009, 121: 175-179.

29. Wichmann D, Panning M, Quack T, et al. Diagnosing schistosomiasis by detection of cell-free parasite DNA in human plasma. PLoS Negl Trop Dis, 2009, 3: e422.

30. Li YS. Diagnosis and Treatment of Schistosomiasis. Beijing: People's Medical Publishing House, 2006. (in Chinese)

31. Ding SY. Village Doctor's Manual of Schistosomiasis Prevention and Control. Changsha: Hunan People's Publishing House, 2004. (in Chinese)

32. Ren GH. Schistosomiasis Clinical Medicine. People's Medical Publishing House, Beijing, 2009, pp.388-391. (in Chinese)

33. Parris V, Michie K, Andrews T, et al. Schistosomiasis japonicum diagnosed on liver biopsy in a patient with hepatitis B co-infection: a case report. J Med Case Rep, 2014, 8: 45.

34. Lyra LG, Recouças G, Andrade ZA. Hepatitis B surface antigen carrier state in hepatosplenic schistosomiasis. Gastroenterol, 1976, 71: 641-645.

35. Berhe N, Myrvang B, Gundersen SG. Reversibility of schistosomal periportal thickening/fibrosis after praziquantel therapy: a twenty-six month follow-up study in Ethiopia. Am J Trop Med Hyg, 2008, 78: 228-234.

36. Moreau R, Durand F, Poynard T, et al. Terlipressin in patients with cirrhosis and type 1 hepatorenal syndrome: a retrospective multicenter study. Gastroenterology, 2002, 122: 923-930.

37. Lebrec D, Hillon P, Munoz C, et al. The effect of propranolol on portal hypertension in patients with cirrhosis: a hemodynamic study. Hepatology, 1982, 2: 523-527.

38. Grace ND, Groszmann RJ, Garcia-Tsao G, et al. Portal hypertension and variceal bleeding: an AASLD single topic symposium. Hepatology, 1998, 28: 868-880.

39. Cirera I, Feu F, Luca A, et al. Effects of bolus injections and continuous infusions of somatostatin and placebo in patients with cirrhosis: a double-blind hemodynamic investigation. Hepatology, 1995, 22: 106-111.

40. Villanueva C, Ortiz J, Minana J, et al. Somatostatin treatment and risk stratification by continuous portal pressure monitoring during acute variceal bleeding. Gastroenterology, 2001, 121: 110-117.

41. Escorsell A, Bandi JC, Andreu V, et al. Desensitization to the effects of intravenous octreotide

in cirrhotic patients with portal hypertension. Gastroenterology, 2001, 120: 161-169.

42. Ottesen LH, Flyvbjerg A, Jakobsen P, et al. The pharmacokinetics of octreotide in cirrhosis and in healthy man. J Hepatol, 1997, 26: 1018-1025.

43. Luketic VA. Management of portal hypertension after variceal hemorrhage. Clin Liver Dis, 2001, 5: 677-707.

44. Westaby D, Macdougall BR, Williams R. Improved survival following injection sclerotherapy for esophageal varices: final analysis of a controlled trial. Hepatology, 1985, 5: 827-830.

45. Waked I, Korula J. Analysis of long-term endoscopic surveillance during follow-up after variceal sclerotherapy from a 13-year experience. Am J Med, 1997, 102: 192-199.

46. Seewald S, Sriram PV, Naga M, et al. Cyanoacrylate glue in gastric variceal bleeding. Endoscopy, 2002, 34: 926-932.

47. D'Amico G, Luca A, Morabito A, et al. Uncovered transjugular intrahepatic portosystemic shunt for refractory ascites: a meta-analysis. Gastroenterology, 2005, 129: 1282-1293.

48. Bureau C, Garcia-Pagan JC, Otal P, et al. Improved clinical outcome using polytetrafluoroethylene-coated stents for TIPS: results of a randomized study. Gastroenterology, 2004, 126: 469-475.

49. Boyer TD, Haskal ZJ. The role of transjugular intrahepatic portosystemic shunt in the management of portal hypertension. Hepatology, 2005, 41: 386-400.

50. Seror J, Allouche C, Elhaik S. Use of Sengstaken-Blakemore tube in massive postpartum hemorrhage: aseries of 17 cases. Acta Obstet Gynecol Scand, 2005, 84: 660-664.

51. Condous GS, Arulkumarah S. The "tamponade test" in the management of massive postpartum hemorrhage. Obstet Gynecol, 2003, 101: 767-772.

52. Yang Z. Surgical strategy of diagnosis and treatment in advanced schistosomiasis. J Surg Concept Pract, 2010, 15: 301-304. (in Chinese)

53. Pal S. Current role of surgery in portal hypertention. Indian J Surg, 2012, 74: 55-66.

54. Zhang Y, Wen TF, Yan LN, et al. Preoperative predictors of portal vein thrombosis after splenectomy with periesophagogastric devascularization. World J Gastroenterol, 2012, 18: 1834-1839.

55. Winslow ER, Brunt LM, Drebin JA, et al. Portal vein thrombosis after splenectomy. Portal vein thrombosis after splenectomy. Am J Surg, 2002, 184: 631-635.

56. Gines P, Cardenas A, Arroyo V, et al. Management of cirrhosis and ascites. N Engl J Med, 2004, 350: 1646-1654.

57. Chen SX. Dwarf subtype of advanced schistosomiasis. In: Ren GH. Schistosomiasis Clinical Medicine. Beijing: People's Medical Publishing House, 2009.

58. Liu JX, Li ZC, Cai DY. Colon proliferative subtype of advanced schistosomiasis. In: Ren GH. Schistosomiasis Clinical Medicine. Beijing: People's Medical Publishing House, 2009.

Chapter 3

Biology and Control of *Oncomelania* Snail in China

Yi Zhang, Dan-dan Lin, Jun Ge, and Shi-zhu Li

3.1 Biology of *Oncomelania* snail

Oncomelania spp. is often referred to as the intermediate host snail of *Schistosoma japonicum*. *Oncomelania hupensis* belongs to polytypic species, and several sub-species of *O. hupensis* are known to transmit *S. japonicum* in China. Adult *O. hupensis* is a small and amphibious snail able to survive for prolonged periods out of water, whereas young or baby snail could not.

3.1.1 Taxonomic category

O. hupensis was the first found in Wuchang county, Hubei Province of China and named by Gredler (1881). Due to the great variance on *O. hupensis* snail morphology, such as shell sculpture, operculum, etc., the taxonomy of *O. hupensis* in mainland of China has been disputed for many years until early twenty-first century.

In general, most of researchers categorize *O. hupensis* as following:

Phylum: Mollusca

Class: Gastropoda

  Subclass: Prosobranchia

    Subclass: Streptoneura

      Order: Mesogastropoda

        Family: Pomatiopsidae

          Subfamily: Pomatiopsinae

            Tribe: Pomatiopsini

Genus: *Oncomelania*

Species: *O. hupensis*

Oncomelania genus is one of eight genera of the Pomatiopsidae. *O. hupensis* polytypic species is comprised of seven subspecies in the world. Three discrete subspecies, including *O. h. hupensis, O. h. robertsoni,* and *O. h. tangi* are distributed in mainland China. On the basis of the knowledge on morhpology, habitat ecology, genetic variation, phylogenetic network, and population genetics including co-evolution relationships between *O. hupensis* and *S. japonicum*, etc., there are seven strains in mainland China (Table 3.1).[1]

Table 3.1 *Oncomelania hupensis* and distribution

Species	Distribution
Oncomelania hupensis (Gredler, 1881)	Mainland of China
O. h. hupensis (Gredler, 1881)	Middle-lower reaches of Yangtze River
O. h. fausti strain	Hilly areas
O. h. hupensis strain	Lake, marshland regions
O. h. tangi (Bartsch, 1936)	Coasts of east and south regions, China
O. h. tangi strain	Fujian Province, China
O. h. guangxi strain	Guangxi autonomous region, China
O. h. subei strain	Coasts of north parts, Jiangsu Province, China
O. h. robertsoni (Bartsch, 1936)	Southwest regions, China
O. h. yunnan strain	Yunnan Province, China
O. h. sichuan strain	Sichuan Province, China
O. h. formosana (Pilsbry & Hirase, 1905)	Taiwan, China
O. h. chiui (Habe & Miyazaki, 1962)	Taiwan, China
O. h. nosophora (Robson, 1915)	Japan
O. h. quadrasi (Möllendroff, 1895)	Philippine
O. h. lindoensis (Davis & Carney, 1973)	Sulawesi island, Indonesia
Oncomelania minima (Bartsch, 1936)	Japan

3.1.2 Morphology

As one kind of freshwater snails, *O. hupensis hupensis* consists of two well-defined parts: the shell and the soft parts. The operculum covers the soft body of the snail, which is placed on the upper side of the posterior part of the foot. The soft body of the snail includes: head, foot, neck, viscera, etc. Mantle is the part of the soft body which is surrounded by a large fold of skin, covering the visceral mass, and the mantle cavity. The mantle border provides for the growth of the shell. The head-foot part of the soft body is capable of stretching the anterior foot forward and lifting it off the substrate while solidly supported by the mid- and hind-foot. Under certain conditions, for example during aestivation, attack by predators, periods of rest, and shell production, the head-foot part is withdrawn into the shell.

Shell

The shell morphology is one of the criteria for species determination. The secreted external shell is composed of calcium carbonate. The fundamental features of the shell include: sculpture, whorls, aperture, spire, apex, etc. The snails increase the size of their shells throughout life.

Shape and size

A shell is a conical tube, spirally coiled around a central axis or columella. The separate coils of the spiral are called whorls. The whorls are usually in close con-tact, each whorl being partially covered by its successor. The line that occurs where two whorls meet is called suture. The last whorl is called body whorl and is found around the opening or aperture, through which the body of the snail can be protruded or retracted. The body whorl is large and rounded, taking up about two-thirds of the height of the shell. The whorls above the body whorl form the spire, the tip of which is called apex. The umbilicus or hole adjacent to the aperture in the axis of the shell may be present if the whorls are not contiguous with the collumella. That is called perforate or umbilicate. There are several axial striae or ribs on each whorl of the shell from the lake regions.

The size of shell varies and depends on the localization of the snail regardless of their stage of growth. The size of the snail is bigger in the lake regions (i.e. 8.64 mm × 3.49 mm – 9.73 mm × 4.24 mm), smaller in mountainous regions (i.e. 5.80 mm × 2.71 mm – 6.93 mm × 2.85 mm), and is about 7.54 mm × 3.13 mm – 7.87 mm × 3.20 mm in marshland regions. Normally, the shell of *O. h. formosana* is smooth and its height is 4 to 6 mm, with six to seven whorls. The shell of *O. h. nosophora* has a fine axial growthline with a height of 5 to 9 mm, and five to six whorls. *O. h. quadrasi* is small in height (i.e. 3 to 5 mm), with six to seven whorls and smooth shell. *O. h. chiui* is the smallest snail (about 4.5 mm) with five whorls, presenting a sculptured shell with numerous growth lines.

Aperture

The aperture is the opening leading to the cavity of the shell and is enclosed by the peristome consisting of four parts. There are the outer lip or outer margin, the inner lip or inner margin, the columellar margin, and parietal wall. When held with the aperture facing the observer and the apex upward, the turing of the coil is clockwise, called dextral shell (opening to the right). That is different from the counterclockwise, called sinistral shell (opening to the left) where the aperture is directed to the left when facing the observer and the apex held upward. Snails with a dextral shell normally have genital openings, anus, and pneumostome placed on the right side of the body.

The adult shells of *O. h. hupensis* are conico-acuminate, right coiled, dextral, with six or eight whorls and pronounced sutures. The aperture is ovate, elongate, and narrowed apically. The inner lip is slightly reflected over the narrow umbilicus and is connected with the outer lip by a long parietal callus. The outer lip is thin and strong. The base of the shell is slightly pointed and appears truncated.

Sculpture

The sculpture of the shell includes growth lines, spiral striae, spiral raised line, and ribs. The more irregular sculpture may be transverse or spiral, the more delicate microsculpture occurs, consisting of transverse lines, dots or ribs, visible only with the aid of a lens or microscope.

In general, *O. h. hupensis* can be separated into two morphotypes of shells (Figures 3.1 and 3.2): smooth or ribbed. The varix, a rib-like thickening at the lip of the shell is the last rib. The varix is one important identification characteristic between *O. hupensis* and other species. It varies on the surface sculpture of the shell among habitats. Usually there is a vertical sculpture protruding wale on the snail shell in lake regions called vertical ribbon (ribbing snail). In mountainous or hills regions, the vertical ribbon is faintness and unclear, categorizing the so-called smooth snail. Most of the snails in the lake and mashland regions and in the plain and water networks regions of the Yangtze River basin are ribbing snails, with robust varix;

whereas other snails, mainly in the mountainous and hilly regions are smooth snails, with varix except *O. h. robertsoni*. There are five sub-species of *Oncomelania* in mainland of China that are mainly located along the Yangtze valley (ribbing snail with 5.5 – 7.5 whorls), and in the mountainous regions (smooth snails with 5.0 – 7.5 whorls).

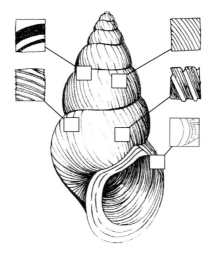

Figure 3.1   Morphological features of *Oncomelania* spp. shell. Left up to down: colour bands and spiral striae; Right up to down: growth line, rib, and varix.

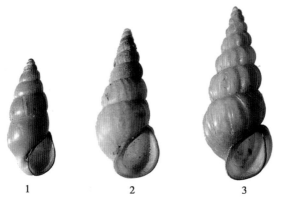

Figure 3.2   *Oncomelania* shells from China. 1, shell from mountianous and hilly regions; 2, shell from the plain and water-net regions; 3, shell from the lake and marshland regions.

The color of the snail shell is slight yellow or yellow palm. But the snails from different habitats have different shell color. The natural color of the shell usually comes from the color of the cuticle and may vary. In order to better observe the natural color and texture of the shell, the extraneous covers, such as diatoms, marl, or iron must be removed. Smooth snail is dark brown. The ribbing snail is light yellow. Snails of different growth stages, for example, baby and adult snails, have different shell color. Young baby color is lighter shade, bright and moise, white or slight yellow, thin and transparent shell. The soft body can be clearly observed from the thin shell. Along with the development, the color of the snail becomes more dark and the shell less polished and transparent. Young shells are more reliable for determining the apical sculpture. In general, the shell of ribbing snail is thick and hard, and the one of smooth snail is thin and easy to break.

Operculum

The operculum is attached to the upper part of the foot. When snails retract their head and foot into the shell, the aperture is closed by a lid called operculum. The growth of the operculum follows the growth of the shell in a spiral direction. An operculum with spiral growth may consist of a few, rapidly increasing whorls. There are one nucleus and the growth lines. *Oncomelania*'s operculum is ovate, a semi-transparent thin slice with the horniness. It can close down the snail mouth to protect the soft parts of the snail.

Soft parts

The soft part of the snail is attached permanently to the columella of the shell by a great retractor muscle. In the body whorl, a number of internal organs can be located in the visceral mass. The visceral mass fills all the whorls of the shell, and normally conforms to the coiling and shape of the whorls. The visceral mass is surrounded by a large fold of skin, called mantle. The mantle border provides for the growth of the shell. The soft part of the snail is divided into four parts as follows: the head, the neck, the foot, and the visceral mass. The parts that extend beyond the aperture are the head, the foot, and the neck. The snail head is located at the front of the soft part, and can move and look for food. The neck is located at rearward of the head and can shrink the head. On the top part of the head there is a pair of tentacles. There is also a pair of eyes dot in the stem of tentacles. Fake eyebrow with yellow spots inside of the two eyes, is a special characteristic of fresh water snail. The mouth is located at the front part of the head, and the two tentacles are separated at the two sides of the head. The foot is located at the lower section of the head and neck.

Mantle cavity

The mantle covers the mantle cavity. Some of anatomical structures in the mantle cavity are of importance in the identification of certain freshwater snails. Several organs are located inside the mantle cavity, such as the gill and osphradium. With regard to male genital, the penis is housed within the cavity. The cavity inside the body is the hemocoel, which is filled with colorless body fluid, or blood.

Eight systems are identified based on the function of visceral organs in snail. They are: sense organ, nervous system, muscular system, respiratory system, excretory system, circulatory system, digestive system, and reproductive system.

Sense organs

Sense organs include skin, tentacles, eyes, osphradium, and statocyst (balance bursa). *Oncomelania* tactile sensation is most sensitive. In order to identify whether the snail is alive or dead, the skin of the head and foot can be stimulated by a needle, and the head might be withdrawn back quickly..

Nervous system

The nervous system of snails is more complex, consisting of the central nervous system and peripheral nervous. In systematic studies, considerable attention is paid mainly on the position of ganglia and their dimensions, the number of nerves and their respective point of origin on a given ganglion, and on the length of the major commissural and connectives.

In *Oncomelania* snails, the central nervous system is composed of several ganglia, connected to each other by strands of nerve tissue called commissures and connectives. Nerves lead to various parts of the body from the ganglia. The ganglia and their joining strands are arranged to form ring, the more important part that encircles the head-neck parts and pharynx. It involves the pairs of cerebral ganglia, pedal ganglia, buccal and pleural ganglia, one supraesophageal ganglion, one visceral ganglion, and one subesophageal ganglion. The paired cerebral ganglia connected by the cerebral commissures are pressed against the mid-posterior curvature of the esophagus where the latter bends ventrally. The pedal ganglia complex consists of three pairs of ganglia, pedal ganglia, propodial ganglia, and metapodial ganglia. The pedal ganglia are quite large and fill the pedal haemocoel beneath the tensor magnus. They are connected by a commissure. From the dorsal aspect, the buccal ganglia are just visible in each angle of the anterodorsal cerebral ganglion and the outer edge of the salivary glands. From the lateral view, these ganglia lie in the depression where the esophagus presses against the posterior buccal mass just after its origin. The pleural gandlia arise from the pleuro-pedal connective immediately at the juncture of the cerebral ganglia and the connective, and are partially pressed beneath the postvern-tral curvature of the cerebral ganglia and intimately associated with them. The pleu-ral ganglia complex is composed of the supra- and sub-oesophageal ganglia and the oesphradial. The visceral ganglion is a single structure exposed by pulling back the columellar muscle of the uncoiled snail.

Muscular system

Muscular system involves columellar muscle and median longitudinal muscle. The columellar muscle is the biggest muscle in soft body. When the muscle shrinks, the snail body can withdraw back the shell, and the aperture is closed by the opercu-lum. The median longitudinal muscle assigns to three pairs of branchings, which are buccal muscles, radular muscles, and proboscis muscle.

Respiratory system

Gills are *Oncomelania*'s mainly respiratory organs. The blood flow through the lacuna between the two layers of the gills.

Excretory system

The kidney consists of a large flattened sac, the wall of which is formed of a single layer of epithelial cells. It is the kidney that connects cheek bursa with short duct. The sac is situated in the roof of the mantle cavity, at its upper end, and touches the pericardium.

Circulatory system

Circulatory system involves heart and blood vessel. The heart is located in front left of the stomach and consists of one auricle, one ventricle, and pericardium. It is located inside an epithelial sac named pericardium. The anterior portion, known as the auricle, which is close to the gills, pumps the blood into the posterior portion, the ventricle. The blood is achromatic and azury liquid. There are few of similarity lam-phocytic small cells in the blood. Muscle fibers running obliquely across each chamber cause the heart chambers to contract alternately. A valve between the chambers and another at the entry into the auricle prevent the backward flow of blood.

Digestive system

The digestive system consists of digestive organs and digestive glands (salivary gland and digestive gland, or liver). The digestive tube opens anteriorly through the mouth. The mouth leads into the buccal mass. At the posterior end of buccal mass is the radula, which is a red globe shaped. This is a ribbon-shaped noncellular cuticle on which there are transverse rows of teeth. The radula or tooth ribbon inside of the mouth is able to fetch food. According to the position and shape of the teeth, a transverse row can be differentiated into a central tooth. The quadrilateral central teeth are provided with some additional cusps on the basal plate (basal denticles), which consist of two rows, lateral teeth, inner marginal teeth, outer marginal teeth on either side of it. The radular formula is comprises of the number of each tooth plate and its teeth in each group (Figure 3.3).

$$\frac{1(2) - 1 - 1(2)}{2(3)(n) - 2(3)(n)} \cdot 2(1) - 1 - 3(2) \cdot 6 - 11 \cdot 4 - 7$$

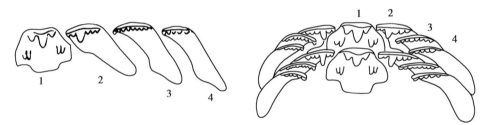

Figure 3.3　*Oncomelania*'s radular formula. 1, central tooth; 2, lateral teeth; 3, inner marginal teeth; 4, outer marginal teeth.

The tubular esophagus proceeds from the top of the buccal mass. The latter leads into the stomach, which in turn is connected to the intestine. The intestine communicates with the exterior through the anus, which is situated anteriorly on the mantle collar. It could be observed that the arranged ovoid fecal pellets are in a rhythm with the intestinal peristalsis into the anus of the gradual shift, and from the anus excreted in the body of living snails, especially in the intestine of the snail.

Secretory glands associated with the digestive tract are the salivary glands, which open into the buccal cavity situated around the esophagus. The digestive gland or liver is a leptospire, puce, or coffee-like in color, able to excrete digest enzyme and deposited nourishment. The digestive gland and gonad accounted for most of the visceral mass. Cercariae and primary sporocysts of schistosome can be seen in the digestive gland of snail infected with *S. japonicum*. The digestive gland tends to swell in pale brown or gray white. The gap between the visceral mass and the shell is filled. When snail shell is cleaned, the color of the digestive gland presents in white. This can be used to identify whether the snail is infected or non-infected with *S. japonicum*.

Reproductive system

The *Oncomelania* are dioecious. After mating, the male and female are fertilized in vivo.

The female snail reproductive system consists of ovary, oviduct, sperm receptacle, seminal receptacle, spermathecal duct, and accessory gland. The size of ovary changed regularly with the change of spawning season. The ovary is yellow and large, and plumps during spawning season, within which the size is 1/3 – 1/2 of the digestive gland (liver), with an average width up to 571.2 μm. However, during the un-spawning season, the ovary is usually pale yellow and the size of the digestive gland (liver) is only 1/3 or less. Thus, 91 – 97% ovary of the female will be atrophied after being infected with *S. japonicum* or other larva, and eggs are only accounted for 2.7 – 4.4%. The oviduct is a direct duct, the upper end is connected with the ovarian tube, and the end is communicated with the accessory gland. The sperm receptacle is an ovoid vesicular tissue, made of epithelial cells with cilla, with about 170 – 310 μm × 0.12 - 0.24 μm in size. The sperms will be seen in the fertillized sperm receptacle of female snail.

The male snail reproductive system consists of testis, spermatophore, deferent duct, prostate gland, and penis. The testis surrounds the digestive gland (liver). The testis's size is bigger than the ovary's one. The size also changed regularly with the change of season. Environmental factors, such as infection with *S. japonicum* or other larva can affect the development of the testes. *Oncomelania*'s penis is usually light gray and the end of the part in red or light red.

In male snail, sperm from the gonad travel via the deferent duct to the prostate, enter the prostate, then leave through the anterior portion of the deferent duct which leads into the base of the penis, and fnallly follow the length of the penis to exit at its tip. While in female snail, oocytes pass from the gonad and travel along the oviduct past the entrance of the seminal receptacle and sperm duct to enter the posterior end of the pallial oviduct. In theory, the eggs travel down the pallial oviduct to emerge over the omniphoric groove. Sperm enter the spermathecal duct that opens into the mantle cavity near the anterior end of the pallial oviduct. They travel to the bursa copulatrix or pass into the sperm duct at the entrance of the bursa, move into the oviduct and then into the seminal receptacle. Removing the ventral epithelium from the digestive gland can reveal the male gonad. The whole gonad appears very bright yellow when all of the testicular lobes are productive. Seven to nine multi-branched units arise from the deferent duct, but the units lack the many finely branched tubes that support testicular lobes at their tips. The female gonad is a plastic tubular structure chareacterized by a few branches with a plastic and variable style. The fully matured ovaries have five or six branched lobes. The posterior end of the gonad ends in one of the multi-branched units. The size of this organ varies depending on the season.

Reproduction and growth

Usually, the copulation of the snail happens the whole year round. The copulation rate depends on the season and factors such as temperature, light intensity, etc. From April to June is the top period, followed by Semptember to November. However, the rate of copulation is very low or stopped in severe cold and intense heat. The optimum temperature of *Oncomelania* Snails[1] mating is 15 – 20℃, whereas temperature greater than 30℃ or less than 10℃ are not suitable. Most of the snails like mating in the waters near wet mud and grass root. The time of egg laying is also related to the climate and temperature. The most suitable temperature for egg laying is 20 – 25℃. The suitable spots of laying eggs are waterside and humidity earth. Eggs are laid singly on solid objects. The shape of the snail egg is like a small mud ball and the diameter is about 0.8 mm. The snail egg is wrapped mud-cake.

The growth and reproduction depend on local temperature and the sub-species of *Oncomelania*. The time of the snail egg hatching to young snail is related to the temperature. If the temperature is high, the time is short. When the average temperature is 13℃, 16℃ and 23℃, the time for hatching of the egg is about 30 – 40 days, 20 – 28 days and 18 days, respectively. The development zero point of the snail eggs is 11.79℃, and the highest limitted temperature is 38.22℃. When the young snail hatches out from the egg, it needs three or five months growth to become adult one. The average duration for the development from eggs hatching to adults is 334.22 ± 7.52 days. Young snails of 2 mm in size or below three whorls live in water. Generally, the longevity of the adult snail in China is about one year. Some snails live much longer, two or three years. Most snails in the lake areas can survive for one to two years.

3.1.3　Ecology

Habitats

Oncomelania species is one of amphibious snails. Its eggs hatching and young stage of the snail need to be in water, whereas adult snails live in wetland or waterside. The most favorable environment for snail habitats is the place with fertility soil in humidity and weed growing. The density of snail is affected by environmental factors such as water, soil, and weeds.[2]

Water

Water is one of the necessary conditions for the growth and reproduction of the snail. Also, water is one of the important conditions that contributs to its activities. Young snails must be living in water to hatch out from eggs and growing up. The snail is always distributed along the water or river system. *Oncomelania* could crawl, looking for food and lay eggs on the humid soil only. Dry land is not suitable for snail survival. When the snail body loses water content by around 40%, the snail will die.

Although the snail can not live away from moisture soil, the adult snail has a certain capability to bear in dry condition. Under the dry condition, the snails stay in a motionless status without eating, either in summer or in winter. Its capacity of resistance to dry is related to the temperature. The higher the ambient temperature in which the snail lives, the shorter the duration of snail resistance to dry. Most of snails can survive for two months, and a few snails can survive for three and four months during the dry condition. However, when the snails are submerged into water for a long time as more than 8 months, they also will die. Usually, the high density of the snail appears in the places submerged in water for two to five months. Based on the characteristics of the snail ecology with a limitation in dry or wet condition, the approach of environment modification was used to control the snails.

The analysis of the water sample from endemic areas and non-endemic areas showed no significant differences in chloride, nitrate, rigidity, pH, color, turbidity, sandiness, and so on. The snail could adapt wide pH, environment but the suitable pH is from 6.8 – 7.8. The snails have a close relationship with dissolution oxygen in the water. It was considered that the dissolution oxygen in the snail habitats was higher than the places free from snails. When the dissolution of oxygen in marshland or ditches was lower than 3.6 mg/L, the death rate of the snail eggs was 96 – 100%, that of the young snails was 56 – 92%, and the adults was 30%.

Soil

The distribution of *Oncomelania* is relative with soil physicochemical property. The snails favor soil rich in nitrogen, phosphorous, calcium and organic materials, and rich decomposing materials in the lake areas. Usually the bigger size and thicker ribbing of snails are distributed in rich soil area, whereas the smaller size of snail is appeared at the sterile soil area.

Vegetation

Vegetation can supply snails a better condition for their survival, such as appropriate temperature, humidity, food, etc. Weeds can greatly affect the distribution of the snail in plain and water-net region in China. In the same area, snail density has been related to weed density. There are more snails in places where the weed density is high. It is very difficult to find snails in places without weeds. The function of the weed is to create humidity situation so that the snails can hide in dark environment. Meanwhile, rusty grass-blade and algae of odd cell can provide food for the snail. Vegetation in the bottomland provides the condition for *Oncomelania* movement and spreading. Flood is one of the factors that lead to snails spreading. When the snails are migrated with the flood to the area where the vegetation environment is appropriate, a new breeding ground for snails wil be formed. In contrast, if the area does not has suitable vegetation, the snails will die.

Temperature

The ambient temperature is one of the most important factors for the growth of *Oncomelania snail*. It affects the snail activities, up growing, longevity, and distribution. The suitable temperature for *Oncomelania* livelihood is around 20 – 25℃, while the best suitable ones are between 13℃ and 20℃. The average temperature of *Oncomelania* spp. distribution in China is either above 14℃ in whole year or above 0℃ in January. The average duration for the development of eggs is 27.29 ± 17.29 days under 15 – 30℃. The developmental threshold temperature of eggs and adults are 11.79℃ and 5.87℃ respectively. The suitable temperature for the development of eggs is 27℃. The development speed and effective accumulated temperature of eggs increase with the temperature under 15 – 30℃. When the temperature is over 30℃ or below 10℃, the snail reduces its movement. In the summer and winter, the snails fall at the grass root. The highest temperature for the snail survival is 35 – 40℃ and the lowest one is from zero to – 5℃.

Water temperature has a close relationship with the snail's movement. When water temperature is from 10 – 12℃, most of snails move, as for water temperature between 20 – 30℃ snail movement become faster; but, two or three hours later, the rate of movement is on the decrease. In general, the suitable time for snail movement is in spring and autumn, infected snails also increase in that period.

Light

Oncomelania is sensitive to light. Light affects the snail activities. Under strong sunlight the snail usually does not move. The most suitable illumination for snail movement is from 3,600 – 3,800 Lx. As the light is over 3,800 Lx, the snail is moving against the light. In conditions, such as at the night, the daybreak, the dark, and the rainy day, the illumination of the ground drops below 4,000 Lx, the snail moved actively. If the snail is put on the dry land and gets direct sunlight for whole day, it would die, because of both high temperature and dryness.

Distribution

Movement and spreading

There are two ways in the snail movement. One is migrating activity by its crawl and swimming, the other one is natant activity following the water flow. The distance of the snail crawl is limited on the dry land; it is about 20 m a year. Usually, the floating swimming time of *Oncomelania* is not longer. The longest is 20 min, during which the snail can floating swim about 32 m, 1.55 m/min. The snails have a habit of moving up and down following the water level fluctuation. Once the adult snails submerged, they could crawl out of water rapidly and spreading following the current to downstream. When the velocity of flow is less than 0.2 m/sec, the snail could move against the current and crawl upward, whereas with a velocity of flow over 0.6 m/sec, the snail could not attach the ground and sweep downward. The juvenile snail has a habit of floating on the surface of water and is carried by the current to downstream. The adult snail could attach floater or grass, and other plant to translate far distance, as long as the place is suitable for its reproduction and growth. Thus, the place will become a new habitat for snail survival.

Environment distribution

Oncomelania is distributed in the east and southeast of Asia, including China, Japan, the Philippines, and Indonesia. In China, the snail is distributed in the Yangtze River basin and the southern part of Yangtze River.

The distribution of the snail is related with the natural factors of temperature and rainfall. Moreover, soil and plant are also involved in a certain relationship. Based on the characteristics of geological environment and the snail habitats in the endemic area of schistosomiasis, the distribution of the snail can be divided into three types in China. They are plain and water network, lake and marshland, and mountainous and hilly regions.

Plain and water network region: The snail in the plain and water network region is linearly distributed along the canal and irrigation system. Usually, the high density of the snail is distributed in slope, shallow, and waterside. Farther from the waterside, the density of the snail is getting lower. The snails located on the waterside have a trend of up and down following the water level change. Tide flood could affect the snail distribution. There are no snails at the area with big difference of tide fluctuation, such as over 1 m, the place of washing out by wave of tide in coast area, and the pond with the river or ditch barrier.

Lake and marshland region: The snail in the lake and marshland region is planarly distributed. The distribution area of the snail is relatively wide. The snail area in this region is accout for 95% of the total snail habitats in China. Most of snails distributed in the place are submerged from two and half months to five months in whole year, especially the high density of the snails focuses on the place where the altitude is submerged in flood season. No snail distributed in the place that is submerged over 7 – 8 months in whole year. The distribution of the snail has a close relationship with the submerge times in the snail habitats on the floodplain. The distribution of the snail has a variance following the altitude of the floodplain. There is a rule of the distribution of the snail in some lakeshore area. The rule showed the state of 'two lines and three zones'. Two lines mean the highest line and lowest line with the snails colonized. Three zones mean there are certain altitude with a high density of the snail, called high density zone. Apart from the high density zone there is a low density zone. There is no snail distribution in the same altitude at some place because of the topography around the site. The study of the snail distribution on the grass plain showed that there were three kinds of model of the snail distribution. They are stochastic, collective, and symmetrical distribution. Also, the distribution of the snail has a relationship with the altitude of bottomland and the vegetation distribution. It has a relationship with reed development in the reed bottomland.

Mountainous and hilly region: The snail distribution in the mountainous and hilly region is a kind of sporadic distribution which is isolated in bulk, distributed along the water system from top to bottom of the mountain. The geographic environment of the snail distribution is complex in this region. The altitude difference is great disparity. The topography is high and low with massif scatter in the area. The snail habitat is mainly in irrigation ditches and the edge of the field. In the hilly area, the snails show dot distribution in some environment because the water system has a boundary with apex of mountain and independent stream distribution from top to bottom. The individual snails are found in some areas at the top of mountain and half way up the mountain where soil humidity is high in whole year.

References

1. Xu XJ, Zhou XN, Zhang Y. Biology and control of *Oncomelania* snail. Editor in chief Chen MG, Zhou XN, Hirayama K *Asia Parasitology Vol.5 Schistosomiasis in Asia*. AAA Committee. The Federation of Asian Parasitologists Department of Infection and Host Defense, Chiba University Graduate School of Medicine Inohana 1-8-1, Chuo-ku, Chiba 260-8670, Schistosomiasis in Asia 2005, Japan: 133-150.

2. Zhang Y, Zhou XN. Taxa and distribution on *Oncomelania*. Editor in chief Zhou Xiaonong, Vice subeditor Zhang Y. *Science on Oncomelania snail*. Beijing: Science Press, 2005.

3.2 Distribution and survey of *O. hupenesis* in China

3.2.1 Distribution characteristics

Oncomelania hupensis is distributed across the Yangtze River basin and the southern part of the Yangtze River, i.e. Shanghai, Jiangsu, Zhejiang, Anhui, Jiangxi, Hubei, Hunan, Sichuan, Yunnan, Guangdong, Guangxi, and Fujian provinces/municipality. In 1950, it was reported that the snail's habitat was 148×10^8 m^2, covering 418 cities and/or counties in 12 provinces; by 2014, the snail's habitat was 36.43×10^8 m^2. The snail's range spans from the northern part of Baoying County in Jiangsu Province (northern latitude 33°15′) to the southern part of Yulin County in Guangxi Province (northern latitude 22°37′), and from the eastern part of Nanhui District in Shanghai (eastern longitude 121°51′) to the western part of Yunlong County in Yunnan Province (eastern longitude 98°41′). The snail hass been found at an altitude range of 0 m (Shanghai) to 2,400 m (Yunnan). Within this range, the annual average temperature is over 14°C and the annual average precipitation is more than 750 mm, indicating that a mild climate and abundant rainfall are necessary for snail survival. The geographic distribution of *O. hupensis* is consistent with that of schistosomiasis endemic areas in China. It is possible that potential snail habitats will extend further to the north in the context of global warming, thus there is a potential to cause the expansion of endemic areas of schistosomiasis.[1-3]

Based on the geomorphological features of snail habitats in endemic areas of schistosomiasis, the distribution of snails can be divided into three types, i.e., plain and water network region, lake and marshland region, and mountainous and hilly region. These types of snail habitat are typically observed within any given county.

Plain and water network region

Plain water network region is mainly located in the Yangtze River delta, covering Shanghai and part of the Jiangsu and Zhejiang provinces. In these areas, watercourses are well developed and form networks with slow water currents, stable water levels, and weeds on the shore. *Oncomelania* snails are often distributed along irrigation canals, while distribution density varies from location to location. Ponds connected to rivers or canals, dikes in ridged fields, bridge pillars, and gaps between stone or bricks can also be occupied by *Oncomelania* snails. Snails are mainly found waterside and at the surface of water, with a vertical range of 1 m along the bank. The spread of snails through irrigation systems occurs via main canals to branch canals, to ditches to branch ditches, and finally to rice fields. The snail usually inhabits the sides of a rice paddy, with no snails present in the middle of the paddy. These snails are typically medium-sized, with a height of 6.5 – 7.5 mm and transverse ribs. By the end of 2014, the snail-infested areas in the plain and water network region only accounted for 0.04% of the national total snail-infested area.[3]

Lake and marshland region

The endemic areas in the lakes and marshland region are mainly distributed across the middle and lower reaches of the Yangtze River and along small lakesides that connect with the Yangtze River, and are mainly located in five provinces, i.e. Hunan, Hubei, Jiangxi, Anhui, and Jiangsu. Currently, snail areas in lake and marshland region account for 96.62% of the total snail habitats in the whole country (Table 3.2). Mild climate, abundant rainfall, fertile and humid soil, and overgrown grassy vegetation contribute to favorable conditions for snail breeding. Snails in these areas generally grow to be larger than those in the mountainous and hilly areas, as well as the plain and water network areas, typically attaining a height greater than 7.5 mm and a width greater than 3.2 mm, with a thick, ribbed shell.[3]

Marshland areas are characterized by large seasonal fluctuations in the water level, typically being flooded during summer and dry during winter. Usually, spring floods appear during the rainy season from April to May, resulting in the submergence of the marshlands of lakes. In June and July, the water level of the Yangtze River and its branches increases rapidly, and all snail habitats in the marshlands are submerged. These marshlands remain submerged until October or November. Afterwards, flooding may move backwards into the lakes and marshlands come out of water. This kind of natural geographical landscape is called flooding in summer and dry land in winter.

At different altitudes and with flooding periods, snail distribution also varies.

Table 3.2 Snail infested areas in China, 2014.

Province/ Municipality	No. of townships infested with snails	No. of villages infested with snails	Total area (hm²)	Lake and marshland region (hm²)		Plain and water network region (hm²)	Mountainous and hilly region (hm²)
				Inside embank-ment	Outside embankment		
Shanghai	11	22	1.74	0.00	0.00	1.74	0.00
Jiangsu	42	124	2,253.75	0.00	2,094.53	145.14	14.08
Zhejiang	91	323	69.47	0.00	0.00	0.40	69.07
Anhui	208	957	27,279.98	0.00	24,341.19	0.00	2,938.79
Fujian	10	16	3.17	0.00	0.00	0.00	3.17
Jiangxi	138	596	78,720.94	0.00	76,907.04	0.00	1,813.90
Hubei	357	2,666	76,165.12	21,516.28	52,219.69	0.00	2,429.15
Hunan	200	924	175,910.47	829.02	174,096.01	0.00	985.44
Guangdong	0	0	0.00	0.00	0.00	0.00	0.00
Guangxi	5	6	5.43	0.00	0.00	0.00	5.43
Sichuan	344	1,682	2,525.29	0.00	0.00	0.00	2,525.29
Yunnan	48	227	1,389.06	0.00	0.00	0.00	1,389.06
Total	1,454	7,543	364,324.42	22,345.30	329,658.46	216.38	12,173.38

The duration of submergence is a very important factor. Snail distribution is closely related to the length of time of the submergence in the snail habitats in the lake and marshland region. Most snails distributed in these areas are submerged from half a month to five months per year. There is an especially high density of snails focused at the altitudes that are submerged between two and four months of the year. Water-level fluctuations can affect the macro- and micro-environments of snail habitats, as well as snail's living activities and distribution status, which in turn affect schisto-somiasis transmission. Snail density is sparser in low-elevation marshlands that are submerged for more than eight months per year, or high-elevation marshlands that are submerged less than three months per year. Thus, snail distribution exhibits high spatial heterogeneity in these vast marshland areas. The feature of snail distribution can be summarized as: "Two lines and three zones". 'Two lines' means the highest and lowest elevation lines where snails can be found, and 'three zones' means upper and lower zones with a low snail density, and a middle zone with a high snail density. As for the distribution altitude of the snails, there are various differences between different areas in the provinces along the Yangtze River. The altitude of snail distri-bution in the Hunan and Hubei Provinces in the middle of the Yangtze River reaches up to 20 – 30 m above sea level. However, on the marshlands of the Poyang Lake in the lower reaches of the Yangtze River, the maximum altitude in which snails may be found is 13 – 17 m, while the altitude of snail distribution in Guichi District of Anhui Province is only 9 – 10 m above sea level. Thus, snail distribution varies in accordance with the altitude of the marshlands.

In addition, the groundwater level is a dominant factor in terms of snail den-sity. A study has revealed that snail density and the appearance rate of having snail frames with snails is highest when the groundwater level is around 32 cm, and that soil moisture content of 28 – 38% is optimal for snail breeding.[3-7]

Mountainous and hilly region

Snail habitats in the mountainous and hilly region can be found in all endemic prov-inces except Shanghai, but only account for 3.34% of the snail habitats in the entire country (see Table 3.2). Complex landscapes, resulting from diverse elevation condi-tions, lead to many small fragments of snail habitats. In hilly areas, the distribution of snails is restricted to specific zones, and is strikingly variable. For example, snails may be found on one side of a mountain and not on the other. Within a given water system, snails can live in both ditches and farmlands along the entire length of the watercourse. In mountainous areas, snails usually live in the undergrowth with a patchy distribution, or along the watercourse with a linear distribution. Some snails may inhabit the mountainside and the foot of the mountain. A few snails may survive in spring water on top of mountains, and thus form the source of snail distribution on and around the mountain. In the basins of mountainous areas, *O. hupensis* is distributed mainly in ditches and farmlands, similar to that of plain network areas.

Less rainfall and lower temperatures in mountainous and hilly areas are factors affecting the development and breeding of snails. This results in the snail's smaller size in these areas than in the marshland and plain region, with a height of $5.8 - 6.9$ mm and a width of less than 2.85 mm. The snail shell is smooth, free of ribs or with only thin rib lines.

In the mountainous and hilly region, the highest density of snails is found along river banks, the second highest density in irrigation ditches, the third highest density on farmland, and the lowest density on wild grass ground. Sand content and soil humidity are the most important factors determining snail presence and survival. Infected snails are mainly found in ditches, followed by river shore land, then pond and river courses.[8]

3.2.2   Factors influencing snail distribution

The *Oncomelania* snail is an amphibious animal, and thus its distribution is significantly influenced by various biological, environmental, and social factors, such as vagetation, water, and soil, etc.

Vegetation

Vegetation can affect snail distribution significantly. The presence of grass is a necessary but not sufficient precondition to snail habitation. Snail distribution and density are closely related to the type and distribution of phytocenosis. The function of vegetation is to create a suitable microclimate and food microenvironment for snail breeding.

In the marshlands around the Yangtze River, the snail's habitat is often characterized by dominant plant species, such as *Cyperus rotundus*, *Carex tristachya*, and *Phragmites communis*. Usually, snail density in the habitats composed mainly of *C. rotundus* is higher than that in habitats composed mainly of *C. tristachya* and Bermuda grass. In these latter habitats, snail density is minimal where Bermuda grass is the predominant community. In the Poyang Lake region, *Carex* spp. and associated plants form the predominant community of snail habitats, and snail distribution has a significant positive correlation with total coverage, height, and species coverage of *Carex* spp. and associated plants. Generally, snail density is higher in the habitats where the coverage of the *Carex* plant community reaches over 60%, with fewer or no snails found in areas where coverage is less than 20%. In the mountainous and hilly region, the environment is suitable for snail breeding where species richness is between 4 and 14, with vegetation coverage of 60% to 100%, and vegetation heights of 20 to 50 cm, respectively. However, once habitats change, snail distribution and density also changes accordingly.[9-10]

Water and flooding

Snail density is closely related to water levels and flooding. Snails crawl, looking for food, and lay eggs on humid soil only. Young snails also need water for hatching and development. It is pretty deadly for the snail if it loses around 40% of water in its body. Snails cannot live away from moist soil, but adult snails have a certain capacity to survive in dry conditions. Under dry conditions, most snails can survive for two months and a few snails may even survive for three to four months when they remain in a motionless state and do not eat anything either in summer or in winter. However, snails perish when submerged in water for a long period of time. Usually there are no snails in marshlands that remain submerged for more 250 days per year. Higher snail densities exist in areas submerged underwater for two to five months of the year.

Based on the characteristics of snail ecology, the approach of environmental modification has been used to control snail populations. The approaches of environmental modification include i) the burial of surface soil harboring snails, ii) the cement-lining of irrigation ditches, iii) the conversion of paddy fields into dry crop farming, iv) the utilization of marshlands for vegetables and crops, v) the blocking of river branches for aquaculture, vi) the reclaiming of uncultivated land, vii) weeding for manure collection, and so on. Environment modification for snail control has played a significant role in the national schistosomiasis control programme in China.

It has been reported that the greatest changes in the water level in a given previous year affect the distribution of snails in the following year in the lake and marshland region. The present rate of having snails frame is negatively correlated with the average monthly water levels in August and the annual maximum water level in the previous year. In flood season, snail easily diffuse with water flow because floodwater may burst through dikes, flooding farmland, damaging water conservancy facilities, and so on. The studies reported that one-off flooding may affect snail-diffused distribution in the following 3 to 5 years.[11]

Soil

Soil is one of the necessary preconditions for snail breeding, reproduction, and distribution. Not all types of soil are suitable for snail habitation. Snail distribution is related to soil physicochemical properties. In terms of the physical properties of soil, snail density shows a positive linear correlation with the total porosity of soil. Therefore, fluffy soil is most suitable for snail breeding. Snails find compacted soil difficult to burrow into in preparation for periods of dormancy, and snails cannot crawl on completely dry soil or on soil lacking weed growth that protects snails from sunlight and cold conditions. All of these kinds of soil are therefore unsuitable for snail survival. Snails favor soil rich in nitrogen, phosphorous, calcium and organic materials, and the rich decomposing materials in lake areas. Usually, snails of larger size and with thicker ribbing are distributed across rich soil areas, whereas snails of smaller size appear in areas with sterile soil.

Water conservancy projects and tourism development

Environmental modification by water conservancy projects can eradicate fundamental snail habitats and thus block schistosomiasis transmission. However, there have also been some reports of schistosomiasis emergence or reemergence following water conservancy projects in Anhui, Hubei and Hunan Provinces. Generally, snail diffusion occurs and epidemics escalate where necessary surveillance fails to take snail habitation into consideration before project implementation. The Three Gorges Dam (TGD) is one of several huge engineering projects transforming China's environment. Construction commenced in 1994, and in 2003 the TGD went into operation. It was anticipated that the TGD will have a significant impact on ecological systems. This will result in large changes to the flow, depth, and sedimentation load of the Yangtze River, such that the distribution and numbers of schistosome-infected *Oncomelania* snails will be altered, potentially increasing transmission of schistosomiasis in some areas and causing its re-introduction into other areas where transmission is currently under control. In any case, continued surveillance should be undertaken to monitor future ecological impacts and effects on schistosomiasis transmission via the dam launched.

In addition, snails will spread and easily cause schistosomiasis epidemics if snail control is neglected in the implementation of tourism development projects in endemic areas. In 2000, more than 100 infected snail areas were found in the Shitai County of Anhui Province, where schistosomiasis transmission had previously been interrupted. One of the reasons, to a certain extent, was the significant contempt for snail control shown by local government in the development of local tourism.

3.2.3 Snail detection

The purpose of snail detection is to obtain information about snail distribution and density, as well as habitat characteristics. Hence, this helps develop snail control plans, aid in choosing control methods, and evaluate the effects of snail control. The targeted areas for snail detection normally include four types of environments, such as known snail habitats where snails exist at present or have existed historically, suspected environments adjoining known snail habitats, and potential environments which may facilitate the spread of snails. Snail detection is an important part of epidemiological surveillance in the national schistosomiasis control programme. The best season and method of snail detection is determined in accordance with the habitat characteristics and the aims of the survey.

Suitable seasons for snail detection

Snail detection is usually carried out in two seasons, one is from March to May (spring), and the other one from September to November (autumn). During these periods, the temperature is appropriate and snails move actively. In the spring, a lot of snails exist on the surface of the mud that is favorable season for the snail survey. However, sometimes snails are difficult to find because of thick weeds in fields in which surveys take place. Therefore, the best time for snail detection is between the end of March and the middle of April. During this period, the weeds are fewer and it is easier to find snails. Suitable weather conditions for detecting snails include: cloudy skies, low rainfall, in the morning, and at dusk. Snails lie around grass roots or under mud in the winter. It is hard to find snails when water levels are high, during heavy rain, and after long periods of dry weather.

Methods of detecting *O. hupensis* snails

Four methods could be applied in snail detection, namely: i) systematic sampling, ii) environmental selective detection, iii) systematic sampling combined with environmental selective detection, and iv) thorough survey. Snail detection is performed using a square frame of 0.1 m^2 and all snails within the frame are collected manually, in order to understand the density of snail distribution (Figure 3.4).

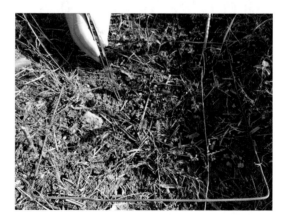

Figure 3.4   The frame for snail detection.

The frame is a square frame sized 0.1 m^2, usually made from iron wire. All snails within the frame are collected manually.

Systematic sampling

This method is suitable for high density and scattered snail distributions. The site of the snail survey is set by point and line. The frames are laid out at an interval of 10 – 20 m along a line. In the survey area, one or several parallel lines should be set at an interval of 10 – 50 m. The interval between frames or lines can be adjusted according to the size of the area surveyed. The space of the point could be decided based on the topography and the size of the environment. Usually, the distance between two points is from 10 to 20 m in lake and marshland areas. When snail detection is carried out on a very large floodplain, the area of the floodplain must be divided into several blocks, each comprising 13.33 h, i.e. 133,340 m^2 (or 200 Chinese mu; one mu equals 667 m^2). One hundred to 200 points are set in each block. Systematic sampling is carried out vertically and horizontally, point by point, and frame by frame. When snail detection is carried out at canals and ditches, the distance between two points is between 5 and 10 m.

All snails found in the point and frame should be collected. The records of snail detection include the localities of the snails discovered, the number of the snails, and the environment of the snail habitats. The collected snails must be brought back to the laboratory for further examination in order to identify whether the snails are dead or alive, and to calculate the rate of infected snails, the average density of live snails, and the present rate of having snails frame. The index of average density of living snails may represent the quantity of the snail hosts in the field. The present rate of having snails frame could reflect both snail distribution and density. These two indexes have a significant correlation and may also be used to evaluate the effects of snail control.

Environmental selective detection

This method is usually used in special environments such as hilly areas, grave mounds, and bamboo forests. The frames are placed in locations that are most likely to harbor snails, such as slot area of an irrigation, wet area with rich weeds, etc. All those selections of snail detecting areas are based on the experiences of the person who is detecting the snails.

Systematic sampling combined with the environmental selective detection

This method is adopted for confirming the snail existing within a snail habitat. In snail habitats where snails cannot be found using the systematic sampling method due to low population, environmental selective detection could be added to increase the opportunities to find. The calculation of snail density is achieved using the results of systematic sampling only.

Thorough survey

This method is usually adopted in suspected habitats that need to be confirmed, or areas where snails have recently been eliminated and need to be certified as snail-free site. In a thorough survey, the snail frames are not used in the survey. The process involves detecting snails in all areas of snail habitats. It cannot be used to calculate snail density and relevant indicators. If snails are discovered, the environmental characteristics and the location of the snail habitat are recorded. This method is time consuming and the cost is high. Thus, it can only be used if snails have been eliminated recently, or in small and complicated areas where the systematic sampling method is difficult to implement. Currently, this method is rarely used.

3.2.4   Snail monitoring and surveillance

In areas where schistosomiasis transmission has been interrupted, or in some endemic areas with very low prevalence, it is necessary to monitor *Oncomelania* snails in existing and historical snail habitats, in order to prevent snails spreading and to consolidate gains achieved by schistosomiasis control. In existing snail habitats, snail detection is conducted in spring or autumn each year. In historical snail habitats where snails have re-emerged within the last three years, one snail survey per year should be carried out during spring, and double surveys should be carried out in the highly suspected environments (for example, close to villages). Thorough snail survey is performed once every three years in the historical habitats where snails have not been found in the last 3 – 9 years, and once every five years in those habitats where snails have not been found in over 10 years. In areas where snails have never been recorded, monitoring sites should be established in suspected environments, and one or two snail surveys should be undertaken each year for two successive years.

Monitoring snails in water bodies

Oncomelania snail is prone to stick to floating objects in water. Thus, one of snails detection is performed with assistance of using floating traps. These traps are usually made of a 0.1 m^2 curtain woven from rice straw. Such traps are put into water near the banks of rivers or canals equidistantly for three days. The retrieved traps are scrubbed twice in clean water and the *Oncomelania* snails are carefully screened using filtered water. This method involves simple operation, low labor intensity, and better performance than systematic sampling, particularly in flowing waterbody. A comparison experiment using two methods, namely, systematic sampling and floating traps attracting snails with rice straw, was conducted in 22 rivers from June to August. The results showed that there were 13.48 snails per 0.1 m^2 (rice straw traps) and 4.67 snails per 0.1 m^2 (frame in systematic sampling) to be detected. Furthermore, the former method is more sensitive to younger snails, since the number of young snails in traps (9.41 snails) was found 11.2 times higher than that in frames (0.84 snails) in systematic sampling. The results also indicated that traps can detect more snails than systematic sampling during May-August and October. This seasonal variation between the effectiveness of the two methods is mainly affected by variations in the movement capabilities of snails.[9]

Monitoring migrated snails

In areas where schistosomiasis transmission is interrupted and in non-endemic areas connected to endemic areas by water courses, potential sources of carrying with snails (e.g. aquatic animals and plants, trees, boats) migrated from schistosomiasis endemic areas should be monitored to avoid the spread of snails. In 2002, acute schistosomiasis cases were reported in two villages around the marshlands of the Gan River basin in Jiangxi Province, where *Oncomelania* snails had never previously been recorded. A subsequent survey confirmed the presence of *Oncomelania* snails in marshlands. Furthermore, 177 fishing boats in this area were investigated. All investigated boats were found to carry with *Oncomelania* snails, with an average number of 13.69 per boat. In addition, 90.9% of crayfish pots and 75.0% of fishing nets in those boats also carried with snails.

In non-endemic areas connected to snail habitat areas by watercourses, floating objects in river systems should be monitored during the flooding season or after the withdrawal of floodwaters. This monitoring can be performed by net-dredge-washing method, that is, using a net to dredge and collect floating objects, including aquatic plants, to screen for snails by washing carefully.

3.2.5   Detection of infected snails

To understand the quantity and distribution of infected snails, and potential risks for schistosomiasis transmission, the detection of infected snails could be carried out by two approaches, such as microscopy and cercariae hatching.

Microscopy

The snails are placed on a glass slide, covered by another glass slide, and the shells of snails are crushed slowly. A drop of water is added to each crushed snail, then the slide is placed under a microscope or dissection scope for observation. The crushed shell is separated with needles or forceps to expose the soft body of the snail, particularly the gland in the posterior part of the soft body where daughter sporocyst located need to be checked carefully. If sporocyst in the gland or cercariae in the drop of water are discovered, the snail is considered to be infected with *S. japonicum*.

Cercariae hatching

Each snail with a diameter less than 15 mm is placed in a small tube. The tube is filled with water up to the upper part of the tube. The tube is covered with a net coating to prevent the snail from escaping. The tube is placed under temperatures of 20 – 25℃ for four to eight hours, and then the surface water of the tube is observed with a magnifying glass to check if cercariae are present at the top surface of water. Sometimes a drop of surface water is taken using an iron ring and put on a slide to identify cercariae with the aid of a microscope.

References

1. Zhou XN. Science on *Oncomelania* snail. People's Medical Publishing House, Beijing. 2005. (in Chinese)

2. Zhou XN, Yang K, Hong QB, et al. Prediction of the impact of climate warming on transmission of schistosomiasis in China. Chin J Parasitol Parasit Dis, 2004, 22: 262-65. (in Chinese)

3. Lei ZL, Zhang LJ, Xu ZM, et al. Endemic status of schistosomiasis in People's Republic of China in 2013. Chin J Schisto Control, 2014, 26: 591-97. (in Chinese)

4. Li ZJ, Chen HG, Liu YM, et al. Studies on relationship between vegetation and snail distribu-

tion inside and outside embankment of Poyang Lake region. Chin J Schisto Control, 2006, 18: 406-10. (in Chinese)

5. Li YP, He Z, He MZ, et al. Impact of the changing water level on the variance of *Oncomelania hupensis* populations in lake area with general additive model. Chin J Epidemiol, 2010, 31: 1148-54. (in Chinese)

6. Wei FH, Xu XJ, Liu JB, et al. Study on the distribution of *Oncomelania hupensis* snail in irrigation schemes of Jianghan Plain. Chin J Schisto Control, 2001, 13: 31-35. (in Chinese)

7. Qiu J, Li RD, Xu XJ, et al. Identifying determinants of *Oncomelania hupensis* habitats and assessing the effects of environmental control strategies in the plain regions with the waterway network of China at the microscale. Int J Environ Res Public Health, 2014, 11: 6571-85.

8. Zhang XD, Qi LH, Huang LL, et al. Influences of soil environmental factors on *Oncomelania* Snail distribution in the hilly and mountainous areas. Acta Ecol Sin, 2007, 27: 2460-67. (in Chinese)

9. Zhang YK, Tao HQ, Liu XT, et al. Research on trap underwater young *Oncomelania* snails by the straw. Chin J Schisto Control, 1989, 1: 37-38,53. (in Chinese)

10. Li ZJ, Chen HG, Gong P, Zeng XJ, Liu YM, Xie SY. Study on relationship between vegetation and spatial distribution of *Oncomlania* snails in Poyang Lake region. Chin J Schisto Control, 2010, 22: 132-35. (in Chinese)

11. Steinmann P, Keiser J, Bos R, et al. Schistosomiasis and water resources development: systematic review, meta-analysis, and estimates of people at risk. Lancet Infect Dis, 2006, 6: 411-425.

3.3 Control of *Oncomelania hupensis*

Oncomelania hupensis is the sole intermediate snail host of *Schistosoma japonicum*.[1,2] Theoretically, then, elimination of the snail can effectively block the *Schistosoma* life cycle, leading to the interruption of schistosomiasis transmission. Practically, it is difficult to eliminate the snail completely in China, especially in the Yangzi River basin, due to unpredictable changes in the climate and environment, and the influence of social and economic factors.[3,7] Nevertheless, an integrated control strategy adapted to local conditions, namely, snail control in combination with other control approaches, has produced a remarkable achievement in the interruption of schistosomiasis transmission in the most part of endemic areas in China.[1,8]

For a long time, snail control has been the key measure in China's schistosomiasis control programme, with an emphasis on eliminating as many snails as possible in every feasible location.[8,9] The great achievements made in the control of *S. japonicum* are to some extent explicable by successful intermediate host snail control. In all transmission-interrupted areas, the success of schistosomiasis control is attributed to active snail control in combination with praziquantel chemotherapy.[8] Moreover, in areas where snails are difficult to eliminate, snail control in infection-susceptible zones is a primary measure to protect people from infection by schistosome.[1,8] Clearly, snail control has played an important role in schistosomiasis control in China. It is still regarded as a rapid and efficient measure to reduce or eliminate transmission, and remains among the methods of choice for schistosomiasis control.[1,8,9]

3.3.1   General concept for snail control

Snail control can be divided into three categories: physical, chemical, and biological apporaches.[1,10,11] The advantages and disadvantages of these methods are summarized in Table 3.3. The concrete measures used in the three types of endemic areas in China—namely, plain and water network region, marshland and lake region, and mountainous and hilly region—are listed in Tables 3.4, 3.5, and 3.6, respectively.[9,12]

The following principles for snail control should be followed when snail control approach is implemented:[1,9]

- Snail control should be well planned according to the local situation and the snail distribution.
- Snail control procedures should be implemented based on habitats according to the water system; for instance, starting from upper stream to lower stream, from simple environments to complicated environments, and from environments near villages to environments far away from villages.
- Snail control should be undertaken in combination with agricultural activities, water conservation and aquatic facilities projects, and the major approaches should be implemented with environmental modification first, supplemented by chemical molluscicides.
- Before carrying out snail control, the snail distribution should be understood through snail detection.

Table 3.3   Comparison of the three methods of snail control.

Control method	Advantages	Disadvantages
Physical	1. Long-term effects: more effective than molluscicides 2. Saving resources: improves local agricultural production through reclaiming of deserted land or wasteland; better utilization of local resources (labor force, materials) 3. Community participation: improving public awareness of diseases prevention by community participation 4. No environmental pollution	1. Large one-off investment: high investment when reclaiming land, construction of flood control projects, and irrigation ditches 2. Slower effect than mollusciciding and needs to be assessed over a long time period 3. Lesser scope of application
Chemical	1. Large-scale application 2. Easy operation, saving time and labor 3. Rapid effect 4. Repeated use	1. High cost 2. Toxic to non-target organisms; for example, fish, other aquatic animals and plants 3. Possible environmental pollution 4. Needs to be used repeatedly
Biological	1. Low cost 2. No toxicity to non-target organism 3. No environmental pollution	1. Difficult to introduce new competitive species 2. Risk of introduced species becoming new hosts for other parasites

Table 3.4   Approaches to snail control in different environments in the plain and water network region in China.

Environment	Approaches	
	November–March	April–October
River-way/ stream-way	1. Filling in an existing river and building a new one 2. Widening and dredging a river 3. Pumping or filling a channel; 4. Repairing and maintenance of river/ stream bank with soil in snail control zones	Repeat molluscicides by spraying or immersion
Pond	1. Filling in of an existing pond with earth 2. Pumping or filling 3. Digging deeply pond for fish culture	Molluscicides by immersion

(Continued)

Environment	Approaches	
	November–March	April–October
Ditch	1. Filling in an existing or open-cut ditch with earth 2. Building closed conduits 3. Earth-burying	Molluscicides by spraying and immersion
Farmland	1. Leveling 2. Soil-burying	Molluscicides by immersion before rice transplantation; spraying repeatedly along ridges of rice fields
Rubble	1. Removing rubble 2. Paving of roads 3. Filling in of holes 4. Burying of soil	Spraying molluscicides repeatedly
Tree stump/ bamboo grove	1. Cleaning 2. Earth-burying	1. Shoveling and burying snail-infested turfs 2. Spraying molluscicides repeatedly
Grave mound/ earth hummock	1. Leveling 2. Earth-burying	Shoveling turf; molluscicides by immersion and spraying repeatedly
Wasteland	1. Embanking for cultivation 2. Digging of ponds for fishing 3. Digging of ditches to drain water away 4. Planting	Molluscicides by immersion and spraying
Wharf	1. Molluscicides in the dry season 2. Cleaning 3. Shoveling of snail-containing soil 4. Cementing	Molluscicides by spraying
Bridge pier/ stone revetment	Filling gaps/crevices with cement or a mixture of mud and molluscicides	1. Molluscicides by repeat spraying 2. Raising water levels for molluscicides by immersion

- During the implementation of snail control, careful attention should be paid to the technical requirements and quality control.
- After snail control, the effectiveness of the snail control must be evaluated in detail. Frequent snails detection is an important matter in the prevention of the further spread of snails.

Table 3.5   Approaches to snail control in combination with agricultural production in the marshland and lake region.

Control method	Suitable environment	Requirements
Building up high embankments for cultivation	1. Marshlands (without impacting flood drainage and storage) 2. Degraded marshlands	1. Totally controlling water levels in the embankment 2. Cultivating drought crops for more than three years 3. Leveling land without keeping dead angle 4. Molluscicides
Building low embankments for cultivation	1. Marshlands used for flood storage 2. Degraded marshlands	1. Digging ditches for drainage 2. Deep plowing and careful cultivation 3. Cultivating overwintering crops for several years 4. Treating peripheral complex environments 5. Considering one-off molluscicides by immersion after the summer harvest, if possible
Cultivation without embankments	1. High-altitude marshlands 2. Non-flooded marshlands in summer 3. Marshlands bordered by dikes	1. Digging ditches 2. Deep plowing and careful cultivation 3. Cultivating overwintering crops for many years
Digging ponds for fishing	Marshlands (without impacting flood drainage)	1. Burying soil with snails in ponds 2. Breeding snail-eating fishes; for example, herring and carp
Blocking lake branches for cultivation	Marshlands without impacting flood drainage	1. Controlling water levels to flood marshlands for more than 10 months per year 2. Breeding of snail-eating fish
Planting trees	High-altitude marshlands (without impacting flood drainage)	1. Planting fast-growing, economical tree species 2. Digging ditches for drainage 3. Deep plowing and careful cultivation 4. Intercropping with other crops in trees

Table 3.6   Approaches to snail control in various environments in the mountainous and hilly region.

Environment	Approaches	
	November–March	April–October
Grasslands	1. Leveling 2. Cultivation 3. Digging ditch and drainage 4. Converting wet paddy fields into drought land 5. Earth-burying 6. Building dikes for water storage	1. Cultivation 2. Digging ditches for drainage 3. Drying out 4. Planting trees 5. Building embankments for molluscicides by immersion 6. Repeat molluscicides by spraying

(Continued)

Environment	Approaches	
	November–March	April–October
Gullies	1. Filling in existing gullies and digging new gullies 2. Widening for drainage 3. Earth-burying to deal with complex environments	1. Building segmented embankments 2. Repeat molluscicides by immersion and spraying
Irrigation ditches	1. Leveling farmland 2. Earth-burying 3. Filling in existing ditches and digging new ditches 4. Cement-lining	Molluscicides by spraying and immersion
Terraces	1. Leveling 2. Earth-burying 3. Digging ditches for drainage 4. Converting wet paddy fields to drought lands	1. Molluscicides by immersion and spray 2. Converting wet paddy fields to drought lands 3. Digging ditches for drainage 4. Cultivation 5. Re-forestation
Small reservoirs	1. Earth-burying 2. Digging deeply for aquaculture	Repeat spraying of molluscicides
Spring ponds	1. Digging deep ditches to introduce flowing spring water flowing 2. Pumping water 3. Earth-burying	1. Shoveling and burying turfs 2. Repeat spraying of molluscicides
Concealed and bamboo riverbanks	1. Digging of ditches for drainage 2. Complete cleaning 3. Earth-burying 4. Converting riverbanks to fruit farms	Repeated molluscicides
Rubble/ripraps	1. Removal of rubble 2. Paving of roads 3. Filling in of holes 4. Earth-burying	Molluscicides after rubble is removed
Crevices	1. Cleaning 2. Earth-burying 3. Filling in with cement	1. Filling in with a mixture of molluscicides and mud 2. Molluscicides 3. Filling in with cement
Wetlands	1. Digging of ditches for drainage 2. Drying out 3. Building of dikes for water storage	Molluscicides by immersion and spraying

3.3.2   Physical control of *Oncomelania*

Physical control of snail means eliminate snail by physical measures or methods.[1] This includes the use of thermal energy, ecological control of the snail in combination with agriculture and water resource projects, and the prevention of snail spread by means of hydraulics.[1,9,11,13] Each method should be used in line with local conditions.

Thermal energy

Physical energy, including heat and microwaves, has been used to directly control snails.[1,11] Like other animals, the *Oncomelania* snail exhibits poor heat resistance, and will only survive 1 s in water of a temperature above 75 degrees Celsius.[1,11,14] Hyperthermia or microwave irradiation can kill snails by increasing temperatures to levels beyond those suitable for the survival of the snail. This is the basis of thermal energy for snail control.[11]

Hot water, hot vapors, and flames

There were some reports of using hot water, vapor, and flames for snail control in Japan in the 1920s. In the 1950s, this heating method was carried out in the field in China, and heating devices and flamethrowers were invented for this purpose. However, it is difficult to kill snails inside soil or in cracks in soil because flames, vapor drops, and the temperature of hot water cannot penetrate the soil. In addition, this method consumes a lot of energy. Due to these disadvantages, this method is not applied in China in the present day.[1,9,11]

Burning

The burning of dry leaves and weeds in snail-infested reed lands or marshlands to kill snails by producing heat had some molluscicidal effects when it was first practiced in China in the 1950s (Figure 3.5).[1,11] However, field studies have shown that this method suffers from the same disadvantages as the hot water method, and is affected by topography and season. According to a study carried out in several reed lands for two years successively by Hubei Academy of Medical Science in 1975, burning for snail control has showed varied efficacy depending on the snail density in the areas.[1] Generally, burning was observed to be more effective in high and flat reed lands, with an average of mortality rate of 81.6% on the soil surface and only

20.1% of mortality rate inside the soil. In another burning study, mortality rates were 77.8 – 96% on the soil surface and 20 – 41.7% in soil cracks respectively. In any case, the effectiveness of burning for snail control is not ideal, and other supplemental measures should be employed to kill all snails. Moreover, burning in lake areas is forbidden due to the need to protect wetlands and the environment.[11]

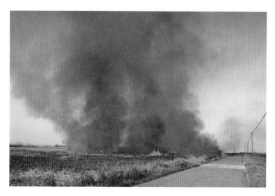

Figure 3.5   Burning grasses in marshlands for snail control (presently forbidden).

Plastic film mulching

Agricultural plastic film can produce high temperatures due to its heat absorption and preservation properties (Figure 3.6). Su *et al.* found that, when snail-infested areas are covered with an agricultural plastic film in summer, the temperature reaches up to 70 degrees Celsius, and the mortality rates of snail at three days, seven days, 10 days, and 15 days were 75%, 93%, 98.3%, and 100%, respectively.[1] This method is

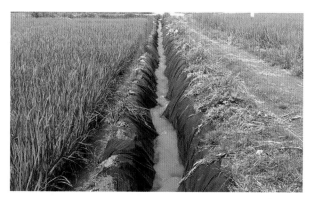

Figure 3.6   Plastic film mulching for snail control in plain water network region.

suitable in plain water network region, the mountainous and hilly region, where connected with fish pound. However, if snails under the film move into water to avoid the high temperatures, the lethal effects on snails will be compromised.[1]

Microwave irradiation

When a snail is irradiated using microwaves, electromagnetic oscillation begins to occur in the cytoplasm of the snail's cells, causing high temperature in the snail's tissue. As a result, the cells of the snail are destroyed. Gu *et al.* used high power microwave sources to irradiate 1,000 cm^2 of snail habitats with the frequency of 2,450 cm/s and 5 kw of output power. The LD50 of the snails was 20 s. The closer to the radiation, the faster the snail would perish. When radiated for 30 s, the mortality rates of snails at the distance of 10 cm, 20 cm, and 30 cm were 100%, 94%, and 54%, respectively. Microwave radiation has the same effect on snails, whether in soil or under stones, or in broken bricks and tiles, such as those found on the surface of soil.[1,11] The disadvantages include the electric power needed, the small range of microwave beams, and harm to the operator's heath. These disadvantages prevent the method from being applied in the field.[1,11]

Ecological control of *Oncomelania*

Ecological snail control refers to the use of various physical methods, based on the biological and ecological characteristics of snails, to forcibly alter the survival and breeding conditions of snails for the purpose of control or elimination.[1,9,11,15] At present, ecological control is the recommended method at home and abroad, as well as the direction of current research.[1,15] Moreover, it is the one of primary snail elimination measures implemented in China.[15] Ecological snail control should be applied in combination with agricultural production, water conservation, and forestry production.[1,9,11,15] Since the 1950s, China has been involved in the study and practice of ecological snail control, and has obtained many successful outcomes. The approach of ecological snail control has a significant and permanent impact. However, it requires huge one-off investment. Therefore, ecological snail control should be well planned and carried out in stages and by steps.[1,9,11,15]

Snail control combined with agricultural activities

Snail control combined with agricultural activities is implemented by means of plowing and cultivation, ditching for drainage, altering agricultural production structure, and so on. It contributes to the development of agricultural production as well as the transmission control of schistosomiasis.[9,11,15,16]

Reclaiming and cultivating snail habitats. In endemic areas infested with *Oncomelania* snails, plowing for cultivation and ditching for drainage can change the environment of snail habitats. It can make the snail habitats dry and reduce sources of snail food. Meanwhile, snails can be buried inside deep soil by plowing.[16-18] Due to the resulting lack of oxygen, activities such as mating and laying eggs are affected, and snails gradually perish.[18] Reclaiming and cultivation are very effective measures for snail control.[16-18] As some studies have shown, following cultivation, the glycogen content of the remaining snails is reduced and the activities of succinate dehydrogenase and lactate dehydrogenase decline, indicating that reclaiming and cultivation of snail habitats can lead to dysbolism, depletion of energy, and decreased fecundity of snails.[16-18] The technical requirements of reclaiming and cultivation include leveling farmland, deep plowing and careful cultivation, ditching and draining, and maintaining cultivation each year. Based on different environmental features, the technical approaches can be divided as follows: reclaiming and cultivation of marshlands that are home to snails, converting paddy fields to dry land, paddy-upland rotation, building terraces on mountainsides, and heightening and thickening the ridges of rice fields (Figure 3.7).[16-18]

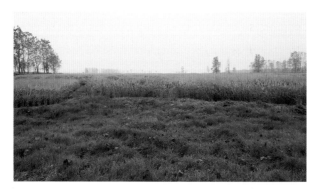

Figure 3.7　Reclaiming and cultivating snail habitats for rice.

Aquaculture for snail control. If snails are submerged in water for a long period of time, mating and egg laying of snails can be affected, and the development of snail egg embryos is inhibited, resulting in damage to its gonad, and irregularities in its substance and energy metabolism.[19] The longer the flooding time, the higher death rate of snails. Snails cannot live in environments submerged in water continuously for more than eight months. Based on these findings, excavating fishing ponds for fish farming in low-lying marshlands and small uncultivated marshlands is a good choice for snail control (Figure 3.8).[19-21]

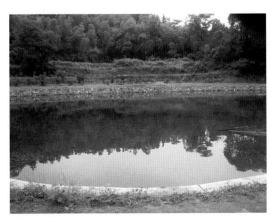

Figure 3.8 Man-made pond for aquaculture snail control.

Snail control combined with water resource projects

Ecological snail control combined with water resource projects is an important method for the control of schistosomiasis.[1,15,22] The construction of water resource projects can alter snail habitats and stop the spreading of snails, resulting in the complete elimination of snails.[15,22]

Building cement pipelines and irrigation ditches. Building cement pipelines and ditches to replace original snail-infested ones alters snail habitats (Figure 3.9). Although these projects need huge investment, significant results can be achieved, and long-term benefits can be attained due to the durability of the pipelines and ditches. These projects not only improve the irrigation capability, but can also control the prevalence of schistosomiasis.[15,21,23]

Widening and dredging river. In combination with projects to widen and dredge rivers, the soil-layer containing snails may be completely dug out and deeply buried, and marshlands containing snails in embankments on both sides of a river may be covered with earth and sand in order to kill snails (Figure 3.10).[15]

Dredging and filling in marshlands with earth at the embankment angle. The surface of the marshland at the embankment angle is filled in and buried with mud

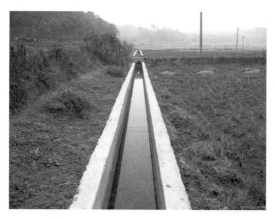

Figure 3.9   Snail control combined with a water resources project: cement-lining ditches.

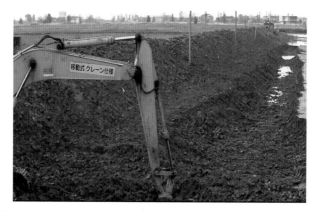

Figure 3.10   Widening and dredging the river for snail control.

and sand at the bottom of the river, and pumped by dredgers for the purpose of killing snails. However, care should be taken with the thickness of the mud and sand, and marshlands should be kept dry when using this method (Figure 3.11).[15]

Snail control combined with agricultural engineering projects

Methods of snail control combined with agricultural projects, e.g. building low embankments, blocking lake branches for aquiculture, leveling marshlands with mud, soil and sand, and so on, can contribute to both snail control and basic agricultural construction.[15,17,20]

Building embankments for snail control. In snail habitats, such as low-lying beaches, marshlands, and lake channels, where the water level cannot be controlled,

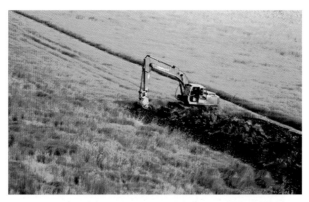

Figure 3.11   Dredging and earth-filling marshland at embankment angle.

a dike encircling these environments for cultivation or aquiculture can be built without significantly influencing flood discharge or storage (Figure 3.12).[5,6,11] These projects create benefits for both snail control and agricultural production, which include building low embankments for cultivation, blocking lake channels for cultivation or aquaculture, and building low embankments with high fishnets for aquaculture.[16,17]

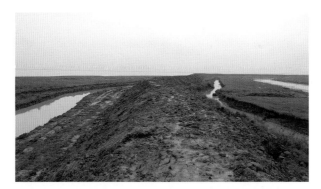

Figure 3.12   Building an embankment for breeding aquatics in lake and marshland areas.

Building reservoirs for snail control. The method of building a reservoir at a cove or small basin among hills may submerge snail habitats underwater for a long period of time so that snails cannot survive or reproduce, and finally die. The reservoir should be repaired and strengthened each year to prevent floodwaters from breaking it, allowing snails to spread with the water flowing (Figure 3.13).[15,21]

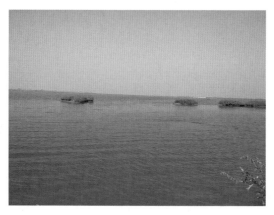

Figure 3.13   Building a reservoir for snail control.

Method of snail control combined with forestry projects

This method is based on changing plant species or the density of phytobiocoenose to inhibit snail survival and breeding (Figure 3.14).[9,24] In nature, it has been observed that snail density exhibits significant differences in different plant communities. Moreover, botanical experts have also found that the growth of plants exhibit, to some extent, promotion or inhibition of other nearby living creatures.[19] This approach forms the theoretical basis for snail control combined with forestry projects. At present, this control method is mainly implemented in schistosome-endemic marshland and lake areas, where water levels cannot be controlled. The method comprises the planting of trees that have an inhibitory effect on snails, such as *Pterocarya stenoptera*, *Sapium sebiferum*, and so on.[25] Altering the ecological

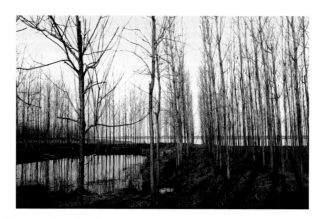

Figure 3.14   Snail control in combination with planting trees.

environments of snail habitats in these regions not only has obvious effects on snail control, but can also yield significant economic and ecological benefits, such as increasing farmer's income and wetland protection.[25]

Preventing snails from spreading by means of hydraulics

The living conditions of snails are closely related to water levels.[3-6,19] Moreover, it is difficult to control snail populations when they extend along the water body, with the consequence that the transmission areas of schistosomes are extended.[24,26] In recent years, researchers in China have determined the biomechanical characteristics of the *Oncomelania* snail according to the principles of hydrodynamics, such as the drifting of snails on the water surface, the suspension of snails in water transportation, the pushing movement of snails in water depths, and the settling rate of snails in water.[26-28] Based on these findings, projects for preventing snails from spreading have been developed and implemented in schistosome-endemic areas in China by means of "intercepting snails by strata", "settling snails", and "blocking snails"; for example, by building tank to settle snail and pumping water for irrigation from the middle level of water body (river, lake or reservoir) to avoid the snails pumped out with water to ditches.[3,4,26-28]

Snail-settling tanks

Snail-settling tanks are built at the gate of irrigation sluices to settle and block snails (Figure 3.15). Then chemical molluscicides are applied to the tank to prevent snails

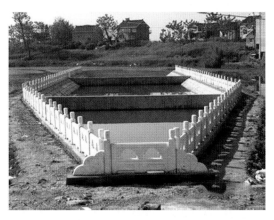

Figure 3.15   Snail control by means of hydraulics: building a snail-settling tank.

from spreading along irrigation ditches. The tank should be built behind the water-drawing sluice (i.e. inside the embankment), and current velocity, depth, width, and length are the key factors in designing snail-settling tanks.[22,23,29] A field snail survey showed that after a snail-settling tank was built in a sluice named Wang-tai in the Jianghan plain, the area populated by snails inside the bank gradually reduced from 536 mu to zero, indicating that snails had been eradicated completely.[23]

Drawing water in the mid-level of water bodies

Based on the fact that snails and their eggs are distributed on the surface or bottom of water bodies, a sealed pipeline system with a bell-like rack for drawing in water at the mid-level of the sluice is used to prevent snails from entering the pipeline (Figure 3.16).[24,26-28] This construction is built at the front of the irrigation sluice (in other words, outside the embankment), guaranteeing the drawing in of water at the mid-level of the water body.[26-28]

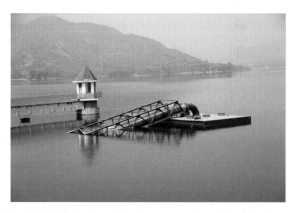

Figure 3.16   Construction used to draw in water at the mid-level of a lake.

3.3.3   Chemical control of *Oncomelania*

Chemical control refers to the use of chemical substances or compounds that are toxic to *Oncomelania* for the purpose of snail transmission control. The use of molluscicides can save time and labor, and is particularly favored as it exhibits a rapid effect and can be deployed repeatedly.[13,30-32]

Molluscicides play an important role in schistosomiasis control in China. Since the 1950s, a variety of chemicals have been employed as molluscicides. Table 3.7 presents a comparison of some of the molluscicides used in China.[11,15,30]

Table 3.7   Various molluscicides implemented in the national schistosomiasis control programme and their mollusciciding features comparison.

Molluscicide	Water solubility (+/−)	Dose (mg/L, g/m²)	Cost (CNY 0.1/m²)	Toxicity		Killing efficacy				Evasion of snail
				Mammal (rat LD50)	*Fish (TLM)*	*Plant*	*Snail*	*Snail egg*	*Cercaria*	
Acetbroma-mide	+	1 – 1.5	2.6 – 4	moderate	moderate	+	+	+	/	/
NaPCP	+	10	2	very high	very high	+	+	+	+	−
Niclosamide	−	1		low	high	−	+	+	+	−
Nicotinanilide	−	1	7	low	low	−	+	±	−	+
Evisect	+	1	2.8 – 3.2	moderate	moderate	−	+	+	+	−
Trifenmoph	−	1		low	moderate	−	+	/	/	/
Metaldehyde	−	2 – 10	6 – 10	low	low	−	+	±	/	−

Formulations

Many formulations of molluscicides have been applied in the field use, including powders, water dispersible powders, diluted emulsions, granules, slow release for mulations, and so on. At present, snail control strategies in the lake and marshland region are focused on killing schistosome-infected snails focalized. This is due to the huge areas of snail habitats in the lake and marshland region. Therefore, certain for-mulations of chemical molluscicides are favored, such as slow-release formulations with the prolonged application of low-dosage, wettable powders integrated with dis-persing or suspending additives and water-floating powders. It is important that cost be considered in the development of novel molluscicide formulations for large-scale application in the field.[15,33-35]

Characteristics of a good molluscicide

The World Health Organization (WHO) has given a list of desired characteristics as a good molluscicide.[10,12,13,32] The minimum requirements need to meet following four points: toxicity for snails at low concentrations; absence of toxicity for mammals, neither presenting acute or chronic problems of toxicity; lack of adverse effects if it enters the food chain; and stability in storage for at least 18 months.[13,32] In addition to these characteristics, judging from the experiences of the large-scale field application of molluscicides in China, following features, such as low cost, water solubility, ease of operation and transport, and proven efficacy with lower dosages are desirable in the field use.[1,8,9]

Molluscicides

Niclosamide (5,2-dichloro-4-nitro-salicylic anilide)

Niclosamide, produced by Bayer, is a yellowish, odorless, crystalline powder with the following characteristics: melting point of 224 – 226 degrees Celsius; not soluble in water; sparingly soluble in ether, ethanol, and chloroform; and soluble in acetone. The commercially available ethanolamine salt (Bayluscide) dissolves in water with 230 mg/L solubility and is formulated as a 70% wettable powder. At present, niclosamide is the only molluscicide recommended by the WHO and registered for commercial use in China for the purpose of snail control.[13,30,32]

Niclosamide is highly toxic to developing and mature *O. hupensis* and its eggs. The compound acts effectively by immersion at a concentration of one part per million for 24 hours. The mortality rate for snails reaches 96.7% in the laboratory at a concentration of two parts per million in a 24-hour period, and is close to 100% in the field. The compound acts effectively by spraying at a concentration of 1 g/m^2 for 24 hours. The mortality rate of the snail is 80% in the laboratory at a dose of 2 g/m^2 for 24 hours, and the mortality of the snail is 97% in the field.[32,34]

Niclosamide exhibits toxicity to fish, shrimps, and other aquatic animals. Another disadvantage of this molluscicide is that the snail may leave water at the lethal dosage, leading to decreased effectiveness. To prevent this happening, a combination with other compounds may increase the efficiency.[13,33,34]

NaPCP (sodium pentachlorophenate)

NaPCP is a white or tan powdered solid with a melting point of 190 – 191 degrees

Celsius. It is soluble in water. NaPCP was the first chemical used widely and extensively with high killing efficacy. Moreover, it has high toxicity to both mature and young snails, as well as to snail eggs. Unfortunately, NaPCP is also highly toxic to humans, livestock, aquatic animals, and hydrophytes, as well as crops, and causes serious environmental pollution. Hence, its use in the field has been forbidden since the 1990s.[1,9,13,32]

Bromoacetamide

Bromoacetamide is made up of needle-like crystals with a melting point of 91 degrees Celsius. It is soluble in water and acetone[31,36]. Bromoacetamide was first synthesized in China in the 1980s. It is highly toxic to snails and has a low toxicity to fish and shrimp. The concentration of one part per million(1 mg/L) by immersion and 1 g/m^2 by spraying may obtain good results of snail elimination when applied in the field.[31,36] No fish die at the rate of six parts per million. However, its high cost limits its large-scale application in the field.[31,36]

Nicotinanilide (N-phenyl-pyridine-3-carboxamide)

Nicotinanilide is a powder with a melting point of 85 degrees Celsius. It is insoluble in cold water but soluble in hot water and ethanol.[30,32] It is formulated as a 50% wettable powder. The compound acts effectively by immersion and spraying at 0.4 mg/L and 1 g/m^2 respectively.[30,32] It is highly effective against both mature and young snails, even at low concentrations. However, snails may escape when contact with the compound occurs.[1,9,32]

Metaldehyde

Metaldehyde is made up of white, needle-like crystals, with a melting point of 246 degrees Celsius. It is an organic solvent and insoluble in water. It was used to kill terrestrial snails and slugs in the garden. The compound acts more effectively by spraying rather than by immersion. The dose is 210 g/m^2 for spraying. It is low toxicity to fish and plants. The effectiveness of this molluscicide is affected by humidity in snail habitats.[1,9,32]

Synergist

Several studies have been conducted for moluscicidal synergist to enhance the efficacy of molluscicides. Mixing niclosamide with a synergistic agent extracted from plants or other chemical compounds can increase the lethal effect on snails and simultaneously decrease toxicity to other aquatic species.[1,9,32]

Operational guidelines for mollusciciding

Field application technologies of mollusciciding

Immersion. Applying molluscicides by immersion is used in environments with a small amount of water or a controllable water level, e.g. ditches, canals, ponds, croplands, etc. Before using molluscicides, dikes should be constructed to contain the flow of water (Figure 3.17). Water volume is calculated according to the following formula: water volume (m^3) = length (m) × width (m) × depth (m).[15] Then, depending on the effective concentration of the compound and water volume, the dosage of the molluscicide is calculated. When applied, the compound is mixed well with a small amount of water and poured into the water body and dispersed. The water is then stirred with sticks. It should be noted that earth around these environments also needs to be shoveled into the water.[15]

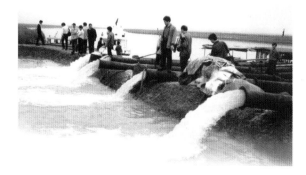

Figure 3.17 Applying molluscicides by immersion.

Two improved molluscicide-immersing methods are adjusted for application to rivers, streams, or ponds with large quantities of water, and lake or riverbanks, respectively. As to the former, there is no need to block the flow of water and maintain the water level. The molluscicide is strewn on both riversides at a range of 30 – 70 cm from the water line. Then, snail-breeding soil with the molluscicides is shoveled into the river to ensure that snails in or on the soil are fully contacted with the mollusicicides, thereby increasing lethal efficacy. As to the later, 2 m high and 1 m high embankments are built 10 – 20 m away from banks and along banks, respectively, to circle floodwater snail habitats. In flood season, water is drawn into the embankment and the molluscicide is applied through the gap in the embankment. The gap is then blocked and keeping the same level of water in the embankment at least three days.[1,15]

Spraying. Applying molluscicides by spraying is widely used in lake or river marshlands. Repeated applications are necessary as grass or soil in marshlands may provide shelter for snails and prevent them from full contact with molluscicides (Figure 3.18). Areas with flourishing and long grass should be mowed before spraying. The water volume for spaying is commonly 1 kg/m^2. However, it can be increased to 2 – 3 kg/m^2 in areas with thick plants.[1,15]

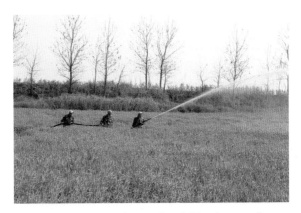

Figure 3.18   Applying molluscicides by spraying.

Dusting powder. Applying molluscicides using dusting powder is carried out in arid environments (Figure 3.19). Depending on the environmental area and the effective dosage, the compound powder is prepared and dusted by machine or manual labor. Personal protection measures are necessary, such as dust-proof masks, gloves, and hats.[1,15]

Integrated mollusciciding. The integrated mollusciciding method is suitable for the plain and water network region with infested *Oncomelania* snails.[9,15] Measures mentioned above, including dealing with complex environments, shoveling soil, and immersion with molluscicides for snail control, are employed in the same area at the

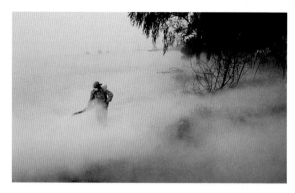

Figure 3.19   Applying molluscicide using dusting powder.

same time to kill all snails in these areas. This method should be conducted in April and May in order to achieve good efficacy of chemical molluscicides before transmission season.[9,15] If the method quality can be well controlled, decreases in snail habitat areas of more than 90% may be obtained.[15]

Slow-release formulation molluscicide. The slow-release formulation method is developed by combining molluscicides with carriers (Figure 3.20). This formulation is deployed in water bodies to release effective components of compounds slowly for sustained snail control efficacy.[37] It is suitable for application in swamps, flooded marshlands, ditches, and other special environments. Experiments have shown the efficacy of slow-release formulations of niclosamide, such as brick-shaped compound of niclosamide, as well as plaster and tablet-like niclosamide coated with polythene film.[37]

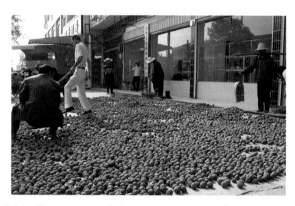

Figure 3.20   Preparation of slow-release formulation of molluscicides.

Delivery systems

Apart from conventional application methods using hand-operated or pressure sprayers, automatic and semi-automatic dispensers have been commonly employed in endemic areas.[1,15]

Compressing sprayer and single pipe sprayer. Snail habitats of 300 m^2/day and 500 – 700 m^2/day may be treated (Figure 3.21).[15]

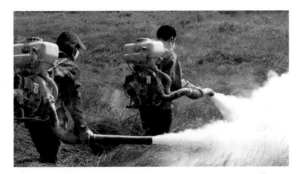

Figure 3.21   Molluscicide apparatus: single sprayer.

Footplate sprayer. The functionality of footplate sprayers is better than that of single pipe sprayers (Figure 3.22). A footplate sprayer can treat 3,000 m^2 of snail habitat per day when sprayed at the canal. One person manages the boat and two persons dispense the chemical and spray the molluscicide from the boat.[1,15]

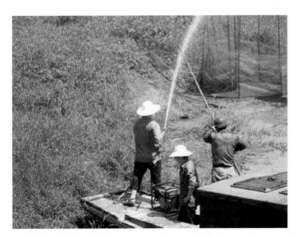

Figure 3.22   Molluscicide apparatus: footplate sprayer on boat.

Machine sprayer. The machine sprayer is refined form of the footplate sprayer (Figure 3.23). It connects to an engine of 0.74 – 1.74 kw, enabling it to treat snail habitats of up to 700 m^2 per day. One machine sprayer, named the Xiangjiang-18, is a gasoline machine weighing 50 kg. Its water capacity is 60 – 80 L/min and its pressure is 0.46 MPa (4.7 kg/cm^3). The width of the spray is 5 – 10 m and the mist emitted by spraying is the same. The sprayer may be operated from boat or on land. The sprayable area is 4,000 – 8,000 m^2/hour. It is suitable for application in the high transmission sites of canals, branches of lakes and small floodplains.[1,15]

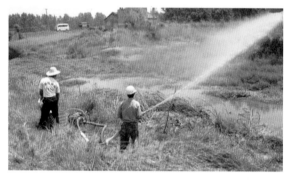

Figure 3.23   Molluscicide apparatus: machine sprayer.

3.3.4   Biological control of *Oncomelania*

Biological control is an environmentally sound method of controlling snails by using other biotic populations in nature, such as natural enemies. It is based on the principle of breaking the balance of the original population and causing an unfavorable environment for snail survival or reproduction by introducing other living organisms into snail habitats. There are three types of biological control of snails: catching and feeding on snails by aquatic and terrestrial animal predators; cultivating and delivering microbial pathogens, such as bacterium and actinomycete, whose metabolin of which has certain toxic effect on snails; and introducing other competitive snails to control *Oncomelania snails*. Currently, utilizing biological competition and parasitism is an important approach worthy of research and development, and is one of the main directions for snail control in China.

Predation for snail control

In nature, the snail-eating qualities of some aquatic animals (such as tortoises, frogs, crabs, crawfish, rice field eels, mosquito larvae, and so on) and of some poultry (such as ducks, geese, birds, and so on) have been reported. Gong *et al*. reported that, when allowing adult ducks and geese to randomly catch and feed 1,000 snails, 60% of the snails were eaten, with the number of snails eaten by ducks being double of that eaten by geese. Zhang *et al*. dissected some aquatic animals, namely, rice field eels, oriental weatherfish, crabs, and crawfish, and snails were found in their intestinal canals. Further experiments showed that a given river crab and eel may eat 418 and 17 snails per day, respectively.[1]

Utilizing microorganisms for snail control

Microorganisms used in snail control may be divided into two groups: bacteria and parasites. Snail control by bacteria involves the infecting and poisoning of snails by artificially cultivating or reproducing snail-sensitive bacterial strains and its metabolin, leading to pathopoiesis and snail deaths. Since the 1950s, China has been researching the effects of microorganisms on snails, isolating hundreds of fungi and bacillus that have depressant and killing effects on snails, such as *Pseudomonas conrexa, Streptomyces griseolus, S. diastatochromogenes*, and so on. Snail control by parasitism refers to the killing of snails using abnormal parasitic trematoda or nematoda to parasitize snails. Trematode infection can lead to a decline in, or complete disappearance of snail reproduction.[1] Jourdane *et al*. observed that when pre-sexually matured *Biomphalaria pfeifferi* were infected with *Echinostoma togoensis*, snails lost the ability to lay eggs. The effectiveness of trematode larvae on snails depends on the number of invading miracidia. Mao *et al*. reported that the more miracidium infected, the higher the mortality rate in snails.[11] Researchers in China also found *Rhabditis cylindric* living in dead snails and the larvae of chironomus, which can eat young snails. However, based on available studies, microorganisms must make contact with snail bodies in order to obtain the greatest effectiveness of snail control, which greatly limits their application. In addition, the application of snail control by microorganism use is also restricted by other factors, such as transportation, storage, temperature, humidity, and so on. At present, virtually all such studies are laboratory-based. Meanwhile, no successful field demonstrations of the efficacy of microorganisms in the control of snails have yet been made.[11]

Intra-molluscan competition

The utilization of intra-molluscan competition in snail control is based on the principle of competition, whereby it is believed that if two snail species are sufficiently similar in their biological profile, the introduced stronger species will inevitably eliminate the original weaker species. This approach is mainly used in the control of aquatic snails. Puerto Rico successful controlled the prevalence of *S. mansoni* by introducing *Melanoides cornuarietis* and *Tarebia granifera* as the competitor of *Biomphalaria glabrata*, the intermediate host of *S. mansoni*. In St. Lucia, *Musa tuberculata* were introduced as the competitor in 1978, which led to the number of *B. glabrata* decreasing to a very low level. In 1981 - 1982, in Martinique, *M. cornuarietis* and *T. granifera* were introduced as the competitor of *B. glabrata* and *B. straminea*. This helped achieve continuous control of the intermediate host of schistosome, with schistosomiasis cases rarely been seen since then. These successful experiences have proved that intra-molluscan competition is an effective and less costly method for snail control. In schistosomiasis transmission-interrupted areas in particular, it has played a great role in further eliminating schistosomiasis. However, there are no reports in China on intra-molluscan competition for the control of *O. hupensis*, the intermediate host of *S. japonicum*.

References

1. Zhou XN. 2005. Science on *Oncomelania* Snail. Beijing: Science Press, 249-316. (in Chinese)

2. Zhao WX. Human Parasitology. People's Medical Publishing House, Beijing. 1983, pp.1-13. (in Chinese)

3. He SY, Shan DC, Liu HS, et al. Study on the correlation between *Oncomelania* snail population and the quantity of the snail detected. Chin J Parastiol Parasitic Dis, 1983,1: 102-105. (in Chinese)

4. Liao LG, Zou XS, Lu LW, et al. The resource of newly found snails in mashland. Chin J Parsi-

tol Parasitic Dis, 1990, 8: 148. (in Chinese)

5. Zhang SJ, Lin ZD, Li GH, et al. Snail distribution and susceptible zones of schistosomiasis in endemic areas around Poyang Lake. Chin J Parsitol Parasitic Dis, 1990, 8: 8-12. (in Chinese)

6. Zhang DS. Compare the effect of the snail survey with systematic and environmental method. Compilation of research data of Schistosomiasis (1986-1990). Publish House of Shanghai Science & technology, Shanghai. 1992, pp.227. (in Chinese)

7. Huang YX, Manderson L. The social and economic context and determinants of schistosomiasis japonica. Acta Trop, 2005, 96: 223-31.

8. Zhou XN, Wang LY, Chen MG, et al. 2005. The public health significance of control of schistosomiasis-then and now. Acta Trop, 2005, 96: 97-105.

9. Yuan Y, Xu XJ, Dong HF, et al. Transmission control of schistosomiasis japonica: implementation and evaluation of different snail control interventions. Acta Trop. 2005, 96: 191-7.

10. WHO, 1998. Report of the WHO informal consultation on schistosomiasis control. Geneva 2-4 December. WHO/CDS/CPC/SIP/99.2.

11. Mao SB. Biology of *Schistosoma* and Schistosomiasis Control. Beijing: Publishing House for People's Health, 1990. (in Chinese)

12. WHO, 2002. Prevention and control of schistosomiasis and soil-transmitted helminthiasis: report of a WHO expert committee, WHO Tech. Rep. Ser. No.912. World Health Organization, Geneva.

13. WHO, 1985. The control of schistosomiasis. Tech Report Ser. No.728. Geneva. WHO, 113,

14. Liu YY, Zhang WZ, Wang YX. Medical malacology. China Ocean press, Beijing. 1993 p.23. (in Chinese)

15. Department of Diseases Control, Ministry of Health in China. Handbook of schistosomiasis control. Publish House of Shanghai Science & Technology, Shanghai. 2000, pp.35-44. (in Chinese)

16. Li Q. Observing the effection on controllong schistosomiasis inside embankment bytransfer of water land into dryland cultivation. Chin J Vet Parasitol. 2002, 10: 40-41. (in Chinese)

17. Nie MC, Wu WB. Observing the effection of administer schistosomiasis in sensitive zone by lakeland cultivation. Chin J Vet Parasitol, 2002, 10: 38-39. (in Chinese)

18. Shi CF, Wang WL, Xiong XQ. Observation of snail control by modification of low output rice field. Chin J Schisto Control, 1998, 10: 179. (in Chinese)

19. Yang GJ, Vounatsou P, Zhou XN, et al. A potential impact of climate change and water

resource development on the transmission of *Schistosoma japonicum* in China. Parassitologia, 2005, 47: 127-34.

20. Lei JQ, Shen HZ, Shao SY, et al. Trial of digging fish pond to control snail at lakes area. Chin J Vet Parasitol, 2000, 8 61-62. (in Chinese)

21. Xia QB. Observation of the snail control with building low dam to keep water for breeding aquatics. Chin J Intern Med, 1976, 1: 11. (in Chinese)

22. Xu XJ, Fang TQ, Yang XX, et al. Trial of preventing the snail spreading with blocking net at the floodgate along the rivers. Chin J Zool, 1993, 28: 12-15. (in Chinese)

23. Xu XJ, Liu JB, Wei FH, et al. Study of a new technique on the prevention of *Oncomelania hupensis* snail dispersal in the irrigation schemes in middle reaches of Yangtze River. Chin J Epidemiol, 2002, 23: 94-98. (in Chinese)

24. Zhu ZJ. Study of regulation on geography distribution of the snail hosts in China. Chin. J. Zool, 1992, 27: 6-9. (in Chinese)

25. Yu FG, Peng WP, Peng ZH, et al. Plant allelopathy effects on *Oncemelania hupensis*. Chin J Appl Ecol. 1996, 7: 407-410. (in Chinese)

26. Xu XJ, Liu JB, Wei FH, et al. Specific gravity and dropping speed in eggs of *Oncomelania hupensis*, a snail intermediate host of schistosomiasis. Molluscan Res, 2000, 20: 31-36.

27. Yang XX, et al. 1992. Experimental study of snail and its egg dropping movement in stable water. Chin J Zool, 1994, 29: 1-3. (in Chinese)

28. Xu XJ, Yang XX, Yu CH, et al. Experimental measurement of specific gravity of *Oncomelania hupensis* and its eggs. Kasetsart J. 1997, 28: 471-475.

29. Yang XX, Xu XJ, Liu JB, et al. Brief introduction of models of preventing the snail spreading through floodgate. Chin J Schisto Control, 1995, 7, 360-361. (in Chinese)

30. Xu XJ, Cai SX, Wei FH, et al. Study on increasing molluscicidal effect by complex nicotinanilide with niclosamide. Chin J Schisto Contr, 2003, 15: 45-48. (in Chinese)

31. Wang GF, Song GM, Becker W. 1991. Mode of action of the molluscicide bromacetamide. Comp Biochem Physiol C, 1991, 100: 373-9.

32. WHO, 1984. Molluscicide screening and evaluation. Bull WHO, 33: 567-581.

33. Zhang, R. Effect of killing the snail and the miracidia with Niclosamide. Chin J Schisto Control, 1990, 8: 60. (in Chinese)

34. Cai SX, Xu XJ, Liu HC, et al. Laboratory and field trials on molluscicidal effect of niclosamide, "shachongding" and metaldehyde. Chin J Schisto Control, 2002, 14: 266-269. (in Chinese)

35. Zhang CS. Study of killing snail by imitation pesticide of Evisect. Compilation of research data of schistosomiasis (1980-1985). Nanjing University Publishing House, Nanjing. 1987. pp.240. (in Chinese)

36. Zhu DP, Gu JR, Yin SY, et al. Study on a new molluscicide, bromoacetamide. Chin J Parasitol Parasitic Dis, 1984, 2: 17-20. (in Chinese)

37. Cai DQ. Study on progress of molluscicides with slow release reagent. Chin J Prev Med. 1985, 19: 171-173. (in Chinese)

Chapter 4

Progress on Schistosomiasis Research in China

**Jian-feng Zhang, Jing Xu, Li-yong Wen, Zheng-yuan Zhao,
Yong-hui Zhu, Hui-lan Wang, Guang-hui Ren, Wei Guan,
Ying-jun Qian, Guo-jing Yang, Le-ping Sun,
Qing-biao Hong, Wei Wang, and Shi-zhu Li**

4.1 Research advances on diagnostics

Schistosomiasis japonica is one of the most important parasitic diseases in China despite a documented history of more than 2,100 years. The study and use of diagnostic techniques play an important role in targeting chemotherapy, assessing morbidity, and evaluating control strategies that have been continuously applied in the national schistosomiasis control programme for more than 60 years. The current widely used diagnostic approaches include two types,[1,2] one is the parasitological techniques (detection of parasite eggs or miracidia in feces), and the other one is immunologic approaches (detection of specific antibodies or circulating schistosome antigens). In addition, two approaches of molecular biotechnology, such as polymerase chain reaction (PCR) and loop-mediated isothermal amplification (LAMP), both of which are based on amplification of DNA fragments have been developed and successfully transferred from the laboratory to the field.[3-5]

When analyzing the efficacy and performance of the main diagnostic techniques currently in use, it is apparent that approaches which worked well in the past are now less suitable. The achievement in successful control of schistosomiasis has shifted the endemic situation towards control and interruption of transmission. The integration of diagnostic tools into national control programmes requires collaboration between researchers, epidemiologists, and control programme managers. This also requires defining assays in terms of sensitivity, specificity and predictive values. Big differences for those indicators aforementioned exist between various endemic areas and stages of control in terms of prevalence and intensity of infection. Diagnostic tools and strategies should therefore vary according to the perceived prevalence level. Attention should also be paid to the prevailing socio-economic situation in endemic areas. This section reviews the development and application of four types of approaches, e.g. parasitological, immunodiagnostic, imaging and molecular diagnostic technology that are currently being used for diagnosis of *S. japonicum* infections in China. It is imperative to choose appropriate diagnostic methods according to different endemic stages or targets.

4.1.1   Historical review of diagnostic tools in China

Parasitological approaches

Stool examination

The detection of eggs or miracidia in stool samples is the traditional way to confirm an infection with *S. japonicum*. For quantification of eggs in feces, the Kato-Katz method, originally developed in the mid-1950s by Japanese researchers Kato and Miura[6], and later standardized by the introduction of 41.7 mg templates by Katz and his colleagues in Brazil[7], is the most broadly used technique in epidemiological surveys pertaining to intestinal schistosomiasis. The number of eggs per gram (EPG) in feces is used as an index of the intensity of infection. As recommended by the World Health Organization (WHO), cases are divided into three categories: light infection (EPG < 100), medium infection (100 ≤ EPG < 400), and heavy infection (EPG ≥ 400). In spite of reduced utility with regard to light infections, the Kato-Katz thick stool smear remains the most commonly used technique for general prevalence mapping and field-based control of schistosomiasis.

Among other traditional tests, the hatching test (HAT),[8] which is based on the positive phototrophic behavior of schistosome miracidia, relies on the observation of miracidia released from parasite eggs in water-diluted feces. The sensitivity of the HAT is supposedly higher than that of the Kato-Katz thick-smear method due to the large volume of feces that is investigated.[9] Sometimes, the HAT followed by microscopic examination of fecal sediment can be implemented to improve sensitivity.[10] However, the result is influenced by several factors, such as temperature, the quality of the water used, and the experience of the examiner. The slight improvement of sensitivity that is achieved may not justify wider use of this method due to the added time and required costs.

Tissue biopsy

When schistosome infection is suspected, but no eggs are found in feces after multiple examinations, proctoscopy combined with rectal biopsy could be attempted to find eggs deposited in intestinal mucosa. However, this is a clinical, hospital-based approach that does not play a role in large-scale control programmes. In addition, the practical use of this approach is limited because of its low level of acceptance by patients and physicians due to associated complications, such as bleeding and the high possibility of sampling error.

Imaging techniques

Radiology, including ultrasonography (US), computer tomography (CT), and magnetic resonance imaging (MRI) must be carried out in a hospital environment when searching for schistosome-induced hepatic, hepatosplenic enlargement or ectopic schistosomiasis. The diagnostic characteristics of all three methodologies are similar in that they are non-invasive and record the damage of intra-abdominal organs in a straightforward way.

US represents a more versatile approach with several advantages. Not only the technology can be adopted for field use, but it is also less costly. Moreover, it is still capable of demonstrating the classical features of periportal fibrosis (appearing as a netlike echogenic pattern in *S. japonicum* infections), hepatic granuloma, and gallbladder thickening. The US approach is especially helpful for documenting advanced schistosomiasis. The technique is not only useful in the diagnosis and differential diagnosis of advanced schistosomiasis, but also for the guidance of treatment and evaluation of therapeutic effects.[11] It is further useful for risk prediction of portal hypertension and upper gastrointestinal hemorrhage. The introduction of portable US equipment has broadened the applicability of diagnostic, imagery investigations in endemic community settings. Although CT and MRI are not routinely used for schistosomiasis diagnosis in resource-poor areas for economic reasons and US is particularly useful in the field, all three techniques require highly qualified users with medical education and special training.

Immunological tests

The intradermal test (ID)

The earliest test based on immune reactions in China is the intradermal test (ID) introduced by Gan.[12] ID has some advantages—such as ease of use, low costs, and high sensitivity (estimated at 90%). These advantages facilitated its application in the early 1950s in the national programme for schistosomiasis control to investigate the distribution and prevalence of *S. japonicum infection*. However, it was soon replaced by other tests because of its low specificity in detection.

The circumoval precipitin test (COPT)

This assay was widely used in China in the remaining part of last century. It has a high sensitivity (94 – 99%) and adequate specificity (2 – 4%). After effective treatment for four or alternatively three to eight years, COPT showed 82.5% and 80 – 83% of negative reversion rates, respectively. However, with repeated treatments in the controlled areas leading to very low rates of prevalence and intensity of infection, the sensitivity of the test declined to 70 – 80%.[13] The technique is comparatively complicated and time-consuming (48 hours for recording result in laboratory), and requires microscopy, thus limiting its wider application in endemic areas these days.

The indirect hemagglutination assay (IHA)

Soluble antigen preparations are necessary for IHA relying on agglutination of micro-particles; for example, sheep erythrocytes. This assay was first employed for the diagnosis of *S. japonicum* in China by Tao.[14] After multiple modifications by Chinese scientists, the diagnostic efficacy and stability of IHA have been improved significantly. The sensitivity of IHA has thus reached 93 – 100%, while the false positive rate in healthy people from non-endemic areas has come down to 2 – 3%. IHA also has diagnostic value in early infection.[15] After effective, periodical treatment for three years or more, most former schistosomiasis patients had negative results in the test. For having been used for more than 50 years, IHA remains a widely used immunoassay in China, second only to COPT.

The enzyme-linked immunosorbent assay (ELISA)

ELISA detects the presence of specific antibodies (or antigens) in samples based on the specific combination of antibody and antigen made visible by the addition of secondary antibodies labeled with an enzyme substrate. Yan and Lv[16] were the first to develop and use ELISA for the diagnosis of schistosomiasis in China. The sensitivity of routine applications of ELISA based on soluble egg antigen (SEA) reaches 95 to 99% in *S. japonicum* egg-positive individuals with a conversion rate of 59 – 60% one to two years after effective treatment. False positive rates in non-endemic area remain as low as 1 – 4%. Special treatment of the antigens or modification of the assay components can improve the diagnostic efficacy of ELISA and extend its application. Various ELISA modifications, including the Falcon assay screening test (FAST-ELISA), the avidin-biotin-peroxidase complex assay (ABC-ELISA), and the fractioned-antigen (FA)-ELISA, have been explored and developed for antibody detection. In the past 20 years, many assays based on recombinant peptide antigens have reported excellent sensitivity and specificity; for example, rSj26GST, rSj23HD, and rSj32. Recently, the rSP13-ELISA developed by Xu[17] shows substantial advantages over simple egg-detection and SEA-ELISA. These include adequate sensitivity and specificity needed in endemic areas where the transmission is at low level. Application of such an assay may allow identification of cases with low-intensity infections for targeted treatment.

With the advent of the hybridoma technique, a number of monoclonal antibodies that reacted with specific schistosome antigens have been developed in China and used for the detection of circulating antigens (CAg). Using nitrocellulose and other paper membranes as a carrier, Yan prepared a monoclonal antibody against *S. japonicum* circulating cathodic antigen (CCA) linked with peroxidise and developed a dot-ELISA kit that detects 90.6% and 83.2% of acute and chronic schistosomiasis patients, respectively.[18] Although various ELISA-based monoclonal antibody assays have been explored by Chinese scientists, most are not put into practical use due to unsatisfactory sensitivity in detecting patients, especially those with light infections.[19] As an ELISA reader is required for most kits, and two to three hours are usually needed to get the results, ELISA is mainly a laboratory-based tool that cannot be easily adapted for large-scale use in field settings.

Rapid diagnostic kits

As application of diagnostic kits in the field needs to be settled at the point of care, this means provides evidences within few minutes rather than hours of waiting for test results. In this regard, ELISA-based assays are inacceptable. To that end, rapid diagnostic kits based on immunofiltration or immunochromatography principles with dyes or colloid metals as markers have been developed. For example, Ding et al.[20] developed the dot immunogold filtration assay (DIGFA) based on SEA, in which the antigen binds to rabbit anti-human IgG labeled with colloidal gold as the probe. Tang et al.[21] developed the assay further by using sheep anti-human IgM immunogold-conjugated as the probe to detect specific IgM anti-*S. japonicum* antibodies that produced positive rates for acute and chronic schistosomiasis at 100% and 96% sensitivity, respectively. The specificity was also good, with only 3% of patients infected with *Paragonimus westermani* reacting positively in the test.

The dipstick dye immunoassay (DDIA)[13,22,23] is another rapid diagnostic approach. It is basically a chromatography technique based on SEA labeled with a dye as the indicator. This test shows high sensitivity for both acute and chronic cases of schistosomiasis (97% and 94 – 97%, respectively) and specificity of 97% when tested on healthy persons from non-endemic communities. This assay has also been adopted for detection of *S. mekongi* infections as dipstick latex immunochromatographic assay (DLIA). The authors have modified the technique and made it capable of detecting specific antibodies in whole blood samples. It has high sensitivity (95% for serum and 94% for whole blood) and specificity (95% for serum and 97% for whole blood), with no cross-reaction with infections of *Clonorchis sinensis* or other intestinal nematodes, including *Angiostrongylus cantonensis*.[24] All of the rapid diagnostic assays referenced above are suitable for general field screenings since they can be read within five to 10 minutes without the need of a microscope or other special equipment.

It should finally be mentioned that recent advances in the detection of CAg have solved the problem of low sensitivity, which has plagued this approach for decades. The up-converting phosphate lateral flow (UCP-LF)[25,26] has presented previously unimaginable sensitivity (a few worm pairs) and specificity. A small-scale field trial conducted in low-endemic areas in China shows that UCP-LF can be used for the diagnosis of *S. japonicum* infections based on the excretion of CCA in urine samples. The assay exhibits much higher sensitivity than that of the Kato-Katz technique and detects a significant number of egg-negative cases.

Techniques based on molecular biotechnology

Better diagnostic tests for schistosomiasis are needed both in the field and in the clinic. Future research for the diagnosis of etiology may depend on molecular tools such as PCR- or LAMP-based approaches. Improved results have been achieved with multiplex PCR (amplification of several different DNA sequences simultaneously) and real-time PCR (monitoring the amplification of a targeted DNA molecule continuously rather than only at its end).

PCR has shown great sensitivity and specificity for the detection of *Schistosoma* DNA in a variety of samples. After Lier *et al.*[27] proved the feasibility of molecular methods for detecting *S. japonicum* DNA, Xia *et al.*[3] developed a specific PCR assay for the highly repetitive retrotransposon *SjR2* of *S. japonicum* DNA based on an animal model infected with *S. japonicum*. The latter detects *S. japonicum* DNA down at 0.8 picogram (10^{-12} g), which approaches the level of 1 EPG of stool. The DNA of *S. japonicum* could be detected in sera at the first week post-infection and became negative 10 weeks post-treatment. Fung *et al.*[28] developed a fecal PCR assay using the same primer to detect *S. japonicum* infection in humans and bovines. The test was highly sensitive, detecting *S. japonicum* DNA at 0.5 EPG of stool.

Based on the sequence of SjR2, a LAMP assay without the requirement of a thermo-cycling machine or electrophoresis equipment was designed and the results show that this assay was able to detect 0.08 femtogram (10^{-15} g) of *S. japonicum* DNA, which was 10^4 times more sensitive than conventional PCR. The test has a high sensitivity of 95 – 97% for the diagnosis of *S. japonicum* infected patients with the lowest intensity (EPG < 10). After treatment with praziquantel (PZQ), the negative conversion rate increased from 23.4% to 83.0% at three months and nine months post-treatment according to LAMP, where the seroconversion rate remained at a low level (25.5% by ELISA and 31.9% by IHA) even nine months after treatment.[4,5]

These studies demonstrate that PCR and LAMP are effective diagnostic tools for early diagnosis and evaluation of therapy effectiveness in schistosomiasis-endemic areas with low-intensity infection. However, the dependence on expensive apparatus and the need for specialized and trained technicians restrict the widespread applications of PCR tests in field conditions. As LAMP has potential value for field use, further studies based on real field settings need to be conducted to evaluate diagnostic efficacy and operational characteristics. However, it should be borne in mind that stool examination may fail depending on the timing of the release of parasite eggs in the stool.

4.1.2 Diagnostic applications in the national schistosomiasis control programme

Since the 1950s when the national campaign against schistosomiasis began in China, the application and development of diagnostic techniques have undergone shifts. An approach that is useful in practice is almost always a compromise between quality and quantity, because the techniques needed for large-scale application must be based on cost-effectiveness, precision, simplicity, and stability.[1] The key of the matter is the required continuous adaption of the diagnostic focus to the different stages of control. According to the criteria for schistosomiasis control and elimination issued by the Chinese government, the targets for schistosomiasis control are identified based on prevalence level[29]. In other words, when prevalence is > 10%, morbidity control is settled as its target; when prevalence is >%, infection control is selected; when prevalence is 1-5%, transmission control is the choice for the target; and when prevalence is <1%, transmission interruption is the target. The absence of local infected cases for five years signifies transmission interruption and the continued absence of cases for another five years means that elimination has been achieved.

Figure 4.1 shows the various stages of the schistosomiasis control programme juxtaposed with the type of diagnostic tools that should be employed for detection.

The morbidity control stage

At the early stage after the founding of the People's Republic of China, there were a large number of people affected by schistosomiasis, and hence a high prevalence and infection intensity were very common, especially during the 30-year period from 1950 to 1980. Treatment of patients with severe illness to save their life and rescue the workforce was the primary task. The etiologic diagnostic techniques,

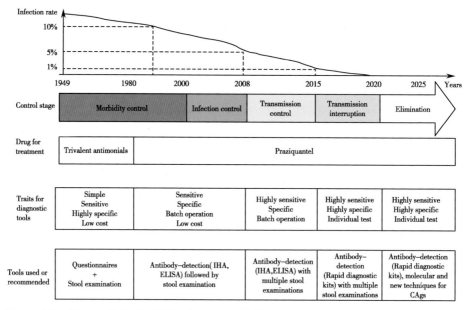

Figure 4.1   Diagnostic tools shift juxtaposed with the control stage and drug used for schistosomiasis control in China.

including direct stool smear examination, sedimentation, concentration, and hatching, combined with a questionnaire approach, were almost compulsory in identifying individuals for mass chemotherapy because of the high infection intensity and the toxicity of the available effective drugs; for example, antimonials for treatment. The parasitological techniques had a better diagnostic efficacy, while the immunodiagnostic approach commonly produced false positive results that increased the number of individuals who were receiving unnecessary chemotherapy. Eventually, the immunodiagnostic approach was only adapted for screening prior to further parasitological examination. In the national survey undertaken in 1956, the strategy of first screening populations by ID followed by stool examination for those who were ID positive made it possible to rapidly understand the distribution and prevalence of schistosomiasis.

The development and release of PZQ for clinical use in the later 1970s was a milestone for schistosomiasis control. PZQ had high efficacy against all species of human schistosomiasis and it could be used in single oral dose, with no or only mild side effects. This made PZQ highly attractive when the cost fell dramatically in the

1990s; then, it was used for mass drug administration (MDA). Along with the reduced intensity of infection that resulted, the limited sensitivity of parasitological diagnosis became apparent. Consequently, control programme managers looked for replacements, such as immunological techniques based on both antigen and antibody detection.[1,2,30,31] During the implementation of the 10-year "World Bank Loan Project for Schistosomiasis Control in China" that was initiated in 1992[32] and aimed for morbidity control, diagnostic approaches varied according to prevalence status and chemotherapy strategies. For instance, in areas of high endemicity (prevalence $\geqslant$ 15%), all individuals between six and 60 years old were given yearly treatment, without examination. In areas of medium endemicity (15% > prevalence > 3%) and low endemicity (prevalence < 3%), residents or special populations were screened using the Kato-Katz method or serological tests (ELISA, COPT, or IHA), and only those positives were given treatment.

Epidemiological surveys differed according to the perceived infection status and the diagnostic techniques that were available. Direct stool examination was the only method to evaluate the prevalence of schistosomiasis in the first national sampling survey in 1989. With the development of immunological techniques and the decrease of infection intensity and prevalence in some endemic areas, direct stool examination was only used in highly endemic areas, while a serological survey followed by confirmation through stool examination were used where morbidity control had been reached. In a recent national survey conducted in 2004 after the World Bank Loan Project terminated, prevalence was estimated using ELISA screening prior to stool examination for confirmation. The endemicity of schistosomiasis had then decreased significantly in most endemic counties.

The infection control stage

Once morbidity is under control, infection control through decreasing prevalence and prevention of reinfection is the next target. This situation, characterized by less MDA and predominantly a low intensity of infections, requires more sensitive diagnostic techniques to support the distribution of chemotherapy. In 2004, a medium- and long-term national strategic plan for schistosomiasis control was initiated in P.R. China to face the challenges after the termination of the World Bank Loan Project. To reach the medium-term goal of infection control by 2008, diagnostic and chemotherapy strategies were determined according to the prevalence of schistosomiasis based on the situation at the administrative village level. Apart from inquiry examinations about the history of contact with infected water conducted in villages with a prevalence higher than 10%, serological methods were used to test annually residents aged 6 to 65 years old in villages with an estimated prevalence of 5 – 10%, 1 – 5%, 0 – 1%, respectively. Once infected snails were detected, a serological survey would be conducted in the same year no matter the estimated prevalence of schistosomiasis.

In areas having reached the stage of infection control, the survey tools shifted from direct Kato-Katz for all residents to initial immunological screening to increase the diagnostic efficiency and compliance rate of residents who were being examined. A system with primary immunodiagnostic screening followed by Kato-Katz tests for the antibody-positive individuals[33] was advised. At present, this approach is widely used in the Chinese national schistosomiasis control programme, as well as for community surveys and field studies.

The transmission control stage

With the implementation of an integrated control strategy for schistosomiasis control, the infection rates of *S. japanicum* has decreased to the lowest level in history and infection control was reached nationwide in 2008.[34] The whole country has to move forward to transmission control; that is, nationwide prevalence is < 1% based at the village level. At this stage of the control programme, selective chemotherapy with PZQ becomes the main strategy due to the significant decrease of infection rate in humans. However, it requires considerably more sensitive diagnostic tools to accurately identify infected individuals at this stage. The Kato-Katz missing rate increases significantly and may reach as high as 80% when the level of prevalence, accompanied by much lower infection intensity, falls to a level below 1%.[35] At egg excretion levels from the host below 100 EPG, it becomes increasingly difficult to determine unequivocally whether there is an infection. Although multiple Kato-Katz thick smears per sample or increasing frequency of stool sample collection would boost diagnostic sensitivity,[36] this approach could not be used on a large scale due to the workload and increased costs, as well as the risk of waning compliance among village residents.

The Chinese criteria of schistosomiasis control and elimination recommend evaluating whether a place has reached the stage of transmission control by an immunological assay followed by the HAT because it is regarded as more sensitive than the Kato-Katz technique. Conducting multiple methods for the same stool sample simultaneously would also increase the sensitivity of the diagnostic strategy. This approach has been integrated into the revised national surveillance system since 2011 when the national control programme entered into transmission control stage at all. An analysis showed that the parasitological final positive rates was increased when two tests were in combined used; for instance, the individuals who show serological positive results have increased from 4.6% by the Kato-Katz method and 5.9% by the HAT to 7.1% when these two methods were used in combination.[37]

The stage of transmission interruption and elimination

The new data from the national schistosomiasis control programme showed that all endemic counties in China had reached the criteria of transmission controlled by 2016, indicating the prevalence rate in all endemic areas is less than 1% with further target to be transmission interruption. So that China has now reached the stage when the priority is shifting from traditional monitoring to surveillance and response, with the focus on reinfection in areas targeted for elimination. The most urgent need at this time is reliable assessment of control efficacy and the determination of target populations for chemotherapy in different areas, as well as certification of elimination using sensitive and specific assays. The immunological techniques needed now must be fast, highly sensitive, and very specific. Various approaches fulfill these requirements; for example, molecular methods such as PCR, real-time PCR, and LAMP. These methods could be conducted in well-equipped hospitals and laboratories, and the latter can even be used in the field.

The UCP-LF test detects CAg at a previously unimaginable sensitivity and specificity, making it possible to detect infection with only a few worm pairs. One of the great advantages of this approach is that it can detect CAg both in serum and urine, the latter being more acceptable. However, further technical improvements may be needed to make the test more convenient, simple, and applicable for large-scale field operations.

4.1.3　Quality control

Diagnosis would supply information for planning control activities and assessing the effects of control measures or strategies. As many factors—such as laboratory conditions, the diagnostic methods or assays that are chosen, technician capacity, and so on—may impact the quality of the final diagnosis, China has strengthened monitoring and management with respect to diagnostic activities. For example, criteria for schistosomiasis diagnosis have been issued to provide guidance for technical staff and standardize diagnostic approaches. Guidelines are regularly updated by the Ministry of Health with consideration to available technology and supplies, as well as the stage of control and clinical symptoms, including history of water contact and previous laboratory examinations. These criteria define the principles and basis for diagnosis and differentiation between acute, chronic, and advanced cases.

Assessment of the efficacy, reliability, and operational characteristics of the assays in use are important for the assurance of diagnostic accuracy. With the development and implementation of CAg assays in China, three collaborative studies were conducted (in 1993, 1995, and 1996) to evaluate all CAg kits. In 1993, eight kits using monoclonal or polyclonal probes were evaluated. The results show that most of them had low sensitivities ranging from 15% to 73% in chronic and light infections, respectively. The evaluation conducted in 1995 indicated that 10 of the 14 kits that were investigated show specificity above 90%, but only four kits show a sensitivity higher than 60%.[19] In 1996, 12 CAg kits displayed a similar diagnostic efficacy as those in 1995. These results demonstrate that the CAg kits that were evaluated were inappropriate for application in the schistosomiasis control programme at that time, especially in low endemic areas. At the same time, nine assays for antibody detection were evaluated. Those results show that most kits demonstrated specificity over 90% and sensitivity higher than 80% in chronic infection. Comprehensive evaluations conducted in 2004 and 2008 also showed that both sensitivity and specificity were above 90% for most reagents.[38] A field evaluation conducted later proves that these antibody-based assays are acceptable as tools for community surveys and for targeting chemotherapy.

The assessments mentioned above demonstrate that many diagnostic methods in use need quality control. When they are investigated, the standards in the laboratory are often not good enough in the field. Before 2008, many assays for schistosomiasis diagnosis were used without having passed certification by the China's State Food and Drug Administration (SFDA). However, the evaluations provided data for manufacturers to apply for license from the China SFDA. Up to now, nine kits have been accredited by the China SFDA, which indicates that the situation is improving and already all those nine registered assays are taking quality controlled in their production (Table 4.1).

Table 4.1   Immunodiagnostic assay kits for schistosomiasis diagnosis registered and accredited by the State Food and Drug Administration of China.

Type of assay	Probe/target	Company
IHA[1]	SEA/IgG	Yueyang Xunchao Biotechnology Co., Ltd.
IHA[1]	SEA/IgG	Anhui Anji Medical Technology Co., Ltd.
DIGFA[2]	SEA/IgG	Yueyang Xunchao Biotechnology Co., Ltd.
DIGFA[2]	SEA/IgG	Sichuan Maike Biotechnology Co., Ltd.
DIGFA[2]	SEA/IgG	Shanghai Jikong Biotechnology Co., Ltd.
DDIA[3]	SEA/IgG	Wuxi Saide Technology Development Co., Ltd.
MPAIA[4]	SEA/IgG	Beijing Beihai Kang Biological Technology Co., Ltd.
ELISA[5]	SEA/IgG	Shenzhen Huakang Biomedical Engineering Co., Ltd.
ELISA[5]	Not clear/circulating antigen	Sichuan Maike Biotechnology Co., Ltd.

[1]IHA; [2]DIGFA; [3]DDIA; [4]Magnetic particle antibody immunoassay (MPAIA); [5]Enzyme-linked immunosorbent assay (ELISA)

To strengthen the capacity in implementing for schistosomiasis diagnostics, since 2009 the Chinese Center for Disease Control and Prevention (China CDC) has organizes a diagnostic platform that is run through a set of reference or sentinel laboratories for external quality control activities. The CDC also holds training courses every year to improve the implementing capacity for each reference laboratory. So far, one national diagnostic center has been established at the National Institute of Parasitic Disease, China CDC based in Shanghai. The center is responsible for assay assessments, external control and improvement of the diagnostic quality control scheme, planning and organizing training activities, and providing technical support for subordinate laboratories. Furthermore, 12 reference laboratories at the provincial level and 16 sentinel laboratories at the county level have been set up. These laboratories are in charge of activities related to schistosomiasis diagnostics.[39] Subsequently, several provinces have established their own diagnostic platforms to enhance management of diagnostics. Chen et al.[40] organized three external control activities focused on the HAT in 2006, 2008, and 2009. The average accuracy rates of the HAT in 18, 28, and 33 laboratories in Zhejiang Province (where transmission was interrupted in 1995) were 88.9%, 100%, and 93.9%, respectively. Diagnostic capacities have been strengthened through repeated training and control activities.

4.1.4　Current challenges

In the process of schistosomiasis control leading to elimination, rapid and reliable diagnostic techniques are essential to accurately identify targets for treatment as well as certification for elimination. Current diagnostic technology for schistosomiasis is useful in China, but big challenges still exist when moving toward elimination.

First, the stability and quality of the diagnostic assays are overestimated. Most diagnostic kits/assays perform excellent diagnostic efficacy based on laboratory evaluation or small-scale field assessments, but their sensitivity and/or specificity normally decreases when they are evaluated in the large-scale field.[10,29] Although there are several immunological kits accredited by the China SFDA, the quality of immunological diagnosis kits available in the market is uneven. Novel approaches, such as PCR and LAMP, which demonstrate excellent sensitivity and specificity mainly in laboratory evaluations, still need multi-center assessment both in laboratories and field settings. This is because more factors, such as storage, transportation, operational issues, etc., may influence their diagnostic efficacy and stability. Because of their high sensitivity, attention must be paid to the possibility of false positive results due to potential pollution in the laboratory.

Second, the endemic status is underestimated due to the current diagnostic strategy. The antibody-based serological assays currently available cannot distinguish active infection from previous infection or reinfection, which makes it difficult to determine prevalence directly. The sensitivity of the current diagnostic strategy, which uses serological screening followed by stool examination, will be lower than that of direct stool examination. This hinders the process of schistosomiasis elimination due to missed infection cases, even though these may be very few. Further studies should be considered to explore assay systems based on defined antigens or particular antigenic epitopes and corresponding isotype-restricted antibody responses in combination with the advantages of antibody or antigen detection, which are dura-tion- and titer-dependent.

Third, the diagnostic capacity in control stations at township or county level is weak and needs to be strengthened. Feng et al.[41] conducted a survey showing the poor capacity in performance quality in the diagnostic laboratories in charge of national surveillance for schistosomiasis. Also, equipment in most laboratories needs to be improved and updated. In addition, the diagnostic capacity varied significantly among different laboratories. Technicians from Hubei and Hunan Provinces exam-ined specimen panels with eight common helminth eggs that were prepared by Zhu et al.[42] schistosome eggs were misdiagnosed by 6% of the technicians and negative smears were misdiagnosed by half of them. This clearly shows that diagnostic capac-ity must be strengthened.

References

1. Bergquist R, Johansen MV, Utzinger J. Diagnostic dilemmas in helminthology: what tools to use and when? Trends Parasitol, 2009, 25: 151-6.

2. Wu GL. A historical perspective on the immunodiagnosis of schistosomiasis in China. Acta Trop, 2002, 82: 193-8.

3. Xia CM, Rong R, Lu ZX, et al. *Schistosoma japonicum*: a PCR assay for the early detection and evaluation of treatment in a rabbit model. Exp Parasitol, 2009, 121(?): 175-9.

4. Xu J, Guan ZX1, Zhao B, et al. DNA detection of *Schistosoma japonicum*: diagnostic valid-ity of a LAMP assay for low-intensity infection and effects of chemotherapy in humans. PLoS Negl Trop Dis, 2015, 9: e0003668.

5. Xu J, Rong R, Zhang HQ, et al. Sensitive and rapid detection of *Schistosoma japonicum* DNA by loop-mediated isothermal amplification (LAMP). Int J Parasitol, 2010, 40: 327-31.

6. Kato T, Miura M. On the comparison of some stool examination methods. Jpn J Parasitol, 1954, 3: 35.

7. Katz N, Chaves A, Pellegrino J. 1972. A simple device for quantitative stool thick-smear tech-nique in schistosomiasis mansoni. Rev Inst Med Trop Sao Paulo, 1972, 14: 397-400.

8. Qiu LZ, Xue HC. 1990. Experimental diagnosis. In: MAO, S. P. (ed.) Schistosome Biology and Control of Schistosomiasis. Beijing: Publishing House for People's Health.

9. Zhu HQ, Xu J, Zhu R, et al. The establishment and use of creteria to gauge proficiency at

detecting common helminth eggs. J Pathogen Biol, 2013, 8: 141-143,154. (in Chinese)

10. Xu J, Chen NG, Feng T, et al. Effectiveness of routinely used assays for the diagnosis of *S. japonicum* in the field. Chin J Parasitol Parasit Dis, 2007, 25: 175-9. (in Chinese).

11. Li L. Value of ultrasound in diagnosis of liver disease for schistosomiasis in different stages. Proceed Clin Med, 2015, 24: 308-310 (in Chinese).

12. Gan HR. The intradermal test for antigen of *Schistosoma japonicum*. Chin Med J, 1936, 1, 387. (in Chinese).

13. Song H, Liang Y, Dai J, et al. Evaluation on dipstick dye immunoassay for screening chemotherapy targets of schistosomiasis in a lower endemic area. Chin J Schisto Contr, 2003, 15: 102-103. (in Chinese).

14. Shi YE, Han JJ, Zhou ZL, et al. Studies on the Indirect hemagglutination test for the diagnosis of *S. japonicum*. Acta Med Wuhan, 1980, 1: 26-31. (in Chinese).

15. Chen NG, Lin DD, Xie SY, et al. Diagnostic efficiency of indirect hemagglutination assay kit for antibody detection of *S. japonicum*. Chin J Schisto Contr, 2011, 23: 377-80. (in Chinese).

16. Yan ZZ, Lv ZY. The preliminary research and application on the immune enzyme marker technology. Chin Med J, 1978, 88: 470-473. (in Chinese).

17. Xu X, Zhang Y, Lin D, et al. Serodiagnosis of *Schistosoma japonicum* infection: genome-wide identification of a protein marker, and assessment of its diagnostic validity in a field study in China. Lancet Infect Dis, 2014, 14: 489-97.

18. Yan ZZ, Wan W, Lu Z, et al. Detection of circulating antigen in schistosomiasis by dot-ELISA with monoclonal antibody. Chin J Parasitol Parasitic Dis, 1990, 8: 161-4. (in Chinese).

19. Guan XH, Shi YE. 1996. Collaborative study on evaluation of immunodiagnostic assays in *S. japonicum* by treatment efficacy assessment. Chin Med J, Chin Med J (Engl), 1996, 109: 659-64.

20. Ding JZ, Gan XX, Shen HY, et al. Establishment and application of dot immunogold filtration assay for detection of anti-schistosome antibodies. Chin J Parasit Dis Contr, 1998, 11: 308-310. (in Chinese).

21. Tang Y, Wang Y, Shi XH, et al. Rapid detection of specific IgM against *Schistosoma japonicum* by dot immune-gold filtration assay. Inter J Epide Infect Dis, 2008, 35: 316-318. (in Chinese).

22. He W, Zhu YC, Hua W, et al. Development of a rapid immunodiagnosis assay for schistosomiasis-colloidal dye strip immunoassay. Chin J Schisto Contr, 2000, 12: 18-20. (in Chinese).

23. Zhu YC, He W, Liang YS, et al. Development of a rapid, simple dipstick dye immunoassay for

schistosomiasis diagnosis. J Immunol Methods, 2002, 266: 1-5.

24. Yu LL, Ding JZ, Wen LY, et al. Development of a rapid dipstick with latex immunochromato-graphic assay (DLIA) for diagnosis of schistosomiasis japonica. Parasit Vectors, 2011, 4: 157.

25. van Dam GJ, De Dood CJ, Lewis M, et al. A robust dry reagent lateral flow assay for diagnosis of active schistosomiasis by detection of *Schistosoma* circulating anodic antigen. Exp Parasitol, 2013, 135: 274-82.

26. van Dam GJ, Xu J, Bergquist R, et al. An ultra-sensitive assay targeting the circulating anodic antigen for the diagnosis of *Schistosoma japonicum* in a low-endemic area, People's Republic of China. Acta Trop, 2015, 141: 190-7.

27. Lier T, Johansen MV, Hjelmevoll SO, et al. Real-time PCR for detection of low intensity *Schistosoma japonicum* infections in a pig model. Acta Trop, 2008, 105: 74-80.

28. Fung MS, Xiao N, Wang S, et al. Field evaluation of a PCR test for *Schistosoma japonicum* egg detection in low-prevalence regions of China. Am J Trop Med Hyg, 2012, 87: 1053-8.

29. Zhou XN, Xu J, Chen HG, et al. 2011. Tools to support policy decisions related to treatment strategies and surveillance of *S. japonicum* towards elimination. PLoS Negl Trop Dis, 2011, 5: e1408.

30. Bergquist R, Yang GJ, Knopp S, et al. Surveillance and response: Tools and approaches for the elimination stage of neglected tropical diseases. Acta Trop, 2015, 141: 229-34.

31. Doenhoff MJ, Chiodini PL, Hamilton JV. Specific and sensitive diagnosis of schistosome infection: can it be done with antibodies? Trends Parasitol. 2004, 20: 35-9.

32. Chen XY, Wang LY, Cai JM, et al. 2005. Schistosomiasis control in China: the impact of a 10-year World Bank Loan Project (1992-2001). Bull World Health Organ, 2005, 83: 43-8.

33. Balen J, Zhao ZY, Williams GM, et al. Prevalence, intensity and associated morbidity of *Schistosoma japonicum* infection in the Dongting Lake region, China. Bull World Health Organ, 2007, 85: 519-26.

34. Wang LD, Chen HG, Guo JG, et al. A strategy to control transmission of Schistosoma japonicum in China. N Engl J Med, 2009, 360: 121-8.

35. Lin DD, Liu JX, Liu YM, et al. Routine Kato-Katz technique underestimates the prevalence of *Schistosoma japonicum*: a case study in an endemic area of the People's Republic of China. Parasitol Int. 2008, 57: 281-6.

36. Huang MJ, Chen NG, Wu ZQ, et al. Comparison of effect of stool hatching method and Kato-Katz in the field examination of schistosomiasis. Chin J Schisto Contr, 2007, 19: 458-459. (in

Chinese).

37. Zhu R, Qin ZQ, Feng T, et al. Assessment of effect and quality control for parasitological tests in national schistosomiasis surveillance sites. Chin J Schisto Contr, 2013, 25: 11-15. (in Chinese).

38. Xu J, Feng T, Guo JG, et al. Comprehensive evaluation of several diagnosis agents of *S. japonicum* in China. Chin J Schisto Contr, 2005, 17: 116-119. (in Chinese).

39. Qin ZQ, Xu J, Feng T, et al. Strategic thinking of the construction of national schistosomiasis laboratory network in China. Chin J Schisto Contr, 2013, 25: 329-32. (in Chinese).

40. Chen W, Zhu MD, Yan XL, et al. Quality control assessments of feces examination for schistosomiasis in province-level laboratories of Zhejiang Province. Chin J Schisto Contr, 2011, 23: 318-320. (in Chinese).

41. Feng T, Xu J, Hang DR, et al. Conditions of schistosomiasis laboratories at county level. Chin J Schisto Contr, 2011, 23: 370-6. (in Chinese).

42. Zhu HQ, Xu J, Zhu R, et al. Comparison of the miracidium hatching test and modified Kato-Katz method for detecting *Schistosoma japonicum* in low prevalence areas of China. Southeast Asian J Trop Med Public Health, 2014, 45: 20-5.

4.2   Advances in treatment

China has made remarkable progress in technological research to control schistosomiasis. This chapter reviews only those representative and major prodcuts relevant to antischistosomal treatment, such as praziquantel (PZQ) and artemisinin, which has affected to the national schistosomiasis control programme.

4.2.1   Praziquantel: A milestone in schistosomicidal treatment

Before the 1970s, antischistosomal pharmacologic agents (such as niridazole, metrifonate, and antimonials) had been used, but were found to be less effective due to the development of toxicities before therapeutic levels were reached. The situation dramatically changed when PZQ was released in 1979.[1] In 1972, the anthelmintic activity of pyrazinoisoquinoline derivatives was first discovered as a result of joint cooperation between E. Merck and Bayer AG, Germany. Subsequently in 1975, a large number of related compounds—PZQ, 2-cyclohexylcarbonyl (1, 2, 3, 6, 7–11b), hexahydro-4H-pyrazino (2, 1–a), and isoquinolin-4-one (MW 312.42)—were devel-

146

oped as a new broad-spectrum anthelmintic against parasitic trematodes and cestodes.[2] Now PZQ is widely used in treatment of human and animal parasitic infections.

Mechanisms of action of PZQ

The efficacy of PZQ on helminthic infections is considered to be due to the polarized metabolite form, which constitutes the majority of PZQ in the plasma. When schistosomes are exposed to PZQ, they immediately undergo an intense muscular paralysis accompanied by a rapid influx of calcium ions, a slower influx of sodium ions, and a decreased influx of potassium ions.[3] Based on these observations, it is suggested that PZQ may interfere with inorganic ion transport. A second notable feature of PZQ treatment is that the worm tegument is quickly disrupted, leading to the exposure of antigens on the parasite surface,[4] which has also been linked to the disruption of calcium ion homeostasis. These results suggested that PZQ might alter the function of a schistosome voltage-operated calcium channel.[5] Chinese scientists have also carried out extensive work in this aspect. The conclusion in the understanding of the mechanisms of antischistosomal *S. japonicum* by PZQ from this research can be summarized in three points: i) stimulation of worm motor activity; ii) induction of Ca^{2+}-dependent spasmodic contraction of the worm musculature; and iii) tegumental disruption.[6] These observations are in agreement with scientific research related to other *Schistosoma* species.

Enantioseparation and schistosomicidal efficacy of PZQ

From the perspective of its chemical structure, PZQ is not a completely consistent drug; rather, it is a racemic compound composed of equal proportions of its optical isomers, levo- and dextro-PZQ (Figure 4.2). Until now, by means of the enantiomeric separation technique, the optically pure PZQ is recovered from the racemic mixture.[7]

A series of PZQ enantiomers and their chiral analogues have been synthesized and evaluated against *S. japonicum*, both in vitro and in vivo. Based on the degree of tegument damage induced by levo-PZQ, research results indicate that d28 and d35 schistosomes are the most susceptible to levo-PZQ, while d14 schistosomula are the least susceptible.[8] At comparable concentrations, levo-PZQ is more active than

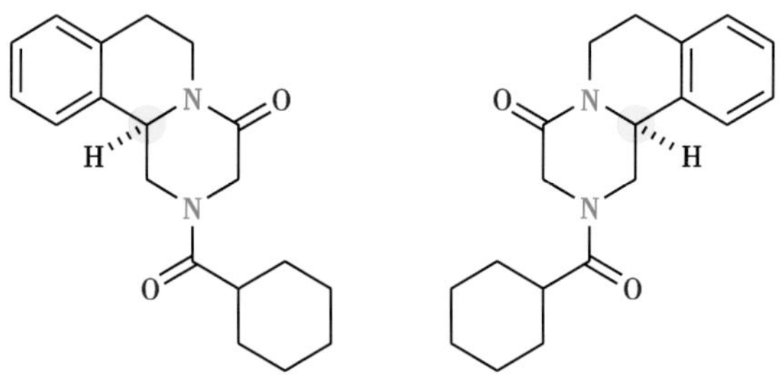

Figure 4.2   Molecular structures of two mirror-image components of PZQ: levo-PZQ (left) and dextro-PZQ (right).

racemic PZQ, even when the concentration of levo-PZQ is reduced to one-half of the minimum effective concentration of racemic PZQ. In contrast, the same concentrations of dextro- PZQ exhibit no apparent in vitro effect on different stages of schistosomes.[8,9]

When infected mice were treated intragastrically with levo-PZQ, racemic PZQ, or dextro-PZQ, only the former two drugs show apparent effects on d0, d21, d28, and d35 schistosomes, and less or much less effects on d3, d7, and d14 schistosomula. Dextro-PZQ only exhibits a negligible effect on d35 adult schistosomes, as compared with levo-PZQ and racemic PZQ. When mice infected with d35 adult schistosomes were treated intragastrically with levo-PZQ 150 mg/kg, the efficacy was similar to that of mice treated with racemic PZQ 300 mg/kg. Hence, this concluded that levo-PZQ is the left isomer of racemic PZQ and an active component of schistosomicidal activity, while dextro-PZQ is almost ineffective.[8-10]

Formulation and route of administration for PZQ

Despite its broad activity spectrum and low toxicity, PZQ still has many shortcomings, such as its rapid absorption into the blood stream one to three hours after ingestion, its low and erratic bioavailability due to its poor water solubility, and extensive first-pass metabolism in the liver, and so on. Based on these factors, scientists at home and abroad have explored many formulations and routes of administration for PZQ to overcome these obstacles.

Lipid-based delivery systems

In recent years, lipid-based delivery systems are finding increasing application in the oral delivery of poorly water-soluble drugs. Liposomes have received considerable attention as drug-delivery systems due to their ability to incorporate hydrophilic and hydrophobic drugs, their good biocompatibility, and their low toxicity.[11] Liposomes are microscopic vesicles consisting of one or more concentric spheres of lipid bilayers separated by aqueous compartments. These spherical structures can have diameters ranging from 80 nm to 100 μm.[12] Clinical and preclinical studies have proven that encapsulation of drugs into liposomes decreases their side effects, targets them to specific sites in the organism, reduces their toxicity, improves their bioavailability, changes their pharmacokinetics, increases their solubility in aqueous systems, and contributes to controlling drug release.[13] It is evidenced that the schistosomicidal efficacy of liposomized PZQ 5 mg/kg is similar to that of PZQ 50 mg/kg. The schistosomicidal efficacy of a 10 mg/kg dose is also significantly higher than that of PZQ 50 mg/kg. Liposomized PZQ could improve schistosomicidal efficacy by five to 10 times than that of PZQ. Moreover, toxicity is also significantly reduced. For liposomized levo-PZQ in a daily dose of 25 and 50 mg/kg for two consecutive days, the worm reduction rates were 55.1% and 74.5%, respectively, while those of liposomized PZQ at same dosage were 20.9% and 55.7%, respectively. There is a significant difference between liposomized levo PZQ and liposomized PZQ groups. The worm reduction rates in PZQ 200 mg/kg and 400 mg/kg groups were 59.2% and 79.1%, respectively.[11,13] These results demonstrate that liposomized PZQ, especially liposomized levo PZQ, is a promising formulation of PZQ to enhance therapeutic efficacy in the treatment of schistosomiasis.

Transdermal delivery of PZQ

Since PZQ is insoluble in water and other common solvents, at present it can be only administered orally. However, the main limitation on the therapeutic effectiveness of PZQ is poor bioavailability, gastrointestinal side effects associated with high peaks, superinfection, etc. Therefore, transdermal delivery of PZQ, which would avoid numerous problems with the oral route, has become the focus of research and is well documented.[14] It is generally accepted that the transdermal absorption of PZQ is related to the partition coefficient and lipophilic characteristics of the solvent. Research finds that the optimal solvent for PZQ transdermal delivery is ethylene glycol monophenyl ether (EGPE). The solubility of PZQ in EGPE is > 400 mg/ml and the apparent partition coefficient of PZQ in the solution is 0.89. After transdermal administration of PZQ in EGPE solution, the bioavailability is 2.85-fold that after oral administration. The serum drug concentration was maintained at 4.0 µg/ml over four hours, which is sufficient for the treatment of schistosomiasis. At the same time, no apparent side effects were found on the skin. EGPE may thus be a promising vehicle for the transdermal delivery of PZQ in the future.[14]

Li explored the effect of PZQ transdermal delivery on *S. japonicum* in-infected mice. It was found that a PZQ transdermal patch has a certain effectiveness in killing *S. japonicum*, with the effects dependent on dosage and frequency. Repeated small dosages of the drug would lead to a better treatment effect.[15] Despite recent progress, one problem frequently encountered in PZQ transdermal delivery is that the concentration of PZQ in penetrating agents is too low for therapy in heavy animals. For maintenance therapy, large volumes of penetrating agents are often needed when PZQ is used for transdermal administration in large animals, such as cattle. This is not feasible because a large volume of penetrating agents is difficult to be absorbed and easily lost.[14] In addition, it is still a challenge to find an ideal solvent in which the solubility of PZQ is sufficiently high to meet the needs of large animals without toxicity.

Injective administration of PZQ

PZQ is the drug of choice for treatment of schistosomiasis in livestock. However, PZQ raw powder is insoluble in water. For large animals, such as cattle, oral administration of PZQ is not easy and its gastrointestinal absorption is slow. After a series of detoxification, decomposition, transformation, and excretion in the liver, the blood-drug concentration is also significantly reduced. Therefore, in recent years, injectable PZQ preparations have been documented in schistosomiasis control. For example, in China, a new oil suspension containing 15% PZQ for intramuscular injection was developed.[16] Corresponding pharmacokinetics-based studies were conducted in swine. The combination product is a white-to-cream-colored oil suspension. Its physical properties, such as settling volume ratio, redispersibility, syringeability, and flowability, are strongly consistent with the technical standards established by the Ministry of Agriculture in China.[17] PZQ concentration in blood was significantly prolonged so that a comprehensive efficacy of controlling schistosomiasis can be achieved with one-single use. In addition, further research indicates that this prolonged administration route can also suppress the formation of schisto-somal egg granulomas, including reduction in the areas of granulomas, suppression of the inflammatory cells, and the hyperplasia of fibroblasts within granulomas.[16,17]

Rectal administration of PZQ

An extensive survey of the literature and patent databases did not reveal much information about the rectal administration of PZQ in schistosomiasis control. There have been only a few similar studies undertaken by Chinese researchers in *S. japonicum* control. It is generally accepted that rectal administration of PZQ cannot only avoid hepatic first pass effect, but also improves the bioavailability of PZQ. It is also especially suitable for those who are unable or unwilling to take the drug orally.[18] Research finds that (in the following indicators, such as bisexual worm reduction rates) the efficacy of PZQ suppositories was better than that of oral PZQ tablets. Histopathologic examination also shows that liver egg granulomas in the rectal suppository PZQ groups were fewer in number and smaller in size than those in the single dose oral PZQ groups. Further, some evidence shows that the relative bioavailability of rectally administered PZQ was 173.2%, compared with oral tablets.[19,20] On the whole, a suppository may be an effective preparation in cases where oral administration is not tolerated.

Sustained-release PZQ tablet

Although approximately 80% of oral PZQ is absorbed in the intestinal tract, only a small proportion reaches the systemic circulation in an unchanged form because of extensive hepatic first-pass metabolism.[21] Moreover, PZQ cannot prevent a reinfection of schistosomiasis in heavy endemic areas. Hence, repeated medication whether for cattle or people, has become the norm. In order to overcome this shortcoming, development of an alternative/modified drug, such asa sustained-release (SRP) PZQ tablet is urgently required. Hong developed a new PZQ tablet formula allowing SRP.[22] In vitro dissolution of SRP tablets shows that PZQ at 300 mg/tablet combined with hydroxypropyl methylcellulose dissolves completely at a constant rate over 10 hours, whereas the conventional PZQ tablet was only 40% dissolved. Pharmacokinetic studies confirmed that SRP is absorbed more slowly than PZQ and has an improved anthelmintic efficacy against parasites in experimental animals, compared with conventional PZQ. In the treatment of clonorchiasis, SRP has entered the clinical phases one and two.[22,23] Hence, there are reasons to believe that SRP could also have broad prospects in schistosomiasis control.

Film-coated PZQ tablets

Globally, chemotherapy by PZQ has been carried out for nearly 40 years in endemic areas of schistosomiasis. The drug has played a key role in controlling both the prevalence and spread of schistosomiasis, as well as in reducing the burden of the disease. However, for population chemotherapy over the long term on a large scale, it is an undisputed fact that chemotherapy compliance has been gradually reducing.[24] The main reason is related to the side effects of PZQ—such as headache, nausea, and vomiting—and its bitter taste.[25] Based on this background, Cao used film-coated PZQ tablets produced by Nanjing Pharm Co. Ltd. to oberserve efficacy and side effectiveness in a filed trial. Results showed that the tablet was more accepted by local patients with lighter side effects; no bad smell and no bitter taste replace traditional PZQ tablets in mass chemotherapy. Overall, patients are more likely to accept film-coated PZQ tablets.[26] Hence, film-coated PZQ tablets also provide an alternative PZQ formulation that can work against increasingly reduced compliance levels.

Meyer found that the disgusting taste of racemic PZQ stems from the nonschistosomicidal component, dextro-PZQ. Therefore, removing the latter from racemic PZQ, which is currently in use, not only offers the chance to halve the dose with the potential to decrease the number or size of the tablets, but also addresses the unpleasant taste of racemic PZQ.[27]

Evolution of chemotherapy model based on PZQ in China

Introduction stage

PZQ was first introduced to China as the clinical treatment drug for schistosomiasis in 1977. For different types of schistosomiasis, the regimen of PZQ was various. For chronic patients, a total dose of 60 mg/kg for one to two days, or total dose of 40 mg/kg for one day was generally used. In treatment of acute cases, total dose 120 – 140 mg/kg for six consecutive days was the standard. As for advanced patients, individuated regiments were offered. Physical status of patients determined the delivery of schistosomicidal PZQ and the level of dosage. The presence of live worms in their bodies as indicated by evidence from medical examinations can help in the chemotherapy.[28]

Clinical use stage

After PZQ had successfully been applied in the clinical treatment of schistosomiasis for several years, and its efficacy and safety had been fully confirmed, the drug was initially tested as a mass population chemotherapeutic drug in some Chinese villages that were seriously endemic for schistosomiasis in 1978–1985. The expectation of this approach was to reduce the prevalence of schistosomiasis among the general population. In its initial stages, this chemotherapy regime was extended from several pilot villages to be used on a more extensive basis in a greater number of villages. A variety of therapeutic regimes for PZQ was applied in the different trial villages in various provinces throughout China. The dose intervals used for chemotherapy ranged from 30 mg/kg to 50 mg/kg.[28,29] Gradually, a nationwide consensus in treatment dosage was reached, with a dosage of 40 mg/kg administered in a single oral dose becoming the standard practice for the mass chemotherapy used in the treatment of chronic schistosomiasis throughout China.

Chemertherapy stage

So far, this chemotherapy regime for the treatment of schistosomiasis has been implemented for more than 30 years in China. During this period, several chemotherapy models have been put forward. These have evolved, been revised, and finally confirmed based on the changing endemicity of schistosomiasis. In addition, some terms relevant to chemotherapy have appeared in the academic literature on schisto somiasis control in China.

According to the active and passive relationship between PZQ providers and its recipients, chemotherapy types are classified as "passive chemotherapy" and "active chemotherapy". Passive chemotherapy refers to that in which experts first determine a targeted population based on historical data. Basic knowledge about the life cycle of *S. japonicum*, as well as the efficacy and safety of PZQ, are then transmitted to local residents by means of media channels and interpersonal communication between well-informed schistosomiasis consultants and their clients or patinets. Public notices are also posted with the locations and timetables for PZQ delivery, and local residents are urged to seek chemotherapy services.[30] During the drug administration process, medical examinations are not done. However, residents who come for chemotherapy are asked about specific physical and medical conditions in order to screen out those individuals in the target areas who have contraindications for PZQ so as to reduce incidences of serious adverse reactions. For this type of chemotherapy, local residents take the initiative and doctors passively accept.[30]

Active chemotherapy refers to that in which doctors from schistosomiasis control agencies take the initiative to look for individuals (medication objects) in order to persuade them to take the drug. Doctors are also responsible for ensuring that considerable coverage rates for schistosomiasis chemotherapy in endemic populations are achieved. In this approach, those to whom PZQ is administered are passive recipients of the drug and doctors are active providers of the drug.

Mass chemertherapy stage

During the World Bank Loan Project on Schistosomiasis Control in China from 1992 to 2001, the scale of mass chemotherapy had been extended to a wider range of villages and chemotherapy models were further evolved. The purpose of carrying out the chemotherapy was clearly stated as "morbidity control". This aims to lowering the infection rate of schistosomiasis, alleviating the intensity of infections, lowering the burden of the disease, delaying or stopping the transformation of chronic cases into advanced ones, and reducing the transmission sources (eggs) to infest the intermediate host, *Oncomelania* snails.[31] In the first several years of the World Bank Loan Project on Schistosomiasis Control in China, mass chemotherapy was mainly used in endemic villages with an infection rate of schistosomiasis greater than 15%. The entire population was treated without regard to individual infection status.[28,31] This measure quickly reduced the endemic situation in those villages seriously endemic for schistosomiasis. The advantage of this model is that it was simple and convenient to operate. This was particularly relevant in heavy endemic villages in marshland areas, which had snail-ridden environments that were complex and not easily amenable to being improved in a timely manner.[32]

Selective chemotherapy stage

However, the continuous application of mass chemotherapy gradually exposed the inherent defects of this model, including high drug consumption, rising costs, and increasing rates of non-compliance among residents. It was further found that the endemic status of schistosomiasis in some villages could only be reduced to a certain extent, beyond which further reductions could not be achieved—even when the chemotherapy model was continuously applied. Based on these considerations, the mass chemotherapy model was adjusted to a selective chemotherapy approach.[28,31,32]

This involved two completely different operational processes. One process was based on selective individual chemotherapy. This entailed fecal examinations, blood tests, and even taking a medical history, including questions about water contact history and medical symptoms. These were needed to screen out those who would receive chemotherapy from the entire population. The advantage of this model is that village residents easily accepted it. However, the operation was more cumbersome and it was difficult to achieve adequate coverage among floating populations.[32,33] The other process was based on selective population chemotherapy. This approach focused chemotherapy on those occupational populations that were at especially high risk for schistosomiasis, such as fishermen, boatmen, and disaster relief personnel who engaged in flood management and response. In this model, medical examinations were not necessary. The advantage of this method is that those occupational populations that received treatment were very clear and there was good compliance with the drug regime. The drawbacks of this approach are the difficulties and complexities that were involved in organizing the participation of a highly mobile occupational population in the chemotherapy regime.[32,33]

Human and animal synchronous chemotherapy stage

According to the components of the measures applied, chemotherapy in China could be divided into two categories: i) simple chemotherapy; and ii) human and domestic animal synchronous chemotherapy.[32,34] Simple chemotherapy refers to a single measure to be implemented among specific populations. Such measures are generally used for those endemic areas with limited funds, and the presence of large snail-ridden areas and complex environments that cannot be modified in a short time.[32] In Africa, this measure is widely used. However in China, it is mainly applied in some areas that are mildly endemic for schistosomiasis. Human and animal synchronous chemotherapy originated in the Dongting Lake regions, Hunan Province, in 1988, which is a heavy endemic area of schistosomiasis.[35] The chemotherapy experience in the Dongting Lake regions was extended to some endemic areas of other provinces, especially marshland areas and plain regions with networks of water. During the World Bank Loan Project on Schistosomiasis Control in China, human and animal synchronous chemotherapy was a primary chemotherapy model to control the transmission of schistosomiasis. The results from the field have proven that this is the most effective method in the control of schistosomiasis in severe endemic areas[36] (Figures 4.3 and 4.4).

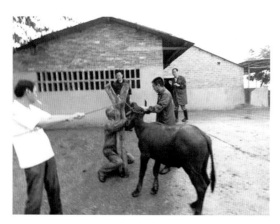

Figure 4.3　Human and animal synchronous chemotherapy.

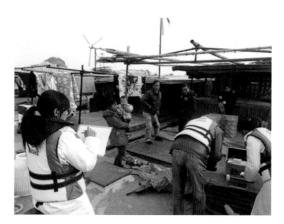

Figure 4.4　Chemotherapy for fishermen and boatmen.

For some mildly endemic areas with lower rates of repeated infection from schistosomiasis, an intermittent chemotherapy model was widely applied. For this model, chemotherapy is generally implemented once every one or two years basis. This approach can be implemented by either mass chemotherapy or selective chemotherapy.

In the late stages of the World Bank Loan Project on Schistosomiasis Control in

China, chemotherapy remained the central focus of attention. However, other measures also supplemented this approach, such as local snail control, health education, supply of safe water, and sanitation improvements in some endemic areas. These various other measures permitted the implementation of control measures that were adapted to local conditions.

Currently, the endemic status of schistosomiasis in China has reached the criteria of transmission control; namely, the infection rate of schistosomiasis in humans and animals is less than 1%. Infectious source control is becoming a more effective and more sustainable model for schistosomiasis control.[37] Nonetheless, it is undeniable that the infection rate of schistosomiasis in some occupational groups, such as migrant fishermen and boatmen in the lake regions, are still maintained at high levels. For these types of groups, the selective chemotherapy model will be continuously applied.

As is indicated throughout the history of schistosomiasis chemotherapy in China, there are several outstanding issues in need of further research in the future. These include: i) how to efficiently and effectively determine target groups for chemotherapy; ii) development of the sustained release PZQ formulation; iii) development of a refined PZQ formulation that has fewer side effects and lower costs; and iv) better understanding of the best timing and interval to carry out chemotherapy on a target population.[32]

4.2.2   Artemisinin: A novel prevention drug for *S. japonicum*

In 1967, China established a national screering group on antimalarial drug research. More than 60 institutes and 500 researchers joined in the project. After screening more than 5,000 traditional Chinese medicines, qinghaosu (anantimalarial principle) was isolated from *Artemisia annua* L in 1972[38,39] (Figure 4.5).

At the end of 1975, the unique chemical structure of *A. annua* was elaborated as a sesquiterpene lactone bearing a peroxy group. It was quite different from that of all known antimalarial drugs. Early pharmacological and clinic studies show that artemisinin (qinghaosu) has a rapid onset of action, low toxicity, and is highly effective on both drug-resistant and drug-sensitive strains of malaria. However, its shortcomings (namely, poor solubility in water or oil; high rate of parasite recrudescence) needed

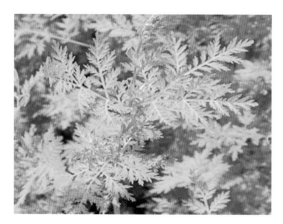

Figure 4.5   Plant of *A. annua*.

to be overcome. In 1976, Shanghai Institute of Materia Medica, Chinese Academy of Sciences, started to carry out research on the relationship between its chemical structure and activity.[40] By mobilizing multi-disciplinary experts and tackling key technical problems, researchers found that some simple peroxides, including monoterpene ascaridol, had no antimalarial activity. These experimental results proved the peroxy group to be an essential, but not sufficient factor. At that time, researchers noted the molecule contained a rare segment, -O-C-O-C-O-C=O, and realized that the whole molecular skeleton might play an important role in antimalarial activity.[41] To improve the pharmacokinetic (solubility and stability) and antimalarial properties of artemisinin, a series of derivatives of artemisinin have been developed. In 1976–1977, more than 50 derivatives of docosahexaenoic acid (DHA) were synthesized and evaluated, among which were artemether and artesunate.[41-43]

The discovery of artemisinin is a collective work of many years of hard work by Chinese medical researchers. Among those medical researchers, Tu Youyou was the most outstanding. She was honored by the Lasker-DeBakey Clinical Medical Research Award in 2011 and was awarded half of the 2015 Nobel Prize in Physiology or Medicine for her discoveries concerning a novel therapy against malaria (that is, extracting artemisinin from *Artemisia annua* mixture).

Artemether

Artemether is the β-methylether derivative of dihydroartemisinin. Its chemical structure is depicted in Figure 4.6. The first report of artemether's activity against *S. japonicum* was published in 1982, just two years after the discovery of the antischistosomal properties of artemisinin.[44]

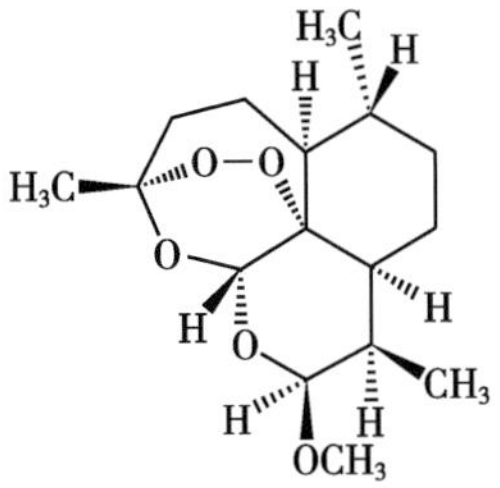

Figure 4.6   Artemether.

Artemether monotherapy

Artemether is active against *S. japonicum*, especially on 5–21-day-old juvenile worms. Clinical trials on artemether against human *S. japonicum* infections found that multiple doses of artemether at 6 mg/kg over 15 day intervals could achieve 60.8% to 100% protection for the prevention of *S. japonicum* infection. Increased doses resulted in improved efficacies. After artemether therapy, only mild, transient treatment-associated adverse events were observed. Repeated dosing of artemether significantly reduced the incidence of *S. japonicum* infections, as compared with the placebo. Trial results also indicated that it is more effective to use multiple doses of artemether with two-week intervals for prevention against *S. japonicum* infection.[44,45]

Artemether–PZQ combination

Since PZQ and artemether act against different developmental stages of *S. japonicum*—PZQ acts against adult worms and artemether acts against juvenile schistosomes —a combination therapy may cover all developmental stages and result in an improved antischistosomal efficacy.[46] To test the hypothesis, animal experiments were performed to evaluate the efficacy of a PZQ-artemether combination against *S. japonicum* infection.

In rabbits infected with 7–14-day-old schistosomula and 42-day-old adult schistosomes, the combined treatment of PZQ and artemether reduced total worm burdens by 79 – 92%. These rates were significantly greater than those resulting from treatment with 50 mg/kg PZQ (28 – 66% total worm burden reduction) or 15 mg/kg artemether alone (44 – 56% total worm burden reduction), using the same dosages and schedules. In another study in rabbits experimentally infected with 42-day-old or 56-day-old adult *S. japonicum*, the PZQ–artemether combination achieved total worm burden reductions of 96 – 99%. At the same time, treatment with PZQ administered at a single dose of 40 mg/kg alone resulted in total worm reduction rates of 87% and a single dose of 15 mg/kg artemether resulted in total worm reduction rates of 25 – 33%.[47] From these results, it has been determined that a PZQ-artemether combination at lower doses is safe and more effective than the administration of PZQ or artemether alone.

In human trials, a randomized, double-blind, placebo-controlled trial in the Dongting Lake regions of China shows that treatment with 60 mg/kg PZQ combined with 6 mg/kg artemether, 60 mg/kg PZQ combined with an artemether placebo, 120 mg/kg PZQ combined with 6 mg/kg artemether, and 120 mg/kg PZQ combined with an artemether placebo achieved treatment efficacies of 98%, 96.4%, 97.7%, and 95.7%, respectively, in the treatment of acute schistosomiasis.[48] The combination of artemether and PZQ chemotherapy did not improve the treatment efficacy compared with PZQ alone. In addition, administration of artemether caused fewer and minor adverse events within four hours of the treatment, including allergy, nausea, vomiting, and abdominal discomfort.[48]

Recommended treatment regimen and contraindications

According to the results from animals and human trials, artemether is currently mainly used for the prevention of schistosome infections. The following regimen is recommended: artemether is administered at a dose of 6 mg/kg, starting one or two weeks after contact with infested water during the transmission season, followed by repeated treatment everyone to two weeks with several doses, and an additional treatment given 15 days post-exposure.[46]

It is noteworthy that the treatment is contraindicated in patients with early pregnancy, severe liver, renal, or hematologic diseases, or with an allergy to artemether. In addition, oral administration of artemether at a dose of 6 mg/kg daily for five to seven days may be given in cases with an allergy to PZQ, since the agent is also active against the adult worms of the parasite.[46,49]

Artesunate

Figure 4.7 shows the chemical structure of artesunate (that is, dihydroartemisinin-10-α-succinate).

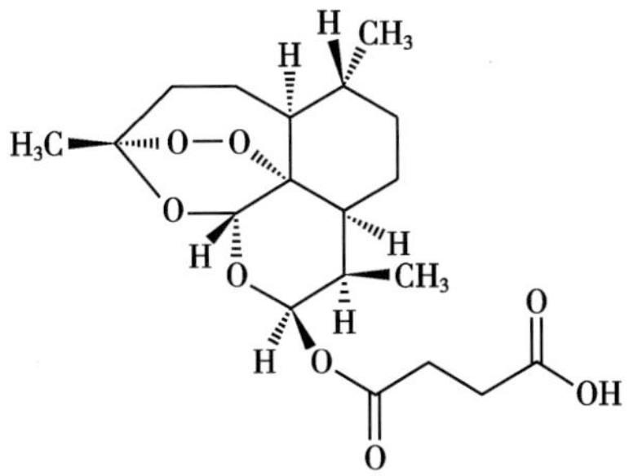

Figure 4.7   Artesunate.

Artesunate monotherapy

Artesunate was found to be active against various developmental stages of *S. japonicum* in experimentally infected mice; notably, seven-day-old schistosomula. After artesunate was given to the infected mice, artesunate was given to experimentally infected rabbits and dogs at doses of 300, 20 – 40, and 30 mg/kg seven days post-infection, once a week for four to six weeks. The treatments resulted in worm burden reductions of 77.5 – 90.66%, 99.53%, and 97.10%, respectively.[50] In addition, in rabbits, treatment with artesunate at a dose of 16 mg/kg, given once a week for four weeks starting at seven days post-infection, was also found to effectively prevent the development of acute schistosomiasis and suppress egg production.[51]

In human trials, it was demonstrated that multiple doses of artesunate at 6 mg/kg, given once a week at seven-day intervals, achieved 68.19 – 100% protection against human *S. japonicum* infection and effectively prevented the development of acute schistosomiasis.[6]

Artesunate-PZQ combination therapy

Co-administration of artesunate and PZQ, or administration of PZQ followed by artesunate, was found to significantly reduce the activities of the artesunate against *S. japonicum* schistosomula. Administration of artesunate first, followed by PZQ, resulted in similar antischistosomal activities to those observed with artesunate alone, while a PZQ–artesunate combination treatment significantly reduced the activities of PZQ against adult worms. However, in experimentally infected rabbits, the administration of artesunate followed by PZQ, was found to achieve a comparative antischistosomal activity to that resulting from treatment with artesunate alone.[49]

A field application of the artesunate–PZQ combination was performed in the major flood of 1998. The administration of artesunate started within seven days of contact with infested water, at an oral dose of 300 mg, given in seven-day intervals four times. Treatment with PZQ at a single dose of 1.2 g within 23 – 25 days of contact with infested water, with an additional dosing seven days post-exposure, significantly improved the protective efficacy compared with the controls[52] (Figure 4.8). The treatment-associated adverse events included mild gastrointestinal reaction in six cases and transient premature heart beats in three cases.[52,53]

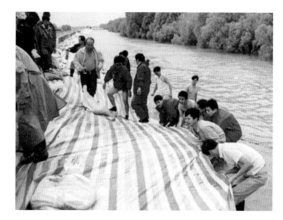

Figure 4.8 Anti-flood personnel in the huge flooding along the Yangtze River Basin in 1998.

Recommended treatment regimen

Currently, artesunate is recommended for the prevention of *S. japonicum* human infection by multiple administrations at 6 mg/kg, starting from within seven days after contact with infested water during the transmission season, with an additional treatment given seven days post-exposure.[54]

Concluding remarks on artemisinin

The combination of artemisinin derivatives with PZQ seems to be the best option for the treatment of schistosomiasis, reflecting their complementary pharmacological profiles against this disease. Although the antischistosomal actions of artemisinin derivatives have been identified for several decades, their exact mechanisms of action remain elusive. The problem of unclear mechanisms of actions of these two artemisinin derivatives severely inhibits the development of other artemisinin analogues. Therefore, elucidation of the mechanisms underlying the antischistosomal activity of artemisinin derivatives is urgently need.

References

1. Andrews P, Thomas H, Pohlke R, et al. Praziquantel. Med Res Rev, 1983, 3: 147-200.

2. Chai JY. Praziquantel treatment in trematode and cestode infections: an update. Infect Chemether, 2013, 45(1): 32-43.

3. Pax R, Bennett JL, Fetterer R. A benzodiazepine derivative and praziquantel: effects on musculature of *Schistosoma mansoni* and *Schistosoma japonicum*. Naunyn-Schmiedebergs Arch Pharmacol, 1978, 304: 309-15.

4. Harnett W, Kusel JR. Increased exposure of parasite antigens at the surface of adult male *Schistosoma mansoni* exposed to praziquantel in vitro. Parasitology, 1986, 93: 401-5.

5. Aragon AD, Imani RA, Blackburn VR, et al. Towards an understanding of the mechanism of action of praziquantel. Mol Biochem Parasitol, 2009, 164: 57-65.

6. Xiao SH. Development of antischistosomal drugs in China, with particular consideration to praziquantel and the artemisinins. Acta Trop, 2005, 96:153-167.

7. Lima RM, Ferreira MA, Ponte TM, et al. Enantioselective analysis of praziquantel and trans-4-hydroxypraziquantel in human plasma by chiral LC-MS/MS: Application to pharmacokinetics. J Chromatogr B Analyt Technol Biomed Life Sci, 2009, 877:3083-3088.

8. Xiao XH, You JQ, Mei JY, et al. In vitro and in vivo effect of levopraziquantel, dextropraziquantel versus racemic praziquantel on different developmental stages of *Schistosoma japonicum*. Zhongguo Ji Sheng Chong Xue Yu Ji Sheng Chong Bing Za Zhi, 1998, 16:335-441. (in Chinese)

9. Liu YH, Qian, MX, Wang XG, et al. Comparative efficacy of praziquantel and its optic isomers in experimental therapy of schistosomiasis japonica in rabbits. Chin Med J (Engl), 1986, 99:935-940.

10. Meister I, Ingram K, Cowan N, et al. Activity of praziquantel enantiomers and main metabolites against *Schistosoma mansoni*. Antimicrob Agents Chemother, 2014, 58: 5466-5472.

11. Mufamadi M.S, Pillay V, Choonara YE, et al. A review on composite liposomal technologies for specialized drug delivery. J Drug Deliv, 2011, 2011: 1-19.

12. Mourau SC, Costa PI, Salgado HRN, et al. Improvement of antischistosomal activity of prazi-

quantel by incorporation into phosphatidylcholine-containing lipossomes. Int J Pharmacol, 2005, 290: 157-162.

13. Frezza TF, Gremiao MPD, Zanotti-Magalhaes EM, et al. Liposomal-praziquantel: Efficacy against *Schistosoma mansoni* in a preclinical assay. Acta Trop, 2013, 128:70-75.

14. Zheng XS, Duan CZ, Xiao ZD, et al. Transdermal delivery of praziquantel: Effects of solvents on permeation across rabbit skin. Biol Pharm Bull, 2008, 31: 1045-1048.

15. Li XH, Zhang DZ, Yang Y, et al. Effect of praziquantel transdermal delivery on infection of *Schistosoma japonicum* of mice. Zhongguo Xue Xi Chong Bing Fang Zhi Za Zhi, 2012, 24:155-159. (in Chinese)

16. Tang S, Chen L, Guo Z, et al. Pharmacokinetics of a new ivermectin/praziquantel oil suspension after intramuscular administration in pigs. Vet Parasitol, 2012, 185:229-235.

17. Tang S, Chen L, Qian M., et al. Pharmacokinetics of a new ivermectin/praziquantel suspension after intramuscular administration in sheep. Vet Parasitol, 2016, 221:54-58.

18. Yang Y, Wang JM, Jiang Yan, et al. Experiment of praziquantel rectal administration in treatment of schistosomiasis in mice. Zhongguo Xue Xi Chong Bing Fang Zhi Za Zhi, 2011, 23:674-676. (in Chinese)

19. Shen XL, Zhang H. Pharmacokinetics of praziquantel liquid suppository in rabbits. J Guangdong Coll Pharm.2006, 22:25-31. (in Chinese)

20. Li G, Qiu J, He G, et al. Phamacokinetics and bioavailability of praziquantel suppository in rabbit. Acta Univ Med Tongji, 1994, 23 (suppl 2): 93-95. (in Chinese)

21. Andrews P. Praziquantel: mechanisms of anti-schistosomal activity. Pharmacol Ther, 1985, 29: 129-156.

22. Hong ST, Lee SH, Lee SJ, et al. Sustained-release praziquantel tablet: pharmacokinetics and the treatment of clonorchiasis in beagle dogs. Parasitol Res, 2003, 91: 316-320.

23. Choi MH, Chang BC, Lee SJ, et al. Therapeutic evaluation of sustained-releasing praziquantel (SRP) for clonorchiasis: Phase 1 and 2 clinical studies. Korean J Parasitol, 2006, 44: 361-366.

24. Cao L, Hu GH, Guo JG, et al. Compliance study on mass chemotherapy with praziquantel in schistosomiasis hyper-endemic area of Poyang Lake region for successive 6 years. Parasito Infec Dis, 2003, 1: 153-155. (in Chinese)

25. Chen CL, You XJ, Zeng XY, et al. Side-effect induced by praziquantel treatment for schistosomiasis. Zhongguo Xue Xi Chong Bing Fang Zhi Za Zhi, 2005, 17:323-327. (in Chinese)

26. Cao CL, Bao ZP, Chen L, et al. Compliance of film-coated praziquantel tablets in schisto-

somiasis transmission-controlled areas. Zhongguo Xue Xi Chong Bing Fang Zhi Za Zhi, 2011, 23:659-663. (in Chinese)

27. Meyer T, Sekljic H, Fuchs S, et al. Taste, a new incentive to switch to (R)-praziquantel in schistosomiasis treatment. PLoS Negl Trop Dis, 2009, 3:e357.

28. Chen MG. Use of praziquantel for clinical treatment and morbidity control of schistosomiasis japonica in China: a review of 30 years's experience. Acta Trop, 2005, 96:168-176.

29. Xiao SH, Keiser J, Chen MG, et al. Research and development of antischistosomal drugs in the People's Republic of China: a 60-year review. Adv Parasitol, 2010, 73: 231-295.

30. Guo JG, Cao CL, Hu GH, et al. The role of passive chemotherapy in schistosomiasis control during maintain and consolidate stage. Chin J Parasit Dis Control, 2003, 16:266-268. (in Chinese)

31. Ross AG, Sleigh AC, Li YS, et al. Schistosomiasis in the People's Republic of China: prospects and challenges for the 21st century. Clin Microbiol Rev, 2001, 14:270-295.

32. Zhu R, Guo JG. Role of chemotherapy with praziquantel in schistosomiasis control. Zhongguo Xue Xi Chong Bing Fang Zhi Za Zhi, 2009, 21:154-157.

33. Chen MG. Chemotherapy in schistosomiasis control program. Zhongguo Xue Xi Chong Bing Fang Zhi Za Zhi, 2003, 15:401. (in Chinese)

34. Cao Z, Huang Y, Wang T. Schistosomiasis japonica control in domestic animals: progress and experiences in China. Front Microbiol, 2017, 8:1-5.

35. Cao MK, Tian ZY, Xiao JW, et al. Effect of synchronous chemotherapy of human and livestock to block schistosomiasis transmission in Changde, Hunan province, P.R.China. Hunan Med, 1989, 6:9-10. (in Chinese)

36. Chen X, Wang L, Cai J, et al. Schistosomiasis control in China: the impact of a 10-year World Bank Loan Project (1992-2001). Bull World Health Organ, 2005, 83:43-48.

37. Wang LD, Chen HG, Guo JG, et al. A strategy to control transmission of *schistosoma japonicum* in China. N Engl J Med, 2009, 360:121-128.

38. Zhang JF. A detailed chronological record of project 523 and the discovery and development of Qinghaosu (Artemisinin). Guangzhou: Yangcheng Evening News Publisher, 2006. (in Chinese)

39. Li Y, Wu YL. A golden phoenix arising from the herbal net - A review and reflection on the study of antimalarial drug artemisinin. Front Chem Chin, 2010, 5: 357-422. (in Chinese)

40. Liu JM, Ni MY, Fan JF, et al. Structure and reactions of arteannuin. Acta Chim Sin, 1979, 37: 129-43. (in Chinese)

41. Li Y. Qinghaosi (Artemisinin): chemistry and pharmacology. Acta Pharmacol Sin, 2012,

33:1141-1146.

42. Li Y, Yu PL, Chen YX, et al. Synthesis of some derivatives of artemisinin. Chin Sci Bull, 1979, 24: 667-9. (in Chinese)

43. Li Y, Yu PL, Chen YX, et al. Studies on analogs of artemisinin I. the synthesis of ethers, carboxylic esters and carbonates of dihydroartemisinine. Acta Pharmaceut Sin, 1981, 16: 429-39. (in Chinese)

44. Le WJ, You JQ, Mei JY. Chemotherapeutic effect of artesunate in experimental schistosomiasis. Acta Pharmaceut Sin, 1983, 18:619-621. (in Chinese)

45. Utzinger J, Xiao SH, Keiser J, et al. Current progress in the development and use of artemether for chemoprophylaxis of major human schistosome parasites. Curr Med Chem, 2001, 8:1841-1860.

46. Utzinger J, Keiser J, Xiao SH, et al. Combination chemotherapy of schistosomiasis in laboratory studies and clinical trials. Antimicrob Agents Chemother, 2003, 47:1487-1495.

47. Utzinger J, Chollet J, You J, et al. Effect of combined treatment with praziquantel and artemether on *Schistosoma japonicum* and *Schistosoma mansoni* in experimentally infected animals. Acta Trop, 2001, 80:9-18.

48. Hou XY, McManus DP, Gray DJ, et al. A randomized, double-blind, placebo-controlled trial of safety and efficacy of combined praziquantel and artemether treatment for acute schistosomiasis japonica in China. Bull World Health Organ, 2008, 86: 788-795.

49. Liu R, Dong HF, Guo Y, et al. Efficacy of praziquantel and artemisinin dervatives for the treatment and prevention of human schistosomiasis: a systematic review and meta-analysis. Parasit Vectors, 2011, 4:201.

50. Wu Lj, Xu PS, Xuan YX, et al. Experimental studies on the prophylactic effect of artesunate in early treatment of schistosomiasis by oral administration. Zhongguo Xue Xi Chong Bing Fang Zhi Za Zhi, 1995, 7:129-133. (in Chinese)

51. Wu LJ Xu PS, Fang JT, et al. Experimental study on the prophylaxis of artesunate against acute schistosomiasis. Zhongguo Xue Xi Chong Bing Fang Zhi Za Zhi, 1997, 9:284-286. (in Chinese)

52. Xiao CS, Zhao XY, Liu NP, et al. Effect of artesunate and praziquantel in the prevention of schistosomiasis. Prev Med J PLA Chin, 2000, 18: 120-121. (in Chinese)

53. Wu L, Li S, Xuan Y, et al. Field application of artesunate in prophylaxis of schistosomiasis: an observation of 346 cases. Zhongguo Xue Xi Chong Bing Fang Zhi Za Zhi, 1995, 7:323-327. (in Chinese)

54. Li SW, Wu LJ, Zhang SJ, et al. Study on the optimal scheme and spreading application of artesunate on prevention of schistosomiasis japonica. Chin Med News, 2002, 10: 14-15. (in Chinese)

4.3 Advances in molluscicides application

The methods for snail control include biological and physical approaches, as well as chemical approaches by using snail-killing compounds or molluscicides. Snail control by using molluscicides is appropriate for large-scale use and more frequently used in the field. They are time-saving and labor-saving, with quick-working effects.[1] Although molluscicides are expensive, having varying degrees of toxicity to humans and animals, and must be repeatedly used to consolidate their effectiveness in killing snails, they remain the main method to control snails in China. Molluscicides that are currently being used in the field in China include chemicals and compounds extracted from plants.

4.3.1 Chemical molluscicides

Effective chemical molluscicides including niclosamide, metaldeyde, lime nitrogen, and *shachongding* have been widely used as one complementary component of the national schistosomiasis control programme in China. Many new chemical molluscicides have also been developed recently in China and are being used against *Oncomelania* in the field. These include: 4% cartap granules, 50% cartap soluble powder, Rongbao (calcium cyanamide powder) and Rongya, O-phenolic compounds of phenolic compounds, and META-Li. However, at present, there are not enough molluscicides available that are ecologically sound and do not cause any pollution effects to the environment.

Sodium pentachlorophenate

Sodium pentachlorophenate is soluble in water. It is highly effective for killing adult snails, young snails, and snail eggs. It has severe toxicity for fish and other aquatic organisms. It also has teratogenic, carcinogenic, and mutagenic effects on human beings. Nowadays, the production of sodium pentachlorophenate has been stopped.

Niclosamide

Niclosamide, first produced by Bayer AG, Germany, has been shown to be highly effective in killing adult snails, young snails, and snail eggs. To improve its solubility, suspension concentrate of niclosamide ethanolamine salt (SCNE) has been developed recently. Thus, niclosamide is applied in the field to kill snails as three formulations, namely wettable powder, suspension agent, and nano agent. A field study on the effectiveness of 50% wettable powder of niclosamide shows that the death rate of snails killed by spraying and sand mixing after 15 and 30 days was 71.9%, 74.34%, 81.08%, and 74.34%, respectively.[2] There was no significant difference between these two methods. Other studies indicated that 25% SCNE was highly effective in killing snails in both laboratory and field tests.[3] Therefore, SCNE is recommended for application as a new formulation and effective molluscicide.

When SCNE and povidone (PVP) were dissolved in a solution of dimethyl sulfoxide to produce a niclosamide nano agent, studies show that the weight ratio of PVP K17 and the niclosamide was within 1:2 – 1:3, the stabilizer could be more resistant to crystallization and the nano sol system was stable.[4] With a specific drug concentration, the mollusciciding effect was similar to that of SCNE.

When niclosamide is applied in the field, it has low toxicity to humans and livestock, but is strongly toxic to fish and other aquatic animals.[5] In an effective concentration, it can even kill fish.

Rongbao and Rongya

Rongbao and Rongya are kind of fertilizer used in agriculture purpose, but they can also be used for mollusciciding as two different molluscicide formulations. Rongbao is solid and predominantly made of nitrolime, while Rongya is liquid and made of cyanamide. An assessment on the effectiveness of Rongbao in mountainous regions shows that this formulation is favorable for use in free plows, as well as in ditches.[6] Other studies have compared the effectiveness of Rongbao in laboratory and field tests. These studies found that the effectiveness of Rongbao increased with higher concentrations. In powder form, Rongbao also proved more durable effects than niclosamide.[7] Moreover, these studies indicated that Rongbao and Rongya were highly effective in killing snails but safe for fish.

Since Rongbao and Rongya have low toxicity to fish, Rongbao can be used as a molluscicide supplement in areas that are predominantly used for aquaculture.[8] Nevertheless, due to their high costs and the large dosages that are necessary to achieve effectiveness, they are inconvenient for delivery and field application. Further, spray nozzles can sometimes become blocked. Therefore, altering the formulation and decreasing the dosage may not only cut down on costs, but extend the application of both Rongbao and Rongya.

META-Li

META-Li is a new water-based product consisting of 40% metaldehyde, which depredates carbon dioxide and does not pollute water. According to laboratory and field tests, META-Li shows better effects in killing snails when compared to other similar products.[9] Other studies indicate that the effect of META-Li in killing snails correlates to the humidity of soil. Using the same dosage, the effect of META-Li is enhanced with higher levels of humidity and raising the soil temperature facilitates the effect of snail killing. In practice, it is therefore important to determine the better season for carrying out snail elimination.

META-Li has the advantages of quick degradation and low toxicity to mammals, fish, clams, silkworms, and plants. This offsets the high toxicity of niclosamide to aquatic animals. As META-Li is soluble in water, it can also be used to spray in the fields.

Other chemical molluscicides

Other chemicals used in eliminating snails such as nicotinanilide, lime nitrogen (calcium cyanamide), quick lime, dipterex, trichlorfon, benzex, copper sulfate, carbamide, and naphthalene were used extensively in the earlier years. However, due to their many disadvantages—for example, toxicity to non-target organisms, complex manufacturing processes, high costs, environmental pollution, and inconvenience in storage and use—these chemical compounds have been phased out.

Chemically synthesized snail-killing compounds are expensive. They also have different degrees of toxicity to humans, animals, plants, and others, such as fish and insects, due to the environmental pollution their use causes. Nonetheless, this range of chemical molluscicides can kill a large number of snails with good levels of effectiveness. Hence, they are still used at present.

4.3.2　Plant-derived molluscicides

A molluscicide made from plant extracts refers to specific plants that possess active ingredients to kill snails. These active ingredients can be extracted from plant roots, stems, leaves, flowers, fruits, and seeds.

Saponins

The calyx budwood of African medicinal plants (*Spathodea campanulata*, also known as the "African lily tree" or the "African tulip tree") and *Phytolacca dodecandra* contain the ingredient saponin. Methanol and water extracted from the roots and leaves of these two plants show mollusciciding activity. The effective ingredient for killing snails is saponin. Turmeric is a type of perennial herbaceous vine that prevails in China. Its rhizomes contain saponins. The compounds extracted from turmeric can effectively suppress snail crawl up. It also has the advantage of being easily degradable in nature and is of medium toxicity to fish.

Alkaloids

The active ingredient extracted from the seeds, branches, and leaves of *Jatropha curcas* is an effective alkaloid-based molluscicide. The 24-hour mortality rate of snails is 90% and the 48-hour mortality rate is 100%, with a 6 mg/L of liquid concentration of jatropha extract—when snail-dipping experiments are conducted indoors. However, after the administration of the molluscicide, the snails show obvious climb up, which impacts the mollusciciding efficacy of the compound. This type of compound has moderate toxicity to fish.

Flavonoids

Several studies indicated that quercetin, 3-O-rhamnose glucoside, and other active ingredients that exist in some plants contain original anthocyanins, flavonoids, and flavonol, which have high molluscicidal activity.

Molluscicidal compounds that are extracted from plants with flavonoids are of low toxicity to fish and other aquatic animals. They are also easily degradable, without damage to the environment. This type of plant molluscicides can make full use of available resources in endemic areas of schistosomiasis, where these kinds of plants are abundant.

However, research on plant-derived molluscicides remains at the stage of laboratory screening to determine active ingredients. Studies on the active ingredients of these molluscicidal compounds and full tests under field conditions are rarely carried out. Due to the slow efficacy of plant-derived compounds, the high costs of extracting the effective components, the risks of limited environmental pollution, etc., research on plant-derived molluscicides has not achieved major breakthroughs yet. Only few are being used in a small scale of the fields.

4.3.3   New types of molluscicidal compounds

Plant-derived molluscicide

By using tea seeds as a raw material (after alkaline hydrolysis and enzymatic treatment, along with desiccation), a product of plant-derived molluscicide is manufactured. It is a plant-derived molluscicide consisting of 4% tea-seed distilled saponins (TDS). This product is soluble in water, methanol, ethanol, and acetonitrile. Its 4% compound is featured as a yellow powder and it is stable in normal conditions. At present, 4% TDS has been widely used in research and field studies.

An evaluation of its molluscicidal effects in both indoor tests and field studies in Hubei Province showed that this product is feasible when applied by spraying or as an immersed solution.[10] Compared to that of 2 g/m^2 50% niclosamide ethanolamine salt (WPN), at 5 g/m^2 TDS in Xingzi County, the snail death rate was 86.53% and 83.04%, respectively, after 15 days. In Huarong County, the mortality rates of snail after treated with TDS and WPN were 88.28% and 93.69%, respectively. In Xingzi County and Huarong County, the decrease in the rate of live snails was 88.86% and 87.99% for TDS, and 85.29% and 93.53% for WPN, respectively. The effect of TDS in lake and marshland areas in Hanchuan show that the mortality rate of snails was 99.33%, 100%, 100%, and 100% in 2.5 g/m^2 and 3.0 g/m^2 TDS, 2.0 g/m^2 50% WPN, and 2.0 g/m^2 26% metaldehyde suspension (MNSC) after a 72-hour immersion. The snail mortality rate was 86.10%, 90.26%, 87.45%, and 90.26%, in 3.0 g/m^2 and 5.0 g/m^2 TDS, 2.0 g/m^2 WPN, and 2.0 g/m^2 MNSC, respectively.

Therefore, the effect of TDS in eliminating snails applied in the field is the same as WPN and MNSC.[11] The recommend dosage for using TDS in the field is 2.5 g/m^2 for immersion and 5.0 g/m^2 for spraying to achieve the molluscicidal effect. The assessment of 5 g/m^2 4% TDS in hill and mountainous regions show killing rates of 56.47%, 57.32%, 90.58%, and 93.41% after one, three, seven, and fifteen days. For 2 g/m^2 50% WPN, the results were 49.22%, 53.37%, 95.92% and 97.26%. The density of live snails reduced from 20.30 ± 16.20/0.1 m^2 to 2.28 ± 2.17/0.1 m^2 and 23.67 ± 21.22/0.1 m^2 to 1.27 ± 0.76/0.1 m^2 for TDS and WPN, respectively, after fifteen days. The rate of decrease in the density of snails for TDS and WPN was 88.77% and 94.63%. With the 4% TDS effect in lake areas in the lower reach of the Yangtze River, the mortality rate of snails was 94.62% and 99.24 for TDS and WPN after seven days. When applied by spraying, the mortality rate was 70.82%, 79.75%, 85.11%, and 91.65% for TDS, and 77.71%, 84.27%, 91.90%, and 95.58% for WPN after one, three, seven, and fifteen days, respectively. In total, the cost of spraying TDS and WPN was CNY 316.71 and CNY 309.71 for every 100 m^2 area.[12]

(Chloroacetyl) catechol

A kind of catechol compounds has been screened for molluscicidal effects. Results showed that with the increase of concentrations of chloroacetyl catechol, the snail mortality was increased as well. Chloroacetyl catechol was effective as a potential molluscicide in low concentrations. The mortality rate of snails was 96.7% in the concentration of the chemical liquid (20.0 mg/L) in 24 hours. The tolerance of the snails to the compounds was enhanced with decreased concentrations of the compounds. Chloroacetyl catechol is more effective than bromoacetyl catechol in killing snails and is worth further study as a potential molluscicide.[13]

Buddleja lindleyana

A kind of fungi was also screened in the laboratory, showing that fungi are a potential molluscicide. The snail mortality rate was 83.3% in a concentration of 2% with endophytic fungi of LL3026 fermentation broth from *Buddleja* after 48 hours.[14] Tests on thermal stability and light stability for the active molluscicidal substance found that LL3026 fermentation broth was stable at high temperatures and in strong light. Screening for active fraction has shown that the molluscicidal active sites of LL3026 were low polar compounds; it was also easy to separate the active substance, and find safe and effective lead compounds for killing snails. At the same time, the application of biotechnology to improve endophytic fungi, and increase the content and yield of the active ingredient, will be of great significance in promoting the screening and sustainable use of biological molluscicides. LL3026 has a good molluscicidal effect, but the impact on non-target organisms and the ecological environment needs to be evaluated. It is also necessary to conduct an in-depth study on the molluscicidal active ingredient and its snail-control mechanism.

4.3.4 Conclusion

Future research priorities on molluscicidal compounds is recommended to focus on the following aspects: i) development of high efficiency, low toxicity chemical compounds, especially ones with low toxicity on aquatic animals and those appropriate to use in mountainous areas; ii) modification of dosage forms in order to reduce toxicity to fish, improve solubility in water, and reduce the costs of producing and applying snail-killing compounds; iii) utilization of plant resources to develop plant-derived compounds that are simple and practical, have high efficiency rates and low toxicity, and minimal environmental impacts; iv) study of molluscicidal active components and their structure-activity relationships to gain insights into new synthetic compounds; and v) exploration of the mechanism of the toxic effect of the molluscicidal compounds to provide a theoretical basis for selecting or screening an effective molluscicide.

References

1. Andrews P, Thyssen J, Lorke D. The biology and toxicology of molluscicides Bayluscide. Pharmac Ther, 1982, 19: 245-295.

2. Tian XG, Pan XP, Ke ZM, et al. Study on molluscicide effect of niclosamide with different methods in the field. J Trop Dis Parasitol, 2007, 5: 97-98. (in Chinese)

3. Dai JR, Li HJ, Shen XH, et al. Study on molluscicidal effect of suspension concentrate of niclosamide ethanolamine salt. Chin J Schisto Control, 2009, 21: 83-86. (in Chinese)

4. Jiang L, Li SF, Li XS, et al. Preparation of niclosamide ethanolamine nano-suspension and its molluscicidal effect. Chin J Schisto Control, 2006, 19: 102-106. (in Chinese)

5. Xi WP, Huang YX. Cute toxicity to brachydanio rerio of qiangluocide powder. Chin J Schisto Control, 2004, 16: 63-64. (in Chinese)

6. Zhu HQ, Zhong B, Cao CL, et al. Molluscicidal effect of Rongbao Powder in schistosomiasis mountainous areas. Chin J Schisto Control, 2007, 19: 212-216. (in Chinese)

7. Lv GL, Wei WY, Li GP, et al. Observation on Long-term field molluscicidal effects of Rong-bao. Pract Prev Med, 2006, 13: 1462-1464. (in Chinese)

8. Li GP, Hu PC, Wei WY, et al. Effect of Rongya in killing *Oncomelania hupensis* and its toxicity to fresh water fish. Chin Trop Med, 2009, 9: 1010-1011. (in Chinese)

9. Zhu D, Zhou XN, Zhang SQ, et al. Study on the molluscicidal effect of META-Li against *Oncomelania hupensis*. Chin J Parasit Dis, 2006, 24: 200-203. (in Chinese)

10. Zhang ZH, Fang R, Yu B, et al. Field evaluation of a novel plant molluscicide "Luo-wei" against *Oncomelania hupensis* snails II Molluscicidal effect in the field of lake areas in Hanchuan City, Hubei Province. Chin J Schisto Control, 2013, 25: 481-484. (in Chinese)

11. Zhou Y, Wang ZM, Zhang B, et al. Field evaluation of a novel plant molluscicide "Luo-wei" against the snail *Oncomelania hupensis* III Molluscicidal effect by spraying method in hilly regions. Chin J Schisto Control, 2013, 25: 495-497. (in Chinese)

12. Shu F, Chen SY, Xie WP, et al. Field evaluation of a novel plant molluscicide "Luo-wei" against *Oncomelania hupensis* IV Molluscicidal effect in field of river beach in Dongzhi County, Anhui Province. Chin J Schisto Control, 2013, 25: 623-626. (in Chinese)

13. Chen L, Guo DY, Ge AQ, et al. Comparison of four kinds of snail-killing compounds. Biotechnology, 2014, 27. (in Chinese)

14. Han BX, Chen J, Hao L, et al. Molluscicidal effect of endophyte LL3026 from *Buddleia lindleyana* against *Oncomelania hupensis*. Chin J Parasit Dis, 2010, 28: 210-213. (in Chinese)

4.4 Surveillance and early warning

The International Health Regulations (IHR) 2005 define surveillance as "the systematic ongoing collection, collation and analysis of data for public health purposes and the timely dissemination of public health information for assessment and public health response as necessary". Public health surveillance is used to prevent and control infectious disease, chronic disease, and injury, as well as to ensure occupational health. While early warning is a major element of disaster risk reduction including reduce the impact of disease outbreak. Early warning systems can be set up to avoid or reduce the impact of hazards such as floods, landslides, storms, and infectious diseases outbreaks. The significance of an effective early warning system to prevent from disease outbreak lies in the recognition of its benefits by local people based on information retrieved from routine surveillance system. Therefore, both surveillance and early warning is an important component in the national schistosomiasis control programme, particularly in the stage when endemicity is at low level.

4.4.1 Surveillance system

According to the definition proposed by the IHR, surveillance consists of three main integrated activities: i) systematic collection of relevant data; for example, case reports of a specific disease; ii) analyses of these data; for example, evaluating disease occurrence and transmission patterns; and iii) timely dissemination of results to guide interventions; for example, reports to public health teams implementing control programmes or to clinicians to guide disease management. Approaches to surveillance can be summarized in terms of six main factors: coverage, intensity, standardization, analysis and interpretation, dissemination, and evaluation.

Coverage

There are two basic strategies employed to achieve coverage. The first is universal surveillance, whereby an entire population or a representative sample is chosen to monitor for a condition of interest, such as acute flaccid paralysis (polio), measles, food poisoning, or bioterrorism agents, and so on. The second is sentinel surveillance, which consists of choosing a key location that is most susceptible to change in order to monitor the condition of interest. Here the word "location" may refer to sites, events, providers, animals, and/or vectors.

Intensity

There are two basic approaches to assess intensity: active surveillance and passive surveillance. i) Active surveillance involves the active periodic solicitation of case reports from reporting sources, such as physicians, hospitals, laboratories, etc.; for example, routine searches of hospital records for schistosomiasis cases in the discharge listings. ii) Passive surveillance relies on health care providers to report cases on their own initiative. Consequently, this reporting process is simple and time efficient. The vast majority of surveillance systems are passive ones.

Standardization

Standardizing case report forms across disease categories allows for improved opportunities to analyze data across nodifiable diseases. Standardization includes several steps:

Case definition

This is a critical decision for surveillance system design because it will impact on the amount, type, and quality of data needed. High sensitivity and specificity are desired. However, case definition should also balance between the costs and benefits associated with false positive and false negative reports. It also needs to decide if laboratory confirmation is required (infectious) or if evidence of an underlying cause is required (chronic). False positive rates must be considered if a positive notification requires investigation.

Data collection

This should be driven by policy decisions. The Health Insurance Portability and Accountability Act of 1996 (HIPPA) regulations will play a role. All forms and processes must be standardized to facilitate data collection. Sometimes "Henderson's Golden Rule" can be followed (although not always) for passive systems: line listing is best; half a page is okay; one side of one page is the maximum. It is important to emphasize the need to think carefully about every data item.

Data processing and management

The format and coding of individual variables, the size and manageability of data files, and the compatibility of the data with other data sources (for example, census files) are some of the issues that need to be considered. Proper management of surveillance data is critical and can often become quite complex. Today's increasingly complex surveillance systems require advanced data analysis and data management support. To adjust for missing data, confounders can be accounted for through multivariate modeling, and formally assessing trends and clusters.

Analysis and interpretation

In the process of data analysis and interpretation, many common questions need to be addressed: "Is the condition reported more frequently than expected? If yes, to what level?"; "Does this constitute 'alert' status?"; "Is there a geographic or time cluster of cases?"; "Does this require an investigation?"; and "Has anything changed in the system to distort the analysis over time?".

Three important factors—person, place, and time—are traditional approaches to data analysis. Focus must be on consistency over time in style of presentation and criteria for "alert" status. Care must be given to interpretations of trends over time, especially in passive systems where actual sensitivity and specificity are not well known.

Dissemination

Primary users of information must be identified during system design. This should include those who contribute information to the system. Dissemination lists should be regularly updated. It is ideal to involve all levels of user in analysis and interpretation, especially if they are primary decision makers for action. It is also important to have feedback systems for information users. A set of recommendations based on the data and other circumstances should be included in each report.

Evaluation

The type and scope of the evaluation should be guided by objectives that are simple, measurable, attainable, realistic, and time-bound (SMART). The relative importance of each of these indicators varies depending on the surveillance system and the disease.

Schistosomiasis surveillance systems in China

Surveillance systems have been set up in China since 1980s, when some of provinces had reached the transmission interruption, such as Guangdong (1985), Shanghai (1985), Guangxi (1986), Fujian (1987) and Zhejiang (1995). At that time, all endemic areas initiated the surveillance programme immediately right after transmission interruption had been reached. The major purpose was to prevent the new infectious sources including human and livestock, as well as *Oncomelania* snails introduced into these areas from neighboring provinces where transmission was still going on.

Since 1985, several national surveillance pilot sites were set up in the endemic areas where transmission intensity ranged from higher to lower areas, in order to understand the effectiveness of interventions in different endemic areas. Gradually, the number of national surveillance sites was increased from 10 to 40 with the time. Also, each province established some of surveillance sites which provide good quality data annually for the estimation of infected cases with *S. japonicum*.

Until 2005, the surveillance systems consisted of two major components: one was the passive surveillance covering all endemic areas, and the other one was the active surveillance in selected sentinel sites. Through passive surveillance, all cases found either in clinics or control stations were reported daily through web-based National Notifiable Infectious Diseases Information System. Active surveillance data will help to understand the changes of epidemic factors and effectiveness of intervention, providing good information to update the control strategy. Therefore, all activities in the surveillance systems from national to local levels became one of important components in the national schistosomiasis control programme. Thus, the endemicity of schistosomiasis became lower and lower. Up to 2015, schistosomiasis transmission had been effectively controlled in all provinces, and the infection rate with *S. japonicum* had been decreased under 1% in almost of all endemic counties in China, in accordance with the surveillance data.

Since 2010, the schistosomiasis surveillance systems were further strengthened by the establishment of reference laboratory at national, provincial and county levels, with more precision on diagnosis and surveillance results. Hence, the surveillance sentinel sites have been extended into all counties that were historically endemic, with better equipment facilities in the laboratory.[1]

4.4.2 Early warning system

Basic concepts

Concept and classification

Early warning is interpreted as before disasters and other dangers occur. An emergency signal is issued to the relevant departments according to past procedures or the precursory signs. Early warning is a major element of disaster risk reduction. It prevents loss of life and reduces the economic and material impact of disasters. Prevention is better than disaster relief or remedy after the fact. Precautionary measures take first place.

Disease early warning is a branch of internal warning that belongs to human disaster warning. Based on the patterns of occurrence and the development of diseases, as well as other relevant factors, disease early warning is designed to predict or forecast the future occurrence and development of diseases through various analytic methods, such as mathematical models. These analytic methods play an important role in improving the predictability of disease and increasing the efficiency and effectiveness of disease prevention and control.

Definitions and features of early warning indicators

Early warning indicators have a potential value to transmit warning signals in advance. The fluctuation magnitude of indicators is associated to epidemics or outbreaks of parasitic diseases. In alliance with the transmission characteristics of parasitic diseases in their different transmission phases, the early warning indicators for parasitic disease epidemics can be classified into three categories: i) prophase indicators of an epidemic or outbreak; ii) indicators of the atypical symptoms phase; and iii) indicators of the typical symptoms phase.

Once the indicator values exceed the fluctuation cordon, an alert is triggered. The appropriate epidemiological investigation or intervention is then launched. Therefore, early warning indicators need to be timely and accurate, and have easy operability. Timeliness refers to indicators that can detect the signals of a parasitic disease occurrence or outbreak as early as possible in order to enable a prompt response. Accuracy refers to indicators that can predict a crisis as precisely as possible so as to avoid unnecessary responses. The information provided by disease early warning indicators should be highly consistent with the actual prevalence of parasitic diseases. Operability refers to the idea that the data and information required for the disease early warning indicators can be easily collected. The establishment of a sensitive and effective early warning indicator system is a prerequisite for a successful early warning system.

The definition, characteristics, and component framework of an early warning mechanism

An early warning mechanism is an early warning system consisting of institutions, regulations, networks, initiatives, etc., that can sense the signals of a parasitic disease outbreak with accuracy and timeliness. It also is the mechanism through which relevant departments and agencies are informed on a timely basis. The primary role of an early warning mechanism is to drive the initiative by leading feedback and responding in a timely manner in order to prevent risks in the first place.

Characteristics of an early warning mechanism system. An effective early warning mechanism system is defined by six characteristics. These include: i) Timeliness: discover an emergency event as early as possible so as to gain enough time for response initiation. Each link within the information flow chain, such as investigation, collection, transfer, analysis, dissemination, and measures taken require timeliness. ii) Efficiency: make predictions as accurate as possible by collecting thorough information with the intention of avoiding unnecessary responses. iii) Operability: based on the national development situation and a realistic assessment of conditions in different regions, the early warning mechanism system should be simple and easy to implement, utilizing appropriate personnel and material reserves. iv) Expansibility: the system has sufficient capacity to increase or decrease the target warning events accordingly. It also has the ability to continually adjust and improve itself. v) Social and corresponding legal efficacy: early warning involves many sectors of society. Having legal efficacy can bring early warning into full play in a short time. vi) Relevance with emergency response systems: early warning and emergency response are two consecutive processes. Without accurate early warning mechanisms, it is difficult to implement emergency response smoothly.

Early warning system in China. Since the prevalence of schistosomiasis in most of endemic areas had been lower than 1%, and the prevention works for schistosomiasis need to be strengthen after 2003, the early warning system for schistosomiasis had been initiated at the national level, with the evidence of a Protocol on Emerging and Response for Schistosomiasis issued by Ministry of Health, China in May 2003, right after SAS outbreak in Beijing. In this document, the concept of outbreak, emerging events as well as the requirements for response actions were clearly described. These ensure that right action can be implemented effectively and in time once outbreak events of schistosomiasis occurred.

Then, several routine activities involved in early warning system for schistosomiasis transmission are documented by the Ministry of Health in following three aspects: i) In the beginning of flooding season every year, the National Institute of

Parasitic Diseases at Chinese Center of Disease Controland Prevention produced an annual risk map of schistosomiasis transmission areas in China based on the epidemiological data, as well as environmental data. This aimed to present the early warning information to provincial institutions that were involved in the schistosomiasis control programme. ii) Whenever an outbreak of acute schistosomiasis is found, intervention should take place as soon as possible and a national expert team should visit the places where the outbreak occurred. More active surveillance in the surrounding areas should be performed including the neighboring counties, and an alarming information and warning maps covering all neighboring counties after active surveillance are produced. iii) At the same time, neighboring provinces were coordinating some of joint activities for the surveillance and response arranged in the high risk areas where linking each other either in spring or fall annually.

Prediction methods

The real world looks complex and chaotic. However, behind haphazard appearances, it often hides regularity. Based on the observation and analysis of history and current situations, on understanding and mastering this regularity, inferences and determinations of the trend of developments can be made. Prediction is a practical science and is a basis for decision-making. Correct prediction is the evidence and basis for correct decision-making.

There are many types of prediction according to different classifications. In terms of length, parasitic disease prediction can be divided into short-term prediction (month, quarter, six months, and one year), mid-term prediction (one to three years) and long-term prediction (more than three years). Short-term prediction is mainly designed for the control of epidemics or outbreaks of disease. Mid- and long-term prediction is normally utilized for the development of long-term prevention and control strategies. The shorter the prediction period, the higher prediction accuracy. According to range, prediction can be classified in terms of macro (global or universal) and micro (regional or local) levels. In accordance with the methodology that is used, prediction can also be categorized as qualitative or quantitative prediction. The latter has a higher prediction accuracy than the former. Different prediction methods are tailored to different prediction purposes in order to develop different types of control programmes.

As a result of the long-term development of prediction theory, progress has been made in qualitative and quantitative modeling. A prediction model abstractly and simply describes the relationships between associated factors and the prediction target, such as interdependence, transformation, and patterns of movement. The model is built up on the basis of certain relatively stable relationships within a fairly steady structure or phenomenon. Model construction in nonlinear systems still lacks a unified method. The traditional approach is to transform a nonlinear system into a linear one, or apply some other special treatment. However, models are often useless in practical prediction systems. Data collection is often inaccurate or may even be wrong. Only if the selected models are tailored to specific environmental settings accordingly, they can achieve better predictions. Traditional prediction methods cannot easily tackle these problems.

Qualitative prediction

Based on the transmission pattern of schistosomiasis and other relevant factors, qualitative prediction determines transmission trends and the intensity of schistosomiasis. Qualitative prediction generally includes epidemic control charts, the Delphi method, and brainstorming.

Epidemic control charts. The epidemic control chart was first developed by Walter Shewhart in 1924 for a variety of infectious diseases. A control chart, also known as a "statistical process control" (SPC), is a statistical tool to identify common causes and special causes of process changes. It has been effectively applied in infectious disease epidemics that have seasonal or periodical patterns. A control chart has a center line (CL), an upper control limit (UCL), and a lower control limit (LCL). Warning levels can be adjusted. For instance, the upper and lower cordon limits of schistosomiasis transmission are set to be $\pm$ 2S. A control chart is one of the statistical quality control (SQC) tools. Technically, an epidemic control chart is the most accurate SQC tool. It is a good early warning method because of its simple operation and easy-to-get indicators.

Different data use different types of control charts and different types of control charts are based on different statistical models. The types of control chart are determined by different classification methods showing below. According to the number of variables, a control chart can be classified as a single-variable control chart or a multivariate control chart. By types of data (i.e. count data or numeric data), count data utilizes an individual X or a moving range control chart (XmR), while numeric data apply XmR or X-Bar control charts, as well as R control charts (when a sample size is large). In terms of control objects, control charts can be divided into a variable control charts (for example, X and R chart; X and S chart; chart of individuals; moving average or moving range chart, etc.) and attribute control charts (for example, p chart; np chart; u chart; and c chart). For any kind of data, control charts can be divided into short-term charts (also known as a "Z map") and group charts (also called a "multiple characteristic chart").

It is believed that a multiple characteristic chart is the simplest traditional problem-solving tool by providing a checklist (or an operation table). When a process is out of control, for example, an attached spreadsheet programme can call an alarm, providing the possibility for automatic warning. Other studies show that Tukey's control chart based on median value analysis is not limited by the hypothesis of data distribution and is not affected by extreme values. It can also be applied to small datasets and does not need to calculate standard deviation or mean. These factors make the application of Tukey's control chart more convenient.

There is another type of SPC chart called a "g and h control chart". This is normally used for monitoring a number of adverse events (such as nosocomial infections or complications after cardiac surgery), in particular to identify the rate changes of rare events, with better prediction effects than traditional methods.

The three commonly used control charts are as follows: i) the Shewhart control chart is the most common one used. But it produces unsatisfactory results when there is a small drift of mean value during the process; ii) the cumulative sum control chart (CUSUM), which is based on the likelihood ratio; and iii) the exponential weighted moving average control chart (EWMA). The latter two have been proven satisfactory in the detection of small drifts. In comparison, CUSUM has more advantages than EWMA. In particular, CUSUM has wider applications.

The Delphi method. The Delphi method is also known as the "expert scoring method" or the "expert consultation". First developed by the RAND Corporation, the Delphi method is the most commonly used prediction method in the world. The

Delphi method is a way to anonymously solicit the opinions of experts, and quantitatively and qualitatively predict and evaluate target objects. During the mid-1970s, the Delphi method began to be applied in the medical field. It is now increasingly used in parasitic diseases surveillance systems.

Brainstorming. Brainstorming meetings (also known as a catch-all for group ideation sessions) organize a group of experts in order to gather a list of ideas spontaneously within a relatively short time. Brainstorming meetings operate through the direct exchange of information, mutual inspiration, and creative thinking.

There are four step to process the brainstorming, including i) Pre-preparation: Participants, hosts, and topics must be agreed in advance. When necessary, flexible thinking training may be useful. ii) Free riding: The host announces the meeting theme and introduces the related references. Free riding requires breaking old modes of thinking and welcoming unusual ideas by looking at a given topic from new perspectives and suspending assumptions. iii) Classification and sorting of ideas: The ideas that emerge as a result of a brainstorming meeting are generally divided into two types; namely, practical and fantasy ones. The former refers to those ideas that current technology can realize. The latter refers to those ideas that current technology cannot achieve. iv) Improve the practical ideas: For practical, tentative ideas, brainstorming is encouraged to conduct feasibility studies for secondary development, so as to further increase the chances that an idea can be realized. v) Redevelopment of fantasy ideas: For fantasy ideas, further brainstorming and development may possibly transform these immature ideas into mature and practical ones. This is a critical step in a second round of brainstorming.

Quantitative prediction

Quantitative prediction uses statistical or mathematical models to quantitatively predict development trends, changes in speed, and levels of development by analyzing historical data. In quantitative prediction, mathematical models are at the core of the variety of prediction methods.

Quantitative prediction methods include regression analysis, time series analysis, gray system prediction, Markov prediction, the artificial neural network method, and so on. These methods all integrate mathematical modeling. The basic steps are: i) assumptions of the model: reasonable assumptions designed to simplify practical problems so as to consider only the most important factors; ii) model establishment: transform the actual problem into a mathematical problem; iii) model solving: find out the answers for the mathematical problems; and iv) testing and application of the model: apply the solutions of the mathematical problems to practical problems.

Quantitative prediction is less affected by subjective factors because it relies more on historical data to quantitatively describe the development of a disease. It uses computer programmes to deal with large amounts of data and therefore is widely used in disease prediction.

Regression analysis. Regression analysis explores the relationship between the disease and the causative factors in order to build a regression model, which is then used to forecast changes in schistosomiasis transmission. According to the number of causative factors, the relationship between the disease and the factors, regression methods can be classified as unary linear regression, multiple linear regression and nonlinear regression. Regression methods have been widely applied in medical statistics. The technology has developed to very mature levels that can predict joint effects by considering multiple factors. The disadvantages of regression methods are larger model error, poor extrapolation, demanding of larger data, and higher requirements of the sample distribution.

Time series analysis. Time series analysis investigates a sequence of data points, typically consisting of successive measurements made over a time interval, and establishes a model varying over time so as to extrapolate to the future forecasting. US and British statisticians George Box and Gwilym Jenkins developed the Box-Jenkins method (also known as the "BJ method" or the "ARMA model" [the autoregressive -moving- average model]). The Box–Jenkins method is the most important and commonly used approach to time series modeling. The ARMA model requires the time series of the prediction target to be stationary. However, many medical cases are non-stationary time series that show a tendency to rise or fall. Therefore, the use of d-order homogeneous non-stationary timing autoregressive integrated moving average model (ARIMA model) is more commonly used in the medical field.

Markov prediction method. Markov prediction is based on dividing the entire time series into a number of states. According to state transition probabilities, the possible state ranges of events are forecasted. It is a prediction interval, which means the final prediction is the range of the actual value. The Markov process states and time are discrete. The Markov chain has no after-effect. It is a stochastic model used to model randomly changing systems where it is assumed that future states depend only on the present state and not on the sequence of events that preceded it (that is, it assumes the Markov property).

Grey system prediction. Grey system theory was first founded by Deng Julong in 1982. Through the original data processing and the establishment of gray model (GM), it is possible to grasp the pattern of disease development and make a quantitative prediction for the future development of the disease. Compared with traditional forecasting models, gray model prediction requires only a relatively small amount of data. It has higher prediction accuracy for an event which requires less data and small fluctuation over a short time. The most common grey system prediction model is GM (1,1), which represents a first-order differential equation of one variable. It only studies the effect of time (a gray variable) on the disease. It is mostly used to conjecture the morbidity or mortality of a disease at one or some time points in the future. The GM (1,1) model is very simple, but it seldom considers risk factors. The sample size is also small, which leads to rough, short-term predictions. It is suitable for exponential growth forecasts, but shows poor fitness for data with larger randomness and volatility. The GM (1, N) model represents a first-order differential equation of N variables. It does not utilize the full range of information and is generally not suitable for multi-factor prediction.

Artificial neural network prediction method. Artificial neural networks (ANNs) imitate biological neural network characteristics. It is a kind of mathematical algorithm model that carries out distributed parallel information processing. It is based on the understanding of how the human neural network functions. From the perspective of information processing using mathematical methods, it is the abstractness of the human brain and establishes a simplified model. ANN has self-adaptive ability, such as nonlinear mistakes tolerance and self-organizing/self-learning. Through the self-learning and data training, it keeps changing the connection weights and the topology of the network so that the output of the network is constantly approaching expectations. It does not analyze the specific relationship between the relevant factors, but through data training, it can summarize the complex internal law, thereby performing disease prediction.

The backpropagation (BP) neural network is currently the most widely used multilayer feed forward network. Epidemiologists can use a BP network to set up disease prediction models. First, this entails collecting the key factors leading to the occurrence of the disease and main consequences. Second, input the influencing factors and the outcomes into the neural network model for repeated training until the desired training error level is reached. Finally, the established model can be used for disease prediction. A BP neural network is a non-traditional nonlinear multivariate model that can identify the complex nonlinear relationships between variables. A BP neural network can be applied to all kinds of variables—normal or not; independent or not. The design of a BP neural network is directly related to the application effect. Therefore, the design of a network should consider every detail based on the data.

Comparison of several quantitative prediction methods. The aforementioned quantitative prediction methods are commonly used in disease prediction. They have their own characteristics. Some have higher accuracy in short- and medium-term forecasting, while others have advantages in long-term forecasting. Some are suitable for more stable data, but others are particularly applicable to data with volatility. Table 4.2 lists the features and disadvantages of these prediction methods, which facilitates better understanding of their advantages and scope of application.

Table 4.2 shows a variety of prediction methods, including: research perspectives, the use of data format, data sample size, and the applicable conditions. In terms of the applicable conditions, the regression prediction method is used for large sample sizes and stable development modes. The grey forecasting method is used to identify patterns through raw data collation, which can be applied to situations with little or unknown information. In terms of data format, grey system theory employs the generated data; the regression analysis method uses the original data; and the Markov method calculates the transition probabilities to predict the future value range.

From the characteristics of the data, the time series, the grey model, and regression forecasting methods require data to be smooth and have low volatility. The Markov prediction method is suitable for larger data with volatility. Regarding the prediction time period, the time series, Markov, and grey model methods are more suitable for the short-term prediction, while the regression method is better for long-term prediction. The artificial neural network method has less limitation. It is a multistructural model. Through sample learning, it constantly changes its own data structure to adapt to changes in the sample. However, the network structure is difficult to determine. It contains complex algorithms and has high knowledge requirements in terms of scientific thinking, artificial intelligence, and computer science. For non-experts, the establishment of a neural network is difficult.

Table 4.2 Comparison of several quantitative prediction methods.

	Characteristics	Disadvantages	Application scope
Regression prediction	Takes into account various factors of the disease and their relationship, but requires a large sample size and better distribution of the data.	When influenced by intricate factors, such as random disturbance, the error level is large and extrapolation is poor.	Suitable for long-term prediction
Time series prediction	No need to consider impact factors. Variable time integrates all these factors. It is simple and easy to grasp, but requires a smooth sequence of samples without too much volatility.	Cannot use the relationship between the factors of disease. When faced with large fluctuations in the data, prediction results are poor.	High accuracy in short-term prediction
Markov prediction	The prediction result is a probability range. Accurate prediction, especially for large fluctuations in data.	Because it is a range prediction, it inevitably leads to relatively low prediction accuracy.	High accuracy in short-term prediction
Grey prediction	A time series prediction method for small sample sizes. Incomplete information with exponential growth.	Poor fitness for data with large randomness and fluctuations.	Suitable for short-term prediction
ANN	Has nonlinear fault tolerance, self-learning, self-organization, and self-adaptive abilities. It is a multistructural model. Through the sample learning and training, it constantly changes its own data structure to adapt to changes in the sample.	Difficult to determine the network structure, algorithm complexity, easy to trap into local minima.	Suitable for both short-term and long-term prediction

Integrated prediction method

Since each single prediction method is not perfect, in 1969 Bates and Granger first proposed a combination of prediction methods. This approach integrates different methods in specific ways that fully use the advantages of the various methods and complement each other in order to maximize the prediction effect. Although the combination can make best use of the advantages and bypass the disadvantages, the theory is not perfect. At present, it is still in the immature stage.

Integrated prediction is the inevitable trend of the development of modern statistical methods. Since first proposed by Bates and Granger, it has received significant attention and has long been a hot topic of discussion because it can effectively improve prediction accuracy. Integrated prediction refers to the application of two or more predictive models for certain parasitic diseases. Utilizing the information provided by various single prediction models, the final combination model is averaged by an appropriate weighting rule.

4.4.3　Application of prediction and early warning methods in schistosomiasis

For schistosomiasis, empirical statistical methods to prediction disease transmission trends are commonly used. Recently, with the introduction of achievements in mathematics and physics, schistosomiasis transmission mechanism models provide a strong theoretical foundation for the study of disease prediction. These models emphasize interpretive and research studies. They are more complex than statistical prediction models, such as the transmission dynamics model, the complex network model, the Bayesian forecasting model, etc.[2,3]

Prediction of transmission status of schistosomiasis japonica at province and county level

With the aim of exploring the usefulness of spatial analysis in the formulation of a strategy for schistosomiasis japonica control in different environmental settings, Yang *et al.* (2005) developed a Bayesian spatio-temporal model based on collected parasitological data of cross-section survey in 47 counties in Jiangsu Province from 1990 to 1998. Climatic factors in the same study region, namely the land surface

189

temperature (LST) and the normalized difference vegetation index (NDVI) were obtained from remote sensing satellite sensors. Bayesian spatio-temporal models were employed to analyze the relationship between prevalence and environmental factors. It showed that spatial autocorrelation in Jiangsu Province decreased dramatically from 1990 to 1992, and increased gradually thereafter. A likely explanation of this finding arises from the large-scale administration of praziquantel morbidity control of schistosomiasis. The analysis suggests a negative association between NDVI and risk of *S. japonicum* infection. However, an increase in LST contributed to a significant increase in the prevalence of *S. japonicum* infections.[4]

By using Geographic Information System, different strata of prevalence were classified and the spatial distribution of human infection with *S. japonicum* was estimated in Dangtu County, China. First, a population-based database was established in Dangtu County. This database, containing the human prevalence of schistosomiasis at the village level from 2001 to 2004, was analyzed by directional trend analysis supported with ArcGIS 9.0 to select the optimum predictive approach. Based on the approach selected, the second-order ordinary kriging approach of spatial analysis was found to be optimal for prediction of human prevalence of *S. japonicum* infection. The mean prediction error was close to 0 and the root-mean-square standardized error was close to 1. Starting with the different environmental settings for each stratum of transmission, four areas were classified according to human prevalence, and different strategies to control transmission of schistosomiasis were put forward. It was concluded that the approach to use spatial analysis as a tool to predict the spatial distribution of human prevalence of *S. japonicum* infection improves the formulation of strategies for schistosomiasis control in different environmental settings at the county level.[5]

Predication of snail-infested areas based on ecological model

Schistosomiasis japonica is a parasitic disease that remains endemic in seven provinces in the People's Republic of China. One of the most important measures in the process of schistosomiasis elimination in China is control of *Oncomelania hupensis*, the unique intermediate host snail of *Schistosoma japonicum*.

Compared with plains and water network region as well as lake and marchland region, the hilly and mountainous region of schistosomiasis endemic areas are more complicated, making the snail survey difficult to conduct precisely and efficiently. There is a pressing call to identify the snail habitats of mountainous regions in an efficient and cost-effective manner. Therefore, an ecological model to predict snail habitats was developed based on the snail surveillance data in Eryuang, Yunnan Province of China. A total of twelve out of 56 administrative villages distributed with *O. hupensis* in Eryuan, were randomly selected to set up the ecological model. Thirty out of the rest of 78 villages (villages selected for building model were excluded from the villages for validation) in Eryuan and 30 out of 89 villages in Midu, Yunnan Province were selected via a chessboard method for model validation, respectively. Nine-year-average Normalized Difference Vegetation Index (NDVI) and Land Surface Temperature (LST) as well as Digital Elevation Model (DEM) covering Eryuan and Midu were extracted from MODIS and ASTER satellite images, respectively. Slope, elevation and the distance from every village to its nearest stream were derived from DEM. Suitable survival environment conditions for snails were defined by comparing historical snail presence data and remote sensing derived images. According to the suitable conditions for snails, environment factors, i.e. NDVI, LST, elevation, slope and the distance from every village to its nearest stream, were integrated into an ecological niche model to predict *O. hupensis* potential habitats in Eryuan and Midu. The evaluation of the model was assessed by comparing the model prediction and field investigation. Then, the consistency rate of model validation was calculated in Eryuan and Midu Counties respectively. Results showed that the final ecological niche model for potential *O. hupensis* habitats prediction comprised the following environmental factors, namely: NDVI ($>/= 0.446$), LST ($>/= 22.70$ degrees C), elevation ($</= 2,300$ m), slope ($</= 11$ degrees C) and the distance to nearest stream ($</= 1,000$ m). The potential *O. hupensis* habitats in Eryuan distributed in the Lancang River basin and *O. hupensis* in Midu shows a trend of clustering in the north and spotty distribution in the south. The consistency rates of the ecological niche model in Eryuan and Midu were 76.67% and 83.33% respectively. Therefore, the ecological niche model integrated with NDVI, LST, elevation, slope and distance from every village to its nearest stream adequately predicted the snail habitats in the mountainous regions.[6]

In addition, the prediction is also able to predict the snail habitats in lake and marshland region. For example, geographic information systems and remote sensing techniques were used to predict potential habitats of *Oncomelania hupensis*. Focussing on the Hongze, Baima and Gaoyou lakes in Jiangsu Province in eastern China, another ecological model was developed using the normalized difference vegetation index, a tasseled-cap transformed wetness index, and flooding areas to predict snail habitats at a small scale, based on remote sensing data. Data were extracted from two Landsat images; one taken during a typical dry year and the other obtained three years later during a flooding event. An area of approximately 163.6 km² was predicted as potential *O. hupensis* habitats around the three lakes, which accounts for 4.3% of the estimated snail habitats in China. In turn, these predicted snail habitats are risk areas for transmission of schistosomiasis, and hence illustrate the scale of the possible impact of climate change and other ecological transformations. The generated risk map can be used by health policy makers to guide mitigation policies targeting the possible spread of *O. hupensis*, and with the aim of containing the transmission of *S. japonicum*.

Prediction of potential transmission areas of schistosomiasis japonica under the scenarios of environmental changes

It is well known that *Oncomelania hupensis* is the unique intermediate host of *S. japonicum*. Therefore, environmental changes, such as Three Goreges Dam (TGD) project and global warming will certainly influence the distribution of *S. japonicum* through changes of *Oncomelania* snail distribution.

It has been noticed that TGD has substantially changed the ecology and environment in the Dongting Lake region. A study was performed to understand the impact of water level and elevation on the survival rate of snail and habitat distribution of snail. Data were collected for 16 bottomlands around 4 hydrological stations, which included water, density of living snails (form the Anxiang Station for Schistosomiasis Control) and elevation (from Google Earth). Based on the elevation, sixteen bottomlands were divided into 3 groups. ARIMA models were built to predict the density of living snails in different elevation areas. Results showed that before closure of TGD, 7 out of 9 years had a water level beyond the warning level of anti-flooding activity initiation at least once in Anxiang hydrological station, compared with only 3 out of 10 years after closure of TGD. There were two severe droughts that happened in 2006 and 2011, with much fewer number of flooding per year compared with other study years. Overall, there was a correlation between water level changing and density of living snails' variation in all the elevations areas. The density of living snails in all elevations areas was decreasing after the TGD was built. The relationship between number of flooding per year and the density of living snails was more pronounced in the medium and high elevation areas; the density of living snails kept decreasing from 2003 to 2014. In low elevation area however, the density of living snails decreased after 2003 first and turned to increase after 2011. Our ARIMA prediction models indicated that the snails would not disappear in the Dongting Lake region in the next 7 years. In the low elevation area, the density of living snails would increase slightly and then stabilize after the year 2017. In the medium elevation region, the change of the density of living snails would be more obvious and would increase till the year 2020. In the high elevation area, the density of living snails would remain stable after the year 2015. Therefore, the TGD initiative influenced water levels and reduced the risk of flooding and the density of living snails in the study region. Based on the prediction models, the density of living snails in all elevations tends to be stabilized. Control of schistosomiasis japonica would continue to be an important task in the study area in the coming decade.

To predict the intensity and scale of impact on transmission of schistosomiasis japonica caused by the climate warming, the climate-transmission model for schistosomiasis was established at national level in China. By using climate data from 193 weather stations in China from 1951 to 2000, the GIS database was created to analyze the tendency of average daily temperature. By using the results from the effective accumulated temperature models on *Oncomelania* snails and *S. japonicum*, the spatio-temporal analysis was performed to create the distribution maps of *Oncomelania* snails and *S. japonicum*, respectively. This was effective by means of GIS approaches based on the ratio of effective accumulated temperature to the snail or the parasite development temperature (ET/SDT) in all 193 stations, under different scenarios of climate changes. The potential distribution maps with the dispersal risk areas of schistosomiasis japonica in 2030 and 2050 were created based on forecast data. The average temperature of the country will increase by 1.7 ℃ in 2030 and by

2.2 ℃ in 2050. Results showed that the average temperature in the last 5 decades inclined, especially after 1990 it increased significantly with its increasing regression formula T = 0.0198X − 28.476. The climate-transmission model for schistosomiasis was established, and it was found that the geographical distribution of *S. japonicum* was much larger than that of *Oncomelania* snails based on the ratio of ET/SDT. The prediction maps for distribution of schistosomiasis in 2030 and 2050 were created respectively, which showed that the sensitive areas were extended with the time. The risk of expansion northward for schistosomiasis will be increasing due to directly the climate warming. It is predicted that a northward expansion of transmission area of schistosomiasis may occur due to the climate warming and the expanded potential area for schistosomiasis transmission will be important for future surveillance.[7]

References

1. Utzinger J, Zhou XN, Chen MG, et al. Conquering schistosomiasis in China: the long march. Acta Trop, 2005, 96: 69-96.

2. Yang GJ, Gemperli A, Vounatsou P, et al. A growing degree-days based time-series analysis for prediction of *Schistosoma japonicum* transmission in Jiangsu province, China. Am J Trop Med Hyg, 2006, 75: 549-55.

3. Zhou XN, Malone JB, Kristensen TK, et al. Application of geographic information systems and remote sensing to schistosomiasis control in China. Acta Trop, 2001, 79: 97-106.

4. Yang GJ, Vounatsou P, Zhou XN, et al. A review of geographic information system and remote sensing with applications to the epidemiology and control of schistosomiasis in China. Acta Trop, 2005, 96: 117-29.

5. Chen Z, Zhou XN, Yang K, et al. Strategy formulation for schistosomiasis japonica control in different environmental settings supported by spatial analysis: a case study from China. Geospatial Health, 2007, 1: 223-231.

6. Yang K, Wang XH, Yang GJ, et al. An integrated approach to identify distribution of *Oncomelania hupensis*, the intermediate host of *Schistosoma japonicum*, in a mountainous region in China. Int J Parasitol, 2008, 38: 1007-16.

7. Zhou XN, Yang K, Hong QB, et al. Prediction of the impact of climate warming on transmission of schistosomiasis in China. Chin J Parasitol Parasit Dis, 2004, 22: 262-265.

4.5　Applicable technology

Applicable technology is defined as a class of practical techniques used to address the difficulties and problems in actual work. During the last several years, professional staff working on the national schistosomiasis control programme in China has developed multiple practical control techniques and tools targeting key points in the transmission and the important epidemiological factors of S. japonicum.[1] These control techniques and tools cover infection source control, snail control, detection of infested water, surveillance and forecasting, rapid screening, and pathological diagnosis. These applicable techniques include the use of novel molluscicides/cercaricides and environmentally friendly, plant molluscicides, new snail control machines, infected snail detection, original approaches to infested water detection, and novel health education materials for schistosomiasis control, all of which have proven effective for schistosomiasis control in the field.[1,2]

4.5.1　Applicable technology for infection source control

Boatmen and fishermen have a high frequency of contact with S. japonicum-infested water and play a dual role in the transmission of schistosomiasis as both victims and transmitters of the disease. Based on the characteristics of boatmen's and fishermen's frequent mobility with relatively fixed anchor points, three-cell harmless toilets have been built in fixed anchor locations to collect and treat the excrement effectively (Figure 4.9). This thereby reduces the contamination of the Yangtze River from schistosome eggs. Two types of public toilets have been constructed: a two-seat toilet with an area of 6 m^2 and four-seat toilet with an area of 13 m^2.[3] A total of 53 harmless latrines have been built in the fixed anchor points along the Yangtze River basin. An estimated 79.62% usage of the harmless public toilets is observed.[3] Currently, this technology has been popularized in the major endemic foci of schistosomiasis in China. It has become an effective method for the management and treatment of feces from boatmen and fishermen in these areas, providing a novel measure for the implementation of an integrated strategy with a focus on infection source control.[3]

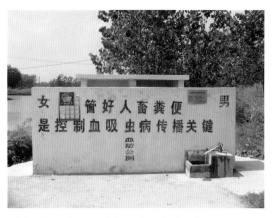

Figure 4.9　Harmless public toilets in the fixed anchor points.

4.5.2　Applicable technology for snail control

A machine simultaneously integrating mechanized environmental cleaning and automatic mollusciciding

Environmental vegetation is a primary factor affecting both the efficiency and quality of snail control. A machine has been developed that simultaneously integrates mechanized environmental cleaning and automatic mollusciciding (Figure 4.10). The machine contains three different systems, including power traction, cutting up and plowing, and automatic mollusciciding. That is, this machine simultaneously cuts down vegetation and cuts it into pieces, plows, and controls snails by spraying niclosamide.[4] In complex marshland regions with vegetation the device can complete a 3,000 m² area of environmental cleaning and mollusciciding per working hour. It has a working efficiency that is similar to 56 workers and an economic cost that is approximately one-sixth of the equivalent in human power. In addition, the snail control effectiveness of this machine is comparative to artificial environmental cleaning plus chemical mollusciciding (86.58% vs. 84.37%, respectively).[4] This device therefore provides a new practical tool for snail control in large marshlands.[4]

A rapid niclosamide detector

Currently, niclosamide is the most widely used chemical molluscicide for snail con-

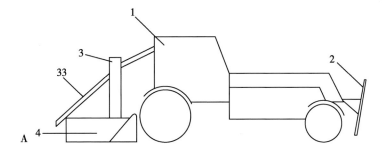

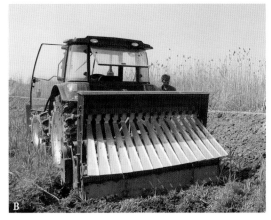

Figure 4.10   Structure diagram (A) and the machine (B). 1, tractor; 2, vegetation-pressing plate; 3, automatic molluscicide releasing apparatus; 33, comb-like molluscicide spraying retainer; 4, plow.

trol in schistosomiasis endemic areas worldwide. A real-time determination of the active concentration of niclosamide is of great importance for ensuring molluscicidal efficacy and reducing the impact of this agent on the environment. A niclosamide detector (Wuxi Runwei Technology Development Co., Ltd.; Wuxi, China) for rapid determination of niclosamide concentrations in endemic areas has been developed (Figure 4.11). It has a linear range of $0 - 8$ g/m^3 and a detection limit of 0.015 g/m^3.[5] This detector is easy to carry (it measures 2.5 cm × 9 cm × 24 cm) and has human-izing design.[5] In addition, the field detection of the niclosamide concentration is simple, rapid, and highly sensitive. It has been widely applied for the quality control of snail control by chemical molluscicides in the schistosomiasis-endemic regions of Jiangsu Province.[4]

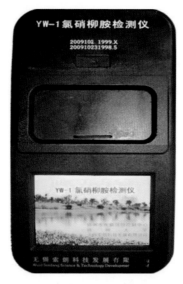

Figure 4.11　A field niclosamide detector.

Snail control with black plastic film coverage

The applicable temperature for snail breeding and reproduction is 15 to 25°C. Snails cannot survive at > 29°C and may die within several hours at > 40°C. To solve the problem of snail control in mountainous and hilly regions, a snail control approach using a black plastic film coverage has been developed (Figure 4.12). In hilly regions, the density of live snails was reduced by 67.71%, 93.06%, and 100% in 7, 10, and 30 days, respectively, post-coverage with black plastic film. In marshland and lake regions, the density of live snails was reduced by 20.77% and 96.92% in 15 and 30 days, respectively, post-coverage with black plastic film. Plastic film coverage is nontoxic to aquaculture. It is also active against snails and snail eggs in the soil layer, which is effective for inhibiting the reproduction and breeding of snails. This snail control approach is applicable for snail control in specific snail habitats, such as fish ponds. Coverage with black plastic film was the predominant snail control approach used for the interruption of schistosomiasis transmission in Sichuan Province in 2015. This approach now has been popularized in other endemic foci of China.[1,6]

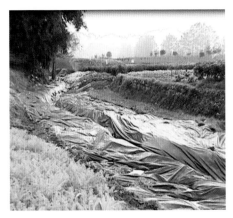 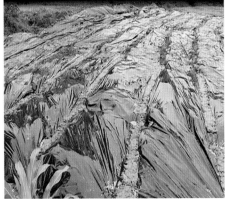

Figure 4.12　Snail control with black plastic film coverage.

4.5.3　Applicable technology for detection and monitoring *S. japonicum* infections

An intelligent detector for *S. japonicum*-infested water using sentinel mice

Based on the biological features of *S. japonicum* cercariae—they float on the water surface and cannot actively migrate—an intelligent detector for *S. japonicum*-infested water has been developed using sentinel mice (Figure 4.13). This method increases the likelihood of detecting *S. japonicum* cercariae through remote-controlled movement in the water body. The detector reduces field detection from eight

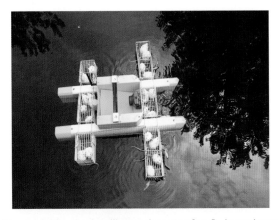

Figure 4.13　An intelligent detector for *S. japonicum*-infested water using sentinel mice.

hours to only one hour. It increases the infection rate of *S. japonicum* in sentinel mice from 15% to 40% and increases the intensity of infection (worm burden) from 0.25 worms per mouse to 2.55 worms per mouse. The intelligent detector has greatly enhanced the efficiency of field detection of infested water. It has also played a critical role in the surveillance-response system for schistosomiasis along the lower reach of the Yangtze River basin.[2]

A kit for detecting *S. japonicum* DNA in snails

To meet the requirement of early detection of *S. japonicum* in snails, a rapid extraction of snail genomic DNA combined with a LAMP assay (National Institute of Parasitic Diseases, Chinese Center for Disease Control and Prevention; Shanghai, China) has been developed. This kit greatly reduces the detection time of infected snails, which is decreased from 60 days (dissection of snails) to approximately one week. As compared to currently available commercial imported reagents, this kit has an equivalent detection efficiency (Figure 4.14). It also costs more than 50% less than other reagents that have been used in China. The kit has been used for the detection of snail infection in all seven schistosomiasis-endemic provinces of China. This assay greatly improves the sensitivity for detection of *S. japonicum*-infected snails in endemic regions relative to conventional approaches, thus providing technical support for the timely eradication of the risk of schistosomiasis transmission.

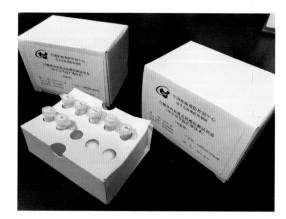

Figure 4.14　A kit for detection of *S. japonicum* DNA in snails.

Internet+ and Google Earth-based surveillance-response system

In the field of schistosomiasis control, the rapid release and sharing of monitoring information is the prerequisite for rapid emergency treatment. A surveillance-response system for schistosomiasis has been developed based on Internet+ and Google Earth (Figure 4.15). This system effectively enhances the use of the monitoring information and achieves the synchronous visualized use of the monitoring information. This system displays the graphs and texts directly and clearly, and is easy and simple to use, playing a critical role in the elimination of schistosomiasis in China.[7,8,9]

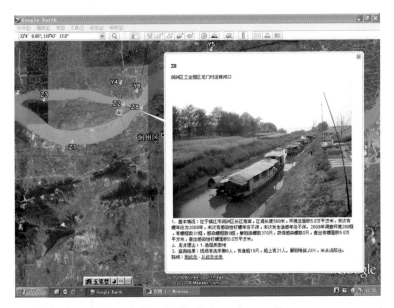

Figure 4.15   Internet+ and Google Earth-based surveillance-response system.

4.5.4   Applicable technology for health promotion

Boatmen and fishermen in China have a high likelihood and a high prevalence of *S. japonicum* infection. Consequently, they are the key target population for health education in schistosomiasis control. However, the conventional distribution of health education materials has an unsatisfactory level of effectiveness due to the high mobility and poor awareness of schistosomiasis prevention among this key target population. A new model of health education for schistosomiasis control therefore has been developed.[10]

This model operates as follows. First, a group of active, respected boatmen and fishermen with high education levels are selected as health education volunteers (one volunteer for 10 boats). Second, these volunteers are trained about schistosomiasis prevention and control by professional staff from local disease control and prevention institutions. This ensures that the volunteers learn and acquire knowledge about the techniques of health education for schistosomiasis prevention and control. Finally, the volunteers transmit the knowledge they have gained about schistosomiasis prevention and control to numerous boatmen and fishermen. In this way, the volunteers actively participate in health education interventions targeting the boatman and fishermen. In addition, the volunteers help professional staff alter problematic behavior. They serve to remind the key target groups about the implementation of self-protective measures and prohibit the pouring of contaminated feces into the water. Volunteers also help to record the use of feces containers in boats and documents the use of the harmless public toilets that have been built at fixed anchor points.

A questionnaire-based survey was conducted to evaluate the effectiveness of this new health education model for schistosomiasis control among boatmen and fishermen. The results show that the three-year (2005 to 2007) implementation period for this health education model increased the awareness of schistosomiasis control knowledge from 23.85% to 95.7%. Over the course of this health education project, the percentage of correct schistosomiasis control behavior increased from 6.59% to 53.42%. The use of harmless public toilets and on-boat fecal containers rose from 0% to 80.21% and 54.52%, respectively. The seroprevalence of *S. japonicum* decreased from 27.95% in 2004 to 19.24%, 12.27%, and 8.15% from 2005 through 2007, respectively.[10] These results demonstrate that the model of health education for schistosomiasis prevention and control that has been developed using trained volunteers to transmit knowledge has played an active role in the prevention and control of schistosomiasis among the key target group of boatmen and fishermen.

It has been proven that applicable technology, which is the basis for schistosomiasis control, promotes and is a driving force for the control, transmission interruption, and elimination of schistosomiasis in China. The development of applicable technology has been integral to the development of effective strategy during the process of schistosomiasis elimination in China. Consequently, the development of applicable technology should be defined as a priority for schistosomiasis research and control. Novel techniques, methods, tools, interventions, and strategies that are suitable for application in the field should continue to be developed. This can provide new technical supports for the implementation of the schistosomiasis control and elimination programme in China, as well as worldwide.[2]

References

1.　Hong QB, Wen LY, Zhong B, et al. Applicable technology: a driver to eliminate schistosomiasis in China. Insights gained from the First Forum on Schistosomiasis Control in China. Chin J Schisto Control. 2015, 27: 447-450. (in Chinese)

2.　Sun LP, Wang W, Hong QB, et al. Approaches being used in the national schistosomiasis elimination programme in China: a review. Int Dis Poverty. 2017, 6: 55.

3.　Gao Y, Yang J, Sun LP, et al. Study on schistosomiasis control measures in mobile boat fishermen I Harmless public toilets at fixed anchor points. Chin J Schisto Control. 2008, 20: 102-105. (in Chinese)

4.　Wang FB, Ma YC, Sun LP, et al. Integration and demonstration of key techniques in surveillance and fore-cast of schistosomiasis in Jiangsu Province Ⅲ Development of a machine simultaneously integrating mechanized environmental cleaning and automatic mollusciciding. Chin J Schisto Control. 2016, 28: 5-10. (in Chinese)

5.　Jiang YF, Wang J, Ji ZP, et al. Development of method and detector for niclosamide detection in field. Chin J Schisto Control. 2009, 21: 209-211. (in Chinese)

6.　Zhu HQ, Zhang GR, Zhong B, et al. Molluscicidal effect of film on ditches in mountainous schistosomiasis endemic regions. Chin J Schisto Control. 2011, 23: 128-132. (in Chinese)

7.　Sun LP, Liang YS, Tian ZX, et al. Surveillance and forecast system of schistosomiasis in Jiangsu Province Ⅱ Establishment of real-time operation and expression platform based on Google Earth. Chin J Schisto Control. 2009, 21: 368-372. (in Chinese)

8.　Sun LP, Liang YS, Wu HH, et al. A Google Earth-based surveillance system for schistosomiasis japonica implemented in the lower reaches of the Yangtze River, China. Parasit Vectors. 2011, 4: 223.

9.　Yang K, Sun LP, Huang YX, et al. A real-time platform for monitoring schistosomiasis transmission supported by Google Earth and a web-based geographical information system. Geospat Health. 2012, 6: 195-203.

10.　Liu XL, Ma YC, Wang FB. Effect of health education on schistosomiasis control in fishermen and boatmen. Chin J Schisto Control. 2009, 21: 424-425. (in Chinese)

Chapter 5

China's Experiences in the Combat of Schistosomiasis

Jing Xu, Hong Zhu, Jian-bing Liu, Jiao-jiao Lin, Jin-ming Liu, You-sheng Liang, Jin-xing Zhou, and Long Wan

5.1 Evolution of schistosomiasis control strategies in China

5.1.1 Introduction

Intestinal schistosomiasis japonica is caused by *Schistosoma japonicum* infection and occurs in Indonesia, the Philippines, and China.[1,2] The amphibious freshwater snail *Oncomelania hupensis* is the only intermediate host of *S. japonicum* but, besides humans, more than 40 mammals can serve as definitive hosts.[3,4] People are infected during water contact due to economic, leisure, and domestic activities. Symptoms resembling early schistosomiasis or Katayama syndrome have been described in ancient Chinese medical publications, in which the disease was called water poison disease. Studies in the 1970s on two exhumed 2,100-year-old corpses from the Western Han dynasty identified schistosome eggs in their inner organs.[5,6] The first modern medical description of schistosomiasis was published by Dr. Logan in 1905 based on a case in Changde city in Hunan Province.[7] By 1949, the disease had been recognized in 12 provinces in mainland China.[8]

Schistosomiasis control was a high priority for the leaders of the People's Republic of China soon after its foundation. Chairman Mao issued the slogan: "Schistosomiasis must be eliminated" in 1955, and a vigorous national control programme was established. More than 60 years of continuous efforts have resulted in the interruption of schistosomiasis japonica transmission in many areas in China and its control in the remaining endemic areas.[9,10] By the end of 2014, 98.9% of all endemic counties (448/453) had interrupted or controlled the transmission of schistosomiasis.[11] The progress of schistosomiasis in China can be attributed to the evolution of schistosomiasis control programmes, and in particular, the shift in strategies from controlling the intermediate host to preventing morbidity in humans, removing non-human definitive hosts, and employing integrated multi-sectoral approaches.

5.1.2 Schistosomiasis control strategies in China

Over all of its 60-year history, schistosomiasis japonica control in China was based on the basic policy of "Prevention first, comprehensive management, mass control and prevention". Based on the insight blocking any step of the schistosome life cycle that would interrupt transmission, control strategies were developed and adapted over time to remain aligned with epidemiological insights, technological advances, and the political environment.

Preparation stage (1950–1955)

In the early stages of the schistosomiasis control programme in China, the treatment of patients with severe illness was the primary task. A manual for schistosomiasis control was issued by the Ministry of Health in 1950, followed by the establishment of a professional control system, treatment of patients, and field surveys, thus providing the basis for future mass campaigns against schistosomiasis.

Preparation for future large-scale control programmes

In order to conduct treatment and control activities on a large scale, a national committee was established to organize the treatment of patients in known endemic regions, and a large number of control teams were formed in a short time.[12] In 1950, the East Branch of the Central Institute of Health was established. This branch moved to Shanghai in 1957 and became the national agency for research and for guiding schistosomiasis control. During 1950–1955, schistosomiasis control stations at provincial, city, and county levels were set up successively. Sixteen stations, 78 substations, and 420 field units were established by 1955.[13] The number of well-trained health workers focusing on schistosomiasis reached 3,000 in East China alone.[14] During this period, field surveys on the distribution of intermediate host snails and human stool examinations were conducted to increase the understanding of the endemic areas and the epidemiology of schistosomiasis in China.[15-19] Knowledge about the schistosome life cycle, morbidity, and prevention was disseminated through meetings, newspapers, leaflets, and so on. This provided rural inhabitants with a basis for reporting the presence of snails or illnesses indicative of schistosomiasis to village leaders in their areas.

Achievements and lessons learnt

During this period, many patients with serious symptoms were able to recover and fatalities caused by schistosomiasis decreased significantly. In 1953 alone, of the 55,355 patients who received treatment, 60% were cured, and health conditions improved in the remaining patients.[14] In addition, pilot studies in different endemic areas were implemented to explore effective approaches for controlling schistosomiasis. However, these achievements did not alter the landscape significantly due to limited manpower and resources, as well as a lack of relevant tools and overall planning.

Mass-campaign stage focused on snail control (1956–1985)

During this stage, the first national plan for schistosomiasis control was drafted and an elimination strategy based on snail control was implemented nationwide. This followed the achievement of a complete understanding of the endemic status of schistosomiasis across China.

Snail control strategy

In 1956, schistosomiasis was listed as one of five major parasitic diseases in the national programme for agricultural development (1956–1967). The objective of eliminating schistosomiasis in all possible endemic areas within 12 years was set, but the complexity of schistosomiasis transmission and its control had been neglected. The key tools to eliminate schistosomiasis were snail control through environmental modification and mollusciciding. The basic strategy of snail control was to implement activities from the upper to the lower reaches of drainage systems, with snail treatment strategies mainly determined by the environmental, available resources, and cost-effectiveness considerations.[20-22] Inter-sectoral cooperation, especially with agricultural and water conservancy projects in endemic areas through reclaiming wetlands, proved efficient in terms of rendering environments unsuitable for the breeding of *Oncomelania* snails. Such cooperation included leveling the land, digging new irrigation ditches with concrete surface and filling up the old ones, changing rice paddies into dry crops, ploughing by machines and afterwards compacting the earth, making fish ponds with stable water levels, lining the river bank with cement, and so on. A large number of people were mobilized to participate in the snail elimination campaign. The most effective drugs at the time: potassium and sodium antimony tartrate, were used to treat patients before the 1980s. The clinical use of praziquantel (PZQ), with its low toxicity and high cure rate, began in 1978. This decreased the mortality and prevalence of late-stage schistosomiasis. By the end of 1984, a total of 11 million patients had received treatment.[23] Other control measures, such as self-protection with chemical repellents or niclosamide-impregnated clothes, and provision of safe water and sanitary toilets were also provided as complementary interventions.[18]

Achievements and lessons learnt

Following three decades of intensive efforts, the prevalence of schistosomiasis japonica and the number of patients with severe illness, as well as the scale of the snail infested area had decreased significantly. By 1981, 11 billion m^2 snail habitats were free of snails.[24] Guangdong Province and Shanghai Municipality had reached the criteria of schistosomiasis elimination in 1985 while Fujian Province and Guangxi Zhuang Autonomous Region eliminated schistosomiasis in 1987 and 1989, respectively.[16,25,26] This experience showed that the elimination of schistosomiasis with snail control could be achieved in areas where the water level was controlled and the economy was relatively developed. However, in 1986–1988 the number of acute cases remained high[27] and the snail-infested area increased from 2.75 billion m^2 in 1980 to 3.47 billion m^2 in 1988.[28] This was attributable to the fact that an elimination strategy focused on snail control could not work well in places characterized by unstable water levels, a complicated environment, or a comparatively undeveloped economy. Such places are found in the middle and lower reaches of the Yangtze River, as well as in the mountainous areas of Sichuan and Yunnan provinces.

Morbidity control stage boosted by international cooperation (1986–2003)

Realizing that the elimination of schistosomiasis was difficult in poor countries, the World Health Organization (WHO) expert consultation committee adjusted its strategy and objective from transmission interruption or elimination to morbidity control in 1984.[29] This strategy focused on people and their behavior rather than the snail and the environment, and had as its objective to reduce morbidity and mortality caused by schistosomiasis rather than focusing on halting transmission.

Morbidity control strategy

Since 1980, China carried out pilot studies on this new strategy in heavy endemic areas.[30,31] In 1986, new policies were formulated that consisted of four items: to actively prevent and treat cases; to consider local and seasonal conditions; to integrate scientific techniques into the mass campaign against schistosomiasis; and to fight against schistosomiasis repeatedly.[32] Since 1987, the morbidity control strategy intended to reduce the prevalence and intensity of infection among local residents and livestock had been inaugurated in Hunan, Hubei, Jiangxi, and Anhui provinces.[33]

The nationwide implementation of morbidity control was boosted by the World Bank Loan Project (WBLP) on schistosomiasis control, which was initiated in 1992 in eight provinces. The project ended in 1998 in five provinces and in 2001 in Hubei, Hunan, and Yunnan Provinces. The key aims of the project were to reduce morbidity caused by schistosomiasis and interrupt transmission in some regions where this was considered possible. Mass chemotherapy was used in endemic areas with a high prevalence (prevalence > 15%), while selective chemotherapy was given to those with positive stool examinations or serological tests in areas with moderate (3 – 15% prevalence) and low (prevalence < 3%) endemicity. PZQ treatment of infected cattle along with chemotherapy for humans was also tested. In the frame of the project, almost 19 million treatments were given to humans, while 1.7 million cattle and buffalo were screened and those infected were treated.[34] Control through molluscicide and/or environmental modification were reinforced as supplementary methods. Areas with infected snails were treated annually with niclosomide. Environmental modification was mainly conducted in low endemic areas with the goal of achieving transmission interruption.[33,34] Health education aimed at changing the behavior of people at high risk was an important intervention measure in this strategy. By the end of 1995, there were more than 4,000 full- or part-time staff conducting health education.[35]

Achievements and lessons

By 2001, 47 of the 219 counties covered by the WBLP had met the criteria of transmission control and 82 had met the criteria of transmission interruption. Zhejiang Province, with 44 formerly endemic counties, reached the target of elimination in 1995.[34] Three national sampling surveys on schistosomiasis conducted before, during, and after the WBLP in 1989, 1995, and 2004, respectively, demonstrated the impact of the WBLP but also showed the shortcomings of this morbidity control strategy. The number of cases decreased from an estimated 1,638,103 in 1989 to 865,084 in 1995, while the average prevalence in humans decreased from 9.7% to 4.9%,[36,37] and the prevalence in cattle and buffalo reduced from 13.2% to 9.1%. However, the third national sampling survey conducted in 2004 after the termination of WBLP indicated that 726,112 individuals were estimated to be infected with schistosomes, and that the prevalence was 3.8% in marshland and lake regions.[38] Schistosomiasis had reemerged in China due to a shortage of financial support following the completion of the WBLP, devastating floods in 1998, important ecological changes caused by water conservancy projects, reforms to the economic and health systems, and so on.[39-43] The chemotherapy-based strategy could quickly decrease the prevalence of schistosomiasis, but failed to interrupt transmission in the hyperendemic areas as it did not prevent reinfection.

Comprehensive strategy to block schistosomiasis transmission (2004–present)

Livestock, especially buffalo, accounted for 70 – 90% of all new schistosomiasis cases in the marshland regions along the Yangtze River at the beginning of new millennium.[44-47] Pilot studies of a new strategy emphasized health education, the removal of cattle from snail-infested grasslands, the provision of farmers with mechanized farm equipment, access to clean water, and adequate sanitation. These approaches aimed at stopping the contamination of the environment with schistosome eggs, and proved that the infection rate could be decreased to less than 1% after three transmission seasons.

Comprehensive strategy of blocking schistosomiasis transmission

With the aim of curbing the rebound of schistosomiasis in the new millennium and realizing the final goal of eliminating schistosomiasis in China, a national strategic plan for schistosomiasis control was issued in 2004. It aimed to reduce the prevalence in humans and livestock in all endemic counties to less than 5% by 2008 and then to below 1% by 2015.[48] Two comprehensive multi-sectoral control projects adopting the comprehensive strategy of blocking the contamination of water bodies with schistosome eggs (and thus preventing snails from being infected) were conducted, covering 164 counties during 2004 – 2008 and 189 counties during 2009 – 2015 respectively.

The intervention approaches varied between counties according to the local conditions: i) in endemic counties targeting infection control, interventions focused on infection resource control. These included: simultaneous chemotherapy of humans and livestock, snail control in high risk regions, agriculture mechanization to replace buffalo with tractors, prohibiting pasturing animals in grasslands inhabited by infested snails, raising livestock in stables or on grasslands free of snails, and so on. Environmental modification to destroy snail habitats was conducted in combination with farmland rehabilitation projects and forestry projects, where possible; ii) in regions aiming to reach transmission control or transmission interruption, in addition to strengthening control interventions as described above, and surveillance of remaining infection resources, snail control focused on eliminating snail breeding areas through agriculture, water conservancy and forestry projects.

Achievements and lessons learnt

After 10 years of implementing the comprehensive control strategy, the medium term goal of reaching infection control nationwide was achieved on schedule. Five provinces which had reached transmission interruption by 1995 consolidated their achievements and no new cases or infected snails had been found during this period. Hubei, Hunan, Anhui, and Jiangxi provinces reached the criteria of infection control by 2008 simultaneously, while Sichuan, Yunnan, Jiangsu, and Hubei Provinces reached the criteria of transmission control in 2008, 2009, 2010, and 2013, respectively. The estimated number of infected patients decreased from 842,525 in 2004 to 184,943 in 2013, a reduction of 78.1%. The number of reported acute cases was nine in 2013.[49,50] Now, the long-term target of the national programme to meet the criteria of the transmission control nationwide drafted in 2004 has been achieved by the end of 2015.

5.1.3   Conclusion

Big differences exist between different endemic areas in China in terms of local epidemiology, environment, and socio-economic conditions. With socio-economic and technological development, strategies for schistosomiasis control have shifted from the initial elimination strategy before the mid-1980s, to morbidity control during the WBLP, to the current comprehensive strategy of blocking transmission. Research pertaining to schistosomiasis was listed as a key research programme in the ministries of health, agriculture, and water resources. The following strategies were developed under the framework of research projects and have promoted the progress of schistosomiasis control in China: the introduction of PZQ, artemether (AM), and artesunate to kill schistosomula; the transfer from laboratory to field of sensitive and easy-to-use diagnostic tools; and new chemicals for mollusciciding and livestock treatment.[20,51-53] Along with the shift in control strategies, criteria for schistosomiasis control and elimination have been formulated and modified six times that provided, guidance for control activities and to assess the effect of interventions.[54] Technical support to different endemic areas has increased the capacity to implement and combine appropriate interventions.

As the whole country has reached the criteria of transmission control by the end of 2015, transmission interruption and then elimination of schistosomiasis must be the next target. In November 2014, the national schistosomiasis control conference at state council level was organized in Hunan Province. Based on existing achievements, a new goal was put forward to eliminate schistosomiasis nationwide in accordance with the approaches laid out in another two consecutive five-year plans.[1] With systematic assessments on the endemic status of schistosomiasis and the efficacy of the current integrated strategy in China, challenges still exist in some regions with complicated surroundings to eliminate schistosomiasis. Precise interventions including chemotherapy, snail control, safe water supply, improving sanitation, environmental modification through water conservancy, agriculture and forestry projects are needed to be encouraged. Intersectoral cooperation must be strengthened. More sensitive and effective diagnostic and surveillance tools and techniques need to be explored to monitor the decline in transmission and verify elimination of schistosomiasis transmission. Risk assessments should be conducted to identify transmission hotspots and guide policymakers. Capacity-building in surveillance should be strengthened to consolidate achievements and prevent the re-emergence of schistosomiasis.

References

1. Gryseels B, Polman K, Clerinx J, Kestens L. Human schistosomiasis. Lancet, 2006, 368: 1106-1118.

2. Ross AG, Bartley P, Sleigh A, et al. Schistosomiasis. N Engl J Med, 2002, 346: 1212-1220.

3. McManus DP, Li Y, Gray DJ, Ross AG. Conquering 'snail fever': schistosomiasis and its control in China. Expert Rev Anti Infect Ther, 2009, 7: 473-485.

4. Wang LD, Utzinger J, Zhou XN. Schistosomiasis control: experiences and lessons from China. Lancet, 2008, 372: 1793-1795.

5. Wei O. Internal organs of a 2100-year-old female corpse. Lancet, 1973, 2: 1198.

6. Ross AG, Li YS, Sleigh AC, McManus DP. Schistosomiasis control in the People's Republic of China. Parasitol Today, 1997, 13: 152-155.

7. Logan OT. A Case of dysentery in Hunan province, caused by the trematoda, *Schistosoma japonicum*. Chin Med J, 1905, 19: 243-245.

8. Ling CC, Cheng WJ, Chung HL. Clinical and diagnostic features of schistosomiasis japonica. Chin Med J, 1949, 67: 347-360.

9. Xu J, Xu JF, Li SZ, et al. Integrated control programmes for schistosomiasis and other helminth infections in P.R. China. Acta Trop, 2015, 141: 332-341.

10. Zhou XN, Wang LY, Chen MG, et al. The public health significance and control of schistosomiasis in China--then and now. Acta Trop, 2005, 96: 97-105.

11. Lei ZL, Zhou XN. Eradication of schistosomiasis: a new target and a new task for the national schistosomiasis control program in the People's Republic of China. Chin J Schisto Contr, 2015, 27: 1-4. (in Chinese)

12. Wang HZ, Jia YD, Guo JP, et al. A histroric review or 40 years' control on schistosomiasis in P. R. China. Chin J Schisto Contr, 1989, 1: 1-4. (in Chinese)

13. Wang GZ. The practice and enlightment of schistosomiasis control by Chinese Communist Party through integrating humanpower in 1950s. Study Teach History Communist Party, 2011, 221: 89-96. (in Chinese)

14. Lu ZH, Zhong HL, Ling ZS, et al. Some aspects of research in the prevention and treatment of schistosomiasis japonica in new China. Chin Med J, 1955, 73: 100-106.

15. Tang CC. Epidemiology of schistosomiasis japonica in Futsing, Fukien Province. Peking Nat Bull, 1951, 19: 225-247. (in Chinese)

16. Sleigh A, Li X, Jackson S, et al. Eradication of schistosomiasis in Guangxi, China. Part 1: Setting, strategies, operations, and outcomes, 1953-92. Bull World Health Organ, 1998, 76: 361-372.

17. Zhuang BJ. History of schistosomiasis control in Zhejiang Province. Shanghai: Shanghai Health Publishing House, 1992. (in Chinese)

18. Wen LY, Tao HQ. Progress and prospect on schistosomiasis control in Zhejiang Province. Int J Epidemil Infect Dis, 2008, 6: 361-364.

19. Chen GX. Endemic status of schistosomiasis in Hunan Province. Data compilation on schistosomiasis reasearch. Shanghai: Shanghai Health Publishing House, 1956. (in Chinese)

20. Yang GJ, Sun LP, Hong QB, et al. Optimizing molluscicide treatment strategies in different control stages of schistosomiasis in the People's Republic of China. Parasit Vectors, 2012, 5: 260.

21. Yang GJ, Li W, Sun LP, et al. Molluscicidal efficacies of different formulations of niclosamide: result of meta-analysis of Chinese literature. Parasit Vectors, 2010, 3: 84.

22. Yuan Y, Xu XJ, Dong HF, et al. Transmission control of schistosomiasis japonica: implementation and evaluation of different snail control interventions. Acta Trop, 2005, 96: 191-197.

23. Zheng G. Progress of schistosomiasis epideiology in P. R. China (1980-1985). Nanjing: Jiangsu Medical Publishing House, 1986. (in Chinese)

24. Guo JG, Zheng J. Epidemiology of schistosomaisis and progress of control and research. Chin J Parasitol Parsit Dis, 1999, 17: 260-263. (in Chinese)

25. Pan HD, Huang DS, Wang KT. Approach to surveillance and consolidation during past 15 years after elimination of schistosomiasis in Shanghai. Acta Trop, 2002, 82: 301-303.

26. Wu XH, Chen MG, Zheng J. Surveillance of schistosomiasis in five provinces of China which have reached the national criteria for elimination of the disease. Acta Trop, 2005, 96: 276-281.

27. Xia C, Wang HZ. The endemic status and control of schistosomiasis. Bull Biol, 1989, 9: 26-27.

28. Yuan HC. Achievements and experience on schistosomiasis control in P. R. China. Chin J Epidemiol, 1999, 20: 3-6.

29. WHO. The Control of schistosomiasis. Report of a WHO Expert Committee 1985.

30. Yuan HC, Zhuo SJ, Zhang SJ, et al. Studies on the epidemic factors and principles in beaches of rivers and lakes. Chin J Schisto Contr, 1990, 2: 14-21. (in Chinese)

31. Zheng J, Gu XG, Qiu ZL, et al. Study on the strategy for schistosomiasis control for mountainous regions. Chin J Schisto Contr, 1996, 8: 65-71. (in Chinese)

32. Mao SP. Epidemiology and control of schistosomiasis in the People's Republic of China. Mem Inst Oswaldo Cruz, 1987, 82: 77-82.

33. Yuan HC, Jiang QW, Zhao GM, He N. Achievements of schistosomiasis control in China. Mem Inst Oswaldo Cruz, 2002, 97: 187-189.

34. Chen XY, Wang LY, Cai JM, et al. Schistosomiasis control in China: the impact of a 10-year World Bank Loan Project (1992-2001). Bull World Health Organ, 2005, 83: 43-48.

35. Guo JG. Historical and current comprehensive control of schistosomiasis in P.R. China. Chin J Prev Med, 2006, 40: 225-228. (in Chinese)

36. MoH. Epidemic status of schistosomiasis in China-a naitonwide sampling survey in 1995. Nanjing: Nanjing University Press, 1998. (in Chinese)

37. MoH. Epidemiological Situation of Schistosomiasis in China: Results from a Nationwide Sampling Survey in 1989. Chengdu: Press of Chengdu Science and Technology University, 1993. (in Chinese)

38. Zhou XN, Guo JG, Wu XH, et al. Epidemiology of schistosomiasis in the People's Republic of China, 2004. Emerg Infect Dis, 2007, 13: 1470-1476.

39. Bian Y, Sun Q, Zhao Z, et al. Market reform: a challenge to public health--the case of schistosomiasis control in China. Int J Health Plann Manage, 2004, 19: S79-S94.

40. Liang S, Yang C, Zhong B, et al. Re-emerging schistosomiasis in hilly and mountainous areas of Sichuan, China. Bull World Health Organ, 2006, 84: 139-144.

41. Xu XJ, Wei FH, Yang XX, et al. Possible effects of the Three Gorges dam on the transmission of Schistosoma japonicum on the Jiang Han plain, China. Am J Trop Med Hyg, 2000, 94: 333-341.

42. Yang GJ, Vounatsou P, Zhou XN, et al. A potential impact of climate change and water resource development on the transmission of Schistosoma japonicum in China. Parasitology, 2005, 47: 127-134.

43. Zhou XN, Lin DD, Yang HM, et al. Use of landsat TM satellite surveillance data to measure the impact of the 1998 flood on snail intermediate host dispersal in the lower Yangtze River Basin. Acta Trop, 2002, 82: 199-205.

44. Guo JG, Ross AG, Lin DD, et al. A baseline study on the importance of bovines for human *Schistosoma japonicum* infection around Poyang Lake, China. Am J Trop Med Hyg, 2001, 65: 272-278.

45. Wang TP, Vang Johansen M, Zhang SQ, et al. Transmission of *Schistosoma japonicum* by humans and domestic animals in the Yangtze River valley, Anhui province, China. Acta Trop, 2005, 96: 198-204.

46. Gray DJ, Williams GM, Li Y, et al. A cluster-randomized bovine intervention trial against *Schistosoma japonicum* in the People's Republic of China: design and baseline results. Am J Trop Med Hyg, 2007, 77: 866-874.

47. Gray DJ, Williams GM, Li Y, McManus DP. Transmission dynamics of *Schistosoma japonicum* in the lakes and marshlands of China. PLoS One, 2008, 3: e4058.

48. Wang LD, Guo JG, Wu XH, et al. China's new strategy to block *Schistosoma japonicum* transmission: experiences and impact beyond schistosomiasis. Trop Med Int Health, 2009, 14: 1475-1483.

49. Lei ZL, Zheng H, Zhang LJ, et al. Endemic status of schitosomiasis in People's Republic of China in 2013. Chin J Schisto Contr, 2014, 26: 591-597. (in Chinese)

50. Hao Y, Wu XH, Xia G, et al. Endemic status of schistosomiasis in P. R. China in 2004. Chin J Schisto Contr, 2005, 17: 401-404. (in Chinese)

51. Xin YT, Dai JR. Progress of research on molluscicide niclosomide. Chin J Schisto Contr, 2010, 22: 504-508. (in Chinese)

52. Zhou Y, Wang Z, Zhang B, et al. Field evaluation of a novel plant molluscicide "Luo-wei" against the snail *Oncomelania hupensis* III molluscicidal effect by spraying method in hilly regions. Chin J Schisto Contr, 2013, 25: 495-497. (in Chinese)

53. Zhang Z, Fang R, Yu B, et al. Field evaluation of a novel plant molluscicide"Luo-wei"against *Oncomelania hupensis* snails II Molluscicidal effect in the field of lake areas in Hanchuan City, Hubei Province. Chin J Schisto Contr, 2013, 25: 481-484. (in Chinese)

54. Zhou XN, Xu J, Lin DD, et al. Role of the new version of the control and elimination criteria for schistosomiasis in acceleration of the schistosomiasis elimination program in China. Chin J Schisto Contr, 2013, 25: 1-4. (in Chinese)

5.2 Development of water conservancy projects for the control of *S. japonicum* in China

5.2.1 Introduction

Schistosomiasis is a waterborne, snail-transmitted parasitic disease. *O. hupensis*, which is an amphibious snail, is the only intermediate host of *S. japonicum*, and plays a crucial role in the transmission of schistosomiasis japonica. The snail must survive and reproduce in a water environment with suitable conditions. Accordingly, the type of water is an important factor that affects the rate of schistosomiasis occurrence. From the aspect of the spread of the disease, water contact behavior is a necessary prerequisite for infection with schistosomes. Because human and animal can be infected by schistosomes once contacted water containing miracidium. Among the factors related to the disease, floods and other natural disasters contribute to the schistosomiasis occurrence. At the same time, it is becoming increasingly more difficult to control schistosomiasis transmission. Therefore, water in nature, like rivers, lakes, as well as snails, which are rely on water as one of the conditions of existence, are two key links in the epidemic of schistosomiasis. Thus, there is a very close relationship between water conservancy and schistosomiasis control.

Moreover, water conservancy is not only the method of schistosomiasis prevention, but also a project represented to affect the livelihood of those areas. Construction is directly related to the vital interests of the general public. The whole society pays huge attention to the influence of water conservancy for schistosomiasis prevention, since it may be a double-edged sword. On the one hand, it can lead to positive results in terms of the control of snails and schistosomiasis through the improvement of the watershed environment with the implementation of the water conservancy project. On the other hand, however, it can increase the risk of the spread of schistosomiasis because of snail diffusion occurring with the flow of water caused by changes in the ecological environment. There has been no shortage of various reports related to the spread of schistosomiasis being attributed to the influence of changes in the ecological environment of water conservancy projects, both domestically and abroad. Some examples include the building of the Aswan Dam in Egypt, the Gezira-Managil water conservancy project in Sudan, the reservoir in Danleng County in the Sichuan Province of China, and the excavation of the north of the Han River in the Hubei Province of China in 1970s, done so without any prevention and control measures of snail diffusion.[1,2] Moreover, in recent years, there have been many studies about whether the Three Gorges Dam,[3-5] currently under construction on the Yangtze River in China, might affect the transmission of *S. japonicum* on the Jiang Han Plain, which is downstream from the dam. Therefore, the various aspects of these influencing factors should be fully considered, and furthermore, corresponding countermeasures must be applied to deal with adverse risk factors in the construction of a water conservancy project.

Over the years, water conservancy development has played an important role in the control of schistosomiasis transmission in China. In July 2004, the Ministry of Health of China along with the National Development and Reform Commission, the Ministry of Finance, the Ministry of Agriculture, the Ministry of Water Resources, and Forestry Bureau issued the "National Programme of Schistosomiasis Control in the Mid- and Long Term (2004–2015)". Three months later, the "National Programme Guidelines for Key Projects of Integrated Schistosomiasis Control (2004 – 2008)" was issued. In 2010, the "National Programme Guidelines for Key Projects of Integrated Schistosomiasis Control (2009 – 2015)" was issued by the seven departments of the State Council, which, in addition to the six groups above, included the Ministry of Land and Resources. The three programmes above specify that water conservancy projects are required to be constructed in schistosomiasis-endemic areas in conjunction with efforts to be taken toward schistosomiasis control. In 2006, the State Council of China issued "The National Regulations of Schistosomiasis Control",[6] in which it specifies that any water conservancy project, together with schistosomiasis prevention, must be undertaken jointly, in the case of water conservancy projects being constructed in schistosomiasis-endemic areas. From then, water conservancy, combined with schistosomiasis prevention, was considered as an important factor at various stages of the construction of water conservancy projects in endemic areas. At present, work involving water conservancy and schistosomiasis control is approaching institutionalization, normalization, and standardization.

5.2.2　The concept of schistosomiasis control through water conservancy

The concept of schistosomiasis control through water conservancy means the construction of a water conservancy project combined with *O. hupensis* control and schistosomiasis control.

Measures for schistosomiasis control through water conservancy projects involve two aspects: one is water conservancy project measures, while the other is water conservancy management measures, which can be taken to control and eliminate *O. hupensis* for anti-schistosomiasis.

218

5.2.3 The guiding principle of schistosomiasis control through water conservancy

Water conservancy and schistosomiasis control involve the two aspects of water conservancy and anti-schistosomiasis. It means combining snail control with the construction of a water conservancy project. To adhere to the principle of "Priority water-control in schistosomiasis endemic areas", and at the same time, "Priority snail-control in the water-control", both should be used as the guiding principle in the stage of planning and designing in documents. Anti-schistosomiasis experts, who participating in the work, not only come from health departments, but also come from water conservancy departments. They should be invited to check the professional schistosomiasis technology in order to check the water conservancy project and schistosomiasis control in a more accurate and effective manner. They have to ensure that water conservancy measures of schistosomiasis control are taking place at the same time as the water conservancy project planning; namely, the two subjects will be considered synchronously, from the stage of design to implementation, to utilization, and to final benefits.

5.2.4 Building water resource projects for schistosomiasis control: current approaches

Measures taken by water conservancy engineering facilities to prevent snail diffusion or barriers erected to prevent people and livestock from entering snail habitats

Preventing the spread of oncomelanid snails through the use of a blocking net
A closed blocking network is installed in the front of or behind sluice gates, or in irrigation canals. There are three forms of blocking networks. The first type is a single-layer blocking network made of nylon or metal, with a specification of 20 holes per square inch for the blocking net. First, it is fixed onto the steel frame, part of a gate-type blocking network, which is suitable for small-sized water transport channels with flat water, with less floating debris and sediment. The second type is a double-layer blocking network, which is suitable for a small- and medium-sized irrigation channel with flat water and less sediment: the first layer is a metal blocking net with

a 2–3 mm diameter coarse mesh for stopping large floating objects; the second layer is a nylon net or metal net with the specification of 20 holes per square inch to block *O. hupensis* from entering. The third type is a multilayer half-range blocking network, which is suitable for an irrigation channel carrying large flow of water (Figure 5.1).

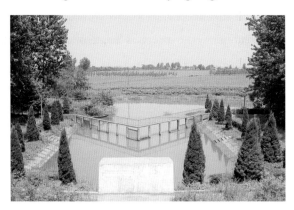

Figure 5.1   Blocking net for preventing the spread of *O. hupensis*.

The settling basin for O. hupensis

The law of motion for snail sedimentation and snail eggs sedimentation in the water reflects the biological distribution characteristics of snails and their eggs in the water. There are two layers for this distribution in the water, the surface and the bottom, using the principle of interception for preventing the spread of snails and their eggs when drawing water from outside embankment to inner embankment. Once the snails and their eggs are drawn from outside embankment to inner embankment with the water, they will be prevented in the settling basin which is connected with the sluice, using the principle of sedimentation for making snails and their eggs deposited in the bottom of the settling basin. Finally, snails and their eggs, which are deposited in the bottom of the settling basin are drowned by water or killed by molluscicides.

The settling basin for the *O. hupensis* is built within a 100-m distance behind sluices or the appropriate location in the irrigation channel that carries a large flow of water. It is composed of three sections, including an upstream connection, a working section, and a downstream connection section. The upstream joint section is called the first pool. There is a blocking network in front of the first pool. There is also a working section, called the second pool, and a downstream joint section, called the third pool. The aim of the settling basin design is to determine the flow speed, depth, width, and length of the pool for meeting the requirements of snail sedimentation in the bottom of the pool. The designed maximum velocity should not exceed 0.2 m/s in the pool. Its cross-sectional area (S) is determined by the water gate diversion flow (Q), and designed maximum velocity (Umax) to meet the S ⩾ Q / Umax. If the cross-section of the pool is trapezoidal, certain width and depth ratios are determined according to the field conditions. The designed length of the pool must be greater than the snail's horizontal sedimentation distance; generally speaking, the length of the pool is 2–3 times that of the snail horizontal sedimentation distance (Figures 5.2–5.6).

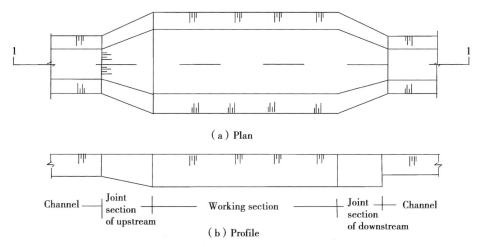

Figure 5.2   Profile map of the settling basin for *O. hupensis*.

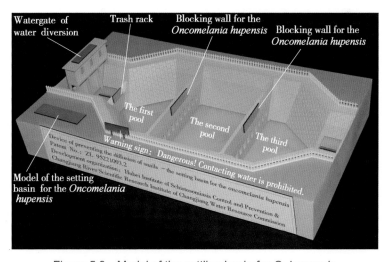

Figure 5.3   Model of the settling basin for *O. hupensis*.

221

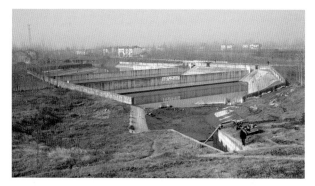

Figure 5.4   Settling basin for *O. hupensis* in Gong'an County, Hubei Province, China (during construction).

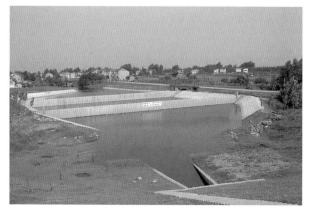

Figure 5.5   Settling basin for *O. hupensis* in Gong'an County, Hubei Province, China (completed).

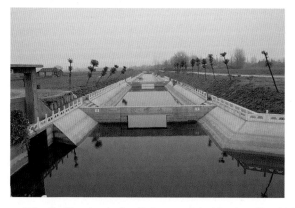

Figure 5.6   Settling basin for *O. hupensis* in Xiantao City, Hubei Province, China (completed).

Removing the middle layer of water without O. hupensis

Based on the biological characteristics of the distribution of snails and snail eggs in the two layers of water (i.e. the surface and the bottom), water is drawn into the middle layer (deep layer water) by use of the deep-water culvert principle. The bell-shaped water sealed pipe system is adapted in order to avoid a water eddy, as well as to stop snails from going into the pipeline with floating adsorption. The basic principles of those designs involve the use of water intake structures via a water pipe from the middle layer of water in front of the sluice (that is, the outer embankment of rivers). The aim of the design is that the altitude of the intake of culvert sluice must be less than the height of the original culvert, which is also below the height of the lowest low water level in the dry season. In addition, an intake of 3 – 5 m must be confirmed under the water during the flood season (Figure 5.7).

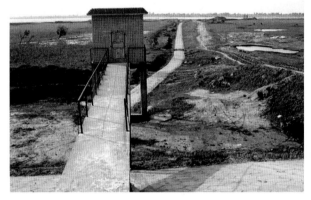

Figure 5.7   Device for removing the middle layer of water without *O. hupensis*.

Building a platform for O. hupensis control

According to the requirements for snail control and snail elimination, dike-dam platforms are set up on both sides of the river embankment. The top elevation of the platforms should not be lower than the highest no snail curve in the local place. In addition, the top width should not be less than 1 m. The surface of the platform should be standard and flat when the platform is wide, in order to avoid the formation of a new pit, where snails may be breeding.

Building an isolation ditch for preventing people and livestock from entering snail habitats

When the width of the bottomland, which is near the embankment of the rivers and lakes, is greater than 200 m in the marshland areas, the isolation ditch for controlling snails can be built at the outer embankment in order to prevent people and livestock from entering the snail habitats. The isolation ditch must be standard and flat, and should be connected to the rivers and lakes. The width of the isolation ditch is 3 – 10 m suitable. The annual submerged time should be kept for more than eight months, and the water depth should not be less than 1 m (Figure 5.8).

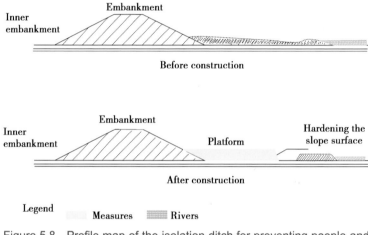

Figure 5.8　Profile map of the isolation ditch for preventing people and livestock from entering the snail habitats.

Measures of water conservancy project combined with snail habitat modification for snail control

There are several necessary condition for the survival and reproduction of *O. hupensis*, such as water, food and oxygen. So they could be killed by hunger or hypoxia. That is the reason of transforming the environment of snail habitats, as being a method for snail control. Secondly, snail mating and oviposition can also be affected because of the above mentioned issues. The growth of embryonic cells in snail eggs is inhibited in this way, so snails cannot grow and develop normally.

The soil or sand burying method for snail control

　　Digging a new trench to fill an old ditch with snails. The method is used along with the construction of an irrigation and drainage system. First, the grass and soil containing snails are shoveled in 10 – 15 cm on both sides of the old ditches. Then, this grass and soil are pushed to the bottom of the ditch, while at the same time sweeping of the area is done 1 – 2 times. Second, a new irrigation and drainage ditch is excavated according to the water conservancy planning. The excavated soil not containing snails is filled into the old ditch with soil at a depth of at least 30 cm, and firmed up by compacting the soil. If there is little water in the old ditch with snails, it cannot be extracted beforehand. Likewise, if there is a significant amount of water in the old ditch, then most of the water will be extracted before. The distance between the old and new ditches should not be less than 1 m, and efforts should be made to avoid crossing or connecting between the old and new ditches. Actions must be taken to prevent the snails in the old ditch from spreading to the new channel, if crossing or connecting occurs.

Burying directly using soil not containing snails. The method of burying directly using soil which does not contain snails can be applied in waste environments for the basic construction of farmland and water conservancies, including pits, ponds, gullies, depressions, and rivers, among others. The soil and grass containing snails is dug out up to about 15 cm, and this soil is then pushed to the bottom. Then the soil which does not contain snails is covered over up to 30 cm, and firmed up by compacting the soil.

Burying directly with sand. The method of burying directly with sand can be applied in some dikes, pits, depressions, and wavebreak forest; for instance, using local materials such as sand to cover snails directly. The sand must have a uniform thickness, and completely cover the area without leaving any gaps. More than 10 cm at least must be covered by sand. Before laying the sand, any remaining grass, reeds, and trees on the ground must be cleared.

Soil cement hardening for snail control

Ditch cement hardening. Together with the construction of a water conservancy project, the ditches with snail habitats are hardened to eliminate snails. The thickness of the cement is generally in the range of 2 – 5 cm. The hardening range of the channel slope should be up to above 0.5 m to the top of the canal or to the designed water level, and extend 1 m down to the bottom of the canal, or the minimum operation water level. Whether or not the canal bottom is hardened depends on the channel construction requirements, operation, and potential snail habitats (Figures 5.9–5.11).

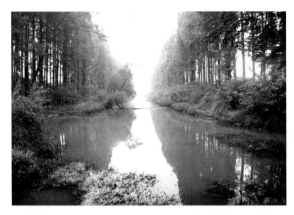

Figure 5.9   Ditch cement hardening in the Huangpi District, Hubei Province, China (before construction).

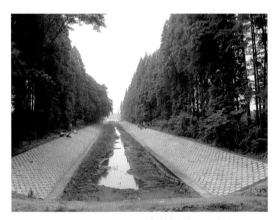

Figure 5.10   Ditch cement hardening in the Huangpi District, Hubei Province, China (completed).

Slope protection using cement hardening for snail control. This method is more suitable for the bottomland, which is less wide and at a lower elevation, or for an embankment engineered without bottomland. Cast-in-place concrete, precast concrete blocks, slurry masonry, etc., are usually applied. The slope should be kept smooth and uniform. The lower edge of the hardened foot should reach the toe line and the top should reach the highest local no snail curve.

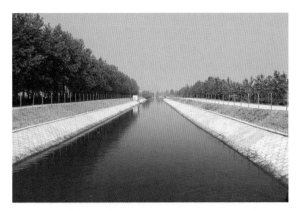

Figure 5.11   Ditch cement hardening in Jiangling County,
Hubei Province, China (completed).

Changing open channels into covered channels for snail control. Combined
with the construction project of water conservancy, channels with snails which are
small flow and small concentration of sand should be changed into pipeline covered
channels. By transforming snail habitats, it can bring a good effect of snail elimination. Covered channels (tubes) can be made by box culvert, prefabricated concrete
pipe or corrugated plastic pipe, etc. The section size, depth of buried snails, and
other measurements should be assessed according to the "Irrigation and drainage
engineering design specification" (GB50288–99).

Falling the bottomland or elevating the bottomland

Bottomland with snails is elevated to an altitude that have rare snails by the method
of covering bottomland with mud. Thus, reaching the altitude that does not have
snails is the best. Alternatively, the marshland with snails is decreasing to the minimum altitude of local no snail curve by the method mud removal.

A comparison of the main water conservancy projects for schistosomiasis prevention is given below (Table 5.1).

5.2.5   Water conservancy cases in the endemic areas of China

Because of the complicated environment in endemic areas in the real world, water
conservancy measures usually require an integrated application, instead of any one
single measure. There are some successful cases of water conservancy in endemic
areas, as shown below.

Table 5.1   Comparison of the main water conservancy projects for schistosomiasis prevention.

Type	Principle	Application environment	Application condition	Advantage	Disadvantage
Settling basin for *O. hupensis*	Measures taken by water conservancy engineering facilities to prevent snail diffusion.	Suitable for medium and small water gates (stations) engineering; large water gates (stations) should be analyzed through test by model to perform before using settling basins for *O. hupensis*.	Building on the downstream channel of irrigation water gates (pump stations); water flow is less than 15 m³/s.	Buildings are not restricted by the terrain. The impact on snail control and prevention is clear.	The investment is large.
Removing the middle layer of water not containing *O. hupensis*		Suitable for water gates (stations) with relatively stable bank lines, a deeper water source, a short distance between the water inlet to the main channel, and a narrow stream segment.	Fixed pumping station: a narrower width of bottomland; deeper water; the water level fluctuation range is not obvious in the intake during the irrigation season; ship navigation is not affected. Non-fixed pumping station: the water level fluctuation range is clear; ship navigation is not affected.	The cost of rebuilding is low, the performance cost is high, and the maintenance cost is low during the period of operation. Buildings are not restricted by the terrain. The impact on snail control and prevention is clear. A large water flow.	A small water flow. The water inlet is easily blocked by the deposition in the "pool". The investment is large, and the maintenance cost is higher during the period of operation.
Decreasing the bottomland or elevating the bottomland	Measures of water conservancy project combined with snail habitat modification for snail control.	Suitable for the engineering of renovation of lakes and rivers.	A fishpond can be built around by the embankment and the bottomland, which has fallen. The requirements with safety and shipping throughout the flood season must be satisfied.	Less investment and cost-effective, the cost performance is high and it is worth being widely used.	Falling the bottomland is regional, so it is advantageous to the *Oncomelania*'s breeding and reproduction, with the seasonal change of water level, which leads to an overgrowth of weeds.
Ditch cement hardening		Suitable for irrigation canals and ditches.	When the irrigation and drainage systems are built, expanded and rebuilt.	Less investment, and simple construction.	The effect of snail control is limited, and the threat of infected snails cannot be eliminated completely.

Snail control and flood control engineering on the Fu River, Yangxin County, Hubei Province, China

Yangxin County which is low-lying and dotted with lakes is located downstream on the Fu River. It had a heavy schistosomiasis epidemic in the past. Snails were mainly spread along the water basin of the Fu River. Because of the water level rising and falling frequently, and its significant characteristic of being dry in winter and flooded in summer, it was the ideal environment for the snail reproduction. During the years from 2000 to 2008, five sections of the Fu River downstream embankment were managed with a comprehensive treatment, as the first phase for both flood control and snail control by the Hubei Province government. Combined with the water retaining structure of Fu River, "snail control by controlling water level" was synthetically applied in the project. Snail control platforms were built and the river channels within the project were smoothed. A bottomland of 3.56 million m^2 was processed, which changed the environment for *Oncomelania* breeding, and prevented the diffusion of *Oncomelania*.[7]

Snail control project for removing the middle layer of water in the West Sluice in Junshan District, Hunan Province, China

This project which started in 2002 and completed in 2004, is located in Junshan District, Yueyang City, Hunan Province. The width of the bottomland of the Yangtze River was approximately 600 m and there was a snail population before 2002.

　　The snails were not eliminated completely because the snails diffused from the outer area of the Yangtze River embankment to the inner area of the embankment. Snail areas along the inner part of the Yangtze River embankment were at about 6.63 hm^2 before the West Sluice modification. A water-pumping wharf used for extracting the middle layer of water was built around the shore of the Yangtze River for the renovation project. A closed water diversion culvert with a cross-sectional area of 5 m^2 and a length of 1,500 m was built in the bottomland containing snails, which were located in the water pumping wharf between the sluices. The middle layer of water, which did not contain the infected water from the Yangtze River, was taken for irrigation into farmland areas along the inner embankment of the Yangtze River.

Snail control engineering of the Wangjiatai sluice in Yingcheng City, Hubei Province, China

The Wangjiatai Sluice is located downstream of the Han River tributaries in Yingcheng City, Hubei Province. The design water diversion flow was 3 m³/s. After the completion of the sluice, diversion and irrigation work was done from the north of the Han River, namely, irrigation from the outer embankment of Han River to the inner embankment. In 1988, a provincial field investigation of *Oncomelania* diffusion from the sluice gate confirmed that *Oncomelania* had diffused from the outer embankment of Han River to the inner embankment with the subsequent irrigation. In 1992, when Wangjiatai sluice was rebuilt, a settling basin for *O. hupensis* which was made of cement precast structures, was built at the gate out flow at the same time, in order to prevent the diffusion of snails caused by irrigation. The engineering structures include the following: the front for a stilling basin, two rows of cement columns for snail control installed at the back, a high blocking net installed on the cement column in the front row, and a low blocking net installed on a cement column in the back row. The impact of the engineering done at the site of the settling basin for *O. hupensis* and the blocking net for snail control were quite clear eventually. On the one hand, the epidemic status of the snail was effectively addressed, and no living snails were found after the settling basin operation inside embankment. However, on the other hand, there was almost no change to the epidemic status of the snail population outside embankment.

5.2.6   Project management and evaluation after completion

Assessment of design and operation management of water conservancy combined with schistosomiasis prevention

Including design and operation, and the later operation management for the project among other steps, several factors were assessed. First, whether the designs abided by the "Technical regulation for water conservancy combined with schistosomiasis prevention" (SL 318–2011). Second, whether construction was done according to the design requirements. Third, whether the actions led to grass overgrowth because of damaged areas from the hardened ditch, which create a breeding ground for *Oncomelania*. Fourth, whether sludge was regularly cleaned for engineering, and whether the effects on snail control are measurable, among others.

Assessment of the effects of water conservancy for snail control

This includes the overall effect of snail control and snail elimination.[8,9] First, it assesses whether there is snail diffusion in rivers, ditches, and channels of the downstream river after the operating of the water conservancy. Second, all the indices of snail surveys on the effect of snail control should be considered after the operation: i) whether or not the density of snails is high in the project, ii) whether the percentage of snail areas has been decreasing annually, iii) whether the percentage of the density of snails has been on a declining trend, among others.

5.2.7 Conclusions and perspectives

Water conservancy, combined with schistosomiasis prevention, is defined as the engineering facilities for snail control and snail elimination. Water conservancy combined with schistosomiasis prevention includes both hydraulic engineering measures and snail control measures. This is done mainly through transforming the environments of *Oncomelania* breeding to achieve the ultimate aim of snail control and snail elimination.

Schistosomiasis control belongs to integrated strategy. Therefore, the strategy of sustainable development of comprehensive control for schistosomiasis must be carried out. This includes the conventional measures of disease surveying, disease treatment, snail surveying and the use of molluscicides, and water conservancy engineering, combined with local social and economic development. Thus, the diffusion of *Oncomelania* can be prevented and the epidemics of schistosomiasis controlled on a fundamental level, and the goal of schistosomiasis elimination can be achieved in the future.

References

1. WHO. The control of Schistosomiasis. Geneva: WHO.1985.22-76.

2. Hunter JM, Rey L, Scott D. Man-made lakes and man-made diseases. Soc Sci Med, 1982, 16: 1127.

3. Xu XJ, Wei FH, Yang XX, et al. Possible effort of the Three Gorges dam on the transmission of *Schistosomiasis japonicum* on the Jiang Han plain, China. Ann Trop Med Parasitol, 2000, 94: 333-341.

4. Xu XJ, Wei FH, Cai SX, et al. Study on the risk factors of schistosomiasis transmission and control strategy in the Three Gorges Reservoir Areas. Chin J Schisto Control, 2004, 25: 559-563. (in Chinese)

5. Wei FH, Wang RB, et al. Risk factors of schistosomiasis transmission after Three Gorges Construction I Possibility of snail breeding with ecological changes in Three Gorges Reservoir Reservoir areas. Chin J Schisto Control, 2007, 19: 81-85. (in Chinese)

6. The State Council of the People's Republic of China, 2006. The national regulations of schistosomiasis control. (in Chinese)

7. Liang XY, Wang JS, Wang NR, et al. Surveilance of schistosomiasis in the first phase project of flood and snail control at the downstream of Fushui River in Yangxin County, Hubei province. Chin J Schisto Control, 2010, 22: 490-492. (in Chinese)

8. Liu JB, Xu XJ, Wei FH, et al. Investigation of snails diffusion for the navigation lock and navigation channel of Sigu in Daye city. Chin J Schisto Control, 2001, 13: 124-125. (in Chinese)

9. Zhu H, Yuan Y, Xu XJ, et al. Risk assessment of the Water Transfer Project from the Yangtze River to Han River in middle scheme of the South-to -North Water Diversion Project on schistosomiasis transmission and intervention measures. Chin J Schisto Control, 2010, 22: 415-419. (in Chinese)

5.3   Countermeasures for controlling schistosomiasis in domestic animals in China

It is well known that *S. japonicum* is a parasitic zoonosis. Besides humans, more than 40 species of mammals, including water buffalo, yellow cattle, goat, sheep, pig and other domestic animals, as well as rats and other wild animals, have been reported as being infected with *S. japonicum*. Schistosomiasis infection causes various degrees of harm to domestic animals' health and considerable economic loss in the area of animal husbandry, and more seriously, the infected animals play an important role in the transmission of the disease. An epidemiological survey reveals that domestic animals, especially bovines, are important carriers in the transmission of schistosomiasis in areas in China where the parasite is most endemic. Therefore, effective intervention into domestic animals suffering from schistosome infection will greatly further the process of controlling the disease in China.

5.3.1 The epidemic status and impact of domestic animal schistosomiasis in China

The epidemic status of domestic animal schistosomiasis in China

Early reports on domestic animal schistosomiasis in China

Faust and Meleney first observed the eggs of *S. japonicum* in the feces of a water buffalo (*Bubalus bubalis*) in Fuzhou City, Fujian Province, in 1924, and Wu Guang first found schistosome worms from two slaughtered yellow cattle (*Bos indicus*) in Hangzhou, Zhejiang Province, in 1937. After that, several clinical reports regarding the infection of *S. japonicum* in yellow cattle, water buffalo, sheep, goats, dogs, and other domestic animals were presented successively. Thus, the role of domestic animals as carriers of *S. japonicum* has been attracting great attention from Chinese parasitologists.[1-3]

The epidemic status of domestic animal schistosomiasis in China in the 1950s

In the 1950s, large-scale epidemiological surveys were carried out to determine the rate of occurrence, incidence, and mortality of *S. japonicum* in bovines and other domestic animals by veterinarians and parasitologists. The results showed that the rate of occurrence was significant and serious in some areas of South China (Table 5.2). According to statistical data from 1958, there were around 1.5 million bovines suffering from schistosomiasis and five million at risk of schistosome infection.[4]

Table 5.2   Reports on the prevalence of domestic animal schistosomiasis in 1950s China.

Areas	Animals	No (+)/No. exam.	Positive rate (%)	Year
Jiangsu/Shanghai	Yellow cattle / water buffalo	2,567/11,034	23.27	1957
Jiangxi	Yellow cattle / water buffalo	3,850/12,096	31.83	1958
Fuqing County, Fujian Province	Yellow cattle	3,047/9,972	30.56	1958
Cheng County, Zhejiang Province	Water buffalo	243/1,641	14.81	1958
Shanghai	Sheep	101/667	15.14	1957
Chenglinji, Hunan Province	Goats	50/90	55.56	1958
Fengyi County, Yunnan Province	Pigs	50/214	23.36	1958
Qichun, Hubei Province	Pigs	67/100	67.00	1958
Yongxiu County, Jiangxi Province	Dogs	34/60	56.67	1958

The current status of schistosomiasis in domestic animals in China

Great achievement in the control of schistosomiasis in domestic animals has been made over the past six decades. By the end of 2012, among 12 endemic provinces (municipality, autonomous regions), the transmission of schistosomiasis had been interrupted in the Guangdong, Fujian and Zhejiang Provinces; Shanghai municipality; and the Guangxi Zhuang Autonomous Region, and no new cases of schistosome infections in local domestic animals have been reported over the past 20 years in these areas. The infection rates of bovine schistosomiasis in the Hunan, Hubei, Jiangxi, Anhui, Sichuan, Yunnan, and Jiangsu provinces were reduced to 1.23%, 0.25%, 1.67%, 0.55%, 0.01%, 0.11%, and 0%, respectively.[5]

The harmful effects of domestic animal schistosomiasis in China

Animals suffering from schistosomiasis usually have visible symptoms, such as high fever; in acute cases, intermittent diarrhea with blood and mucus in the stool, serious anemia; and emaciation in chronic cases. The infected animals develop slowly, and some of the infected calves become gnome cattle. There was report that 73 out of 137 calves were infected with schistosomiasis in Boyang and Yugan Counties, in Jiangxi Province, and that the average body weight detected in infected animals was less than half of uninfected ones. The farming capacity of the infected livestock was also reduced.[6] Abortion is often observed in pregnant animals; for example, 10 out of 14 pregnant cows were reported as having been given an abortion due to schistosome infection on Nanjiao farm, in Jiujiang County, Jiangxi Province. Milk production of infected dairy cows also declined.[6] The severity of the disease is influenced mainly by the degree and duration of the infection, as well as the susceptibility and immune system status of the hosts to the parasite infection. Moreover, there are several reports showing that a large number of domestic animals died due to schistosomiasis infection (Table 5.3).[3,7] All of the above mentioned factors reveal that the death of schistosome-infected animals, the production losses caused directly by *S. japonicum* infection, such as the reduction of growth, milk production, and farming capacity, as well as abortion and effects on reproduction, lead to a tremendous loss in the raising of livestock.

Table 5.3 Evidence on the death of domestic animals caused by *S. japonicum* infection.

Farms	Animals	No. (of animal breeding)	No. of animals that died	Year
Fuxing farm, Susong County, Anhui Province	Yellow cattle	1,292	416	1957
Donghu farm, Changba County, Jiangxi Province	Yellow cattle	47	42	1962
Chenglingji farm, Yeyang County, Hunan Province	Goat	140	More than 60	1957
Two farms in Hukou and Jiujiang, Jiangxi Province	Sheep	1,100	90%	1960

The susceptibility of different species of domestic animals to *S. japonicum* infection in China

More than 40 species of mammals belonging to 28 genera and seven orders have been found naturally infected with *S. japonicum* in China, but the susceptibility of different species of domestic animals to schistosomes is variable. Generally speaking, yellow cattle, sheep, goat, rabbit, and dogs are susceptible hosts, while water buffalo, pig, horse, and donkeys are less susceptible to the infection. Artificial infection tests showed that the developing rate of *S. japonicum* in yellow cattle is around 40 – 65%, but only 5 – 16% in water buffalo.[8] The infection rate in yellow cattle is usually higher than that in water buffalo in the same endemic areas, even though water buffalo are more frequently in contact with infested water than yellow cattle. Also, there is no obvious difference in susceptibility to *S. japonicum* infection among different age ranges in yellow cattle, but the infection rate in water buffalo aged below three years is obviously higher than in those aged more than three years. Water buffalo and pigs have the tendency of self-cure in one to two years post infection, and the duration of excreting eggs in the feces in water buffalo is shorter than in yellow cattle. In addition, the clinical symptoms caused by *S. japonicum* infection in yellow cattle are more severe than those in water buffalo.[9-11]

The role of domestic animals as carriers in the transmission of *S. japonicum*

Taking into consideration all of the main factors that may play an important role in the transmission of schistosomiasis, such as the number of the animals, the infection rate and daily egg output of the hosts, as well as the fecal egg hatching rate, and the chance for eggs to spread to and contaminate water sources and snail habitats, schistosome-infected domestic animals, especially bovines, are regarded as the most important carriers in the transmission of schistosomiasis in the most endemic areas in China.[7,10]

Firstly, there are a large number of bovines that graze freely in endemic areas due to the rich grass pastures in the marshland and lake regions. As the area of movement of the bovines is wide, they are frequently in contact with infested water and become easily infected, leading to high infection rates.[7-12] The investigation of Liu also showed that in some endemic areas, the number of goats and sheep has been increasing in recent years, and the infection rate of these two animals is higher. Thus, goats and sheep also play an important role in the transmission of schistosomiasis in some regions and should be closely monitored.[9] Also, it is quite difficult to treat those animals that are mobile in grazing areas. Secondly, bovines randomly spread the eggs into water sources with snail habitats through contaminated feces. An investigation of the feces of wild animals in these areas has revealed that in most endemic areas, more than 90% of collected schistosome egg-positive feces are from domestic animals, especially bovines. Bovines have a long life with larger amounts of fecal excretion and high daily egg output. The feces in the environment do not dry out easily; as a result, the eggs in the stool do not die easily.[7,10,11] Thirdly, epidemiological surveys have also revealed that there is a positive correlation between the infection rate of bovines and that of humans in the marshland and lake regions. Guo et al. compared human and water buffalo infection rates, as well as the degree of infection rates in a targeted village (Jishan), where both residents and water buffalo were treated with PZQ, and a control village (Hexi), where only residents were treated, in the Poyang Lake Region. Their results revealed that chemotherapy for water buffalo resulted in a decrease in buffalo infection rates in Jishan, which coincided with the reduction in human infection rates there in the last two years of the study. Mathematical modeling predicted that buffalo are responsible for 75% of human transmission in Jishan.[13] Gray et al. carried out a cluster-randomized intervention trial (2004 – 2007) undertaken in Hunan and Jiangxi provinces. Their results supported the previous experimental evidence by Guo, and the authors confirmed that bovines were the major reservoir hosts of human schistosomiasis in the lake and marshland regions of southern China.[14]

5.3.2 Countermeasures for the control of schistosomiasis in domestic animals in China

The comprehensive measures for controlling schistosomiasis in domestic animals were generally formulated and adopted based on the differences in epidemiological factors and characteristics in different endemic areas and different seasons.

The processes for controlling schistosomiasis in domestic animals in China

A national programme for controlling schistosomiasis in domestic animals in China has been underway since the 1950s, and has included three main phases.

Phase one was between the 1950s and early 1980s, and was based on large-scale baseline epidemiological surveys of human and domestic animal schistosomiasis. Comprehensive approaches including agricultural and water conservancy projects with emphasis on snail elimination were carried out, and were complemented with screening and giving chemotherapy to schistosome-infected animals, as well as the use of animal waste management. The drugs used in the treatment of domestic animals in this period include potassium antimony tartrate, sodium antimony gallate, hexachloroparaxylol, metrifonate, and nithiocyamine. The selection of this control strategy was in line with the historical context and scientific limitations that exist at the time when there were no effective, safe, low cost anti-schistosomiasis drugs available, and no other better control measures could be applied. The implementation of this control strategy during that period was successful: large snail habitats became snail free areas, the number of endemic areas shrank, the number of infected bovines and other domestic animals as well as people reduced significantly, and the transmission of schistosomiasis had been interrupted in some plain regions with waterway network areas and in hilly regions.

Phase two was from middle 1980s to early 21th century. With the development of a new anti-schistosomiasis drug, PZQ, which possesses the benefits of high efficacy, low toxicity, acceptable cost and being easily administered; the establishment and application of several sensitive serological diagnostic techniques, such as indirect hemagglutination assay (IHA), circumoval precipitin test (COPT), enzyme-linked immunosorbent assay (ELISA), etc.; and the initiation of the World Bank Loan Project (WBLP) on Schistosomiasis Control in China, schistosomiasis control strategies applied in this period mainly involved chemotherapy supplemented with snail elimination in areas with high transmission potential. During this time, large-scale screening and chemotherapy of schistosome-infected bovines, sheep, goats, and pigs were carried out in each of the endemic provinces. PZQ was provided for free to those domestic animals who grazed on the grassland with snails, and bovines were treated at the same time as people infected with schistosomiasis in some endemic areas. Results showed that the rate of occurrence and degree of the infections were significantly decreased; for example, 47.08% reduction of the number of schistosome-infected bovines was obtained by 2001. However, the strategy cannot prevent re-infection of domestic animals in order to consolidate the achievements of control efforts.

During this period, beginning from 1991 to 1994, the Agriculture Ministry of China carried out a pilot project in Qianjiang, Xiantao, Jianli, Honghu, and Jiangling Counties (Cities) in Hubei Province. The objectives were exploring the comprehensive control measures for control of the transmission source among schistosome-infected domestic animals, in combination with local agricultural activities. To this end, a series of effective measures were put forward. These included: replacing bovine plowing with tractor plowing; replacing schistosome-sensitive ruminants (bovine, sheep, goat, and other similar animals) with non-susceptible poultry (duck, goose, and other similar fowl); the construction of biogas pools and septic-tanks or stacking fermentation for the treatment of feces from domestic animals; building up feeding pens or safe pastures; as well as advocating for safe grazing for domestic animals. All of these measures have been confirmed to be effective against protecting animals from coming into contact with infested water and becoming infected. Also, they significantly reduce the contamination of *S. japonicum* eggs from domestic animal waste to the environment. Since then, these measures have been widely applied in different endemic areas in China.[7,15]

Phase three was from 2004 to the present. In 2004, the State Council of China came up with a comprehensive control strategy for schistosomiasis, mainly focusing on transmission control. The strategies for domestic animal schistosomiasis control in this period emphasized the comprehensive control of schistosomiasis in heavily affected villages. It focused on the replacement of bovine plowing with tractor plowing, the construction of biogas pools for fermenting the feces of animals, and the control of domestic animal transmission sources. The implementation of this strategy resulted in the further decrease of the schistosomiasis infection rate and the degree of infection in domestic animals.[5,7,15]

After continued efforts over the past six decades, schistosomiasis has been successfully eliminated in the Guangdong, Fujian, and Zhejiang provinces; Shanghai municipality; and Guangxi Zhuang Autonomous Region. The remaining seven endemic provinces have all reached the criteria of transmission control, that is, both the schistosomiasis infection rate in bovines and residents being reduced to less than 1% by the end of 2015.

Diagnosis of domestic animal schistosomiasis

Diagnosis is always a central issue in disease control. Since the 1950s when the national campaign against schistosomiasis began in China, the application and development of diagnostic techniques for domestic animals have been highlighted in the national programmes of schistosomiasis control. During the 1950s to the early 1970s, etiologic diagnosis was the main technique used in the identification of individuals for chemotherapy because of the high toxicity of the available effective drugs for treatment. Since the wide application of a safe and effective anti-schistosomiasis drug, PZQ, in the late 1970s, the serological technique has been widely applied in screening targeted individuals for treatment. Generally, for the diagnosis of domestic animal schistosomiasis, a preliminary diagnostic assessment could be made according to the clinical symptom and the epidemiological survey data of the animals. However, a definitive diagnosis can only result from etiological examination, and a serologic diagnosis is usually applied as a technique that assists in identifying the target individuals for treatment.

Etiological diagnosis

Etiological diagnosis consists of stool examination and biopsies of animal tissues. The techniques applied mainly include fecal egg examination, miracidia hatching, biopsies of rectal mucosa, as well as an anatomical diagnosis. Because the fecal quantity excreted from bovines and other domestic animals is larger, and the egg density is rarer, the efficacy of detecting is lower when direct examination of fecal eggs is applied. Thus, the miracidia hatching test is a major technique used under field conditions. The procedures included in the miracidia hatching test are: i) moving large particles of debris and undigested fibers through a 40 mesh copper sieve used for detecting fecal samples (50 – 100 g for bovines, 20 – 30 g for pigs, 5 – 10 g for sheep, goats, and dogs); ii) precipitated dung slag rinses and sediments for several times in a conical flask or washes in a 260 mesh nylon tissue bag to remove the tiny dung slag and concentrate fecal eggs; iii) miracidia hatching is taken under 20–30°C, and miracidia is usually observed in 1, 3, and 5 hr post-hatching periods for bovines, sheep, and goats, and in 5 - 8 hr post-hatching periods for pigs, respectively.[16] The number of miracidia in each testing sample can serve as a point of reference for estimating the degree of infection of the animals. Three consecutive hatching tests for one sample are generally carried out. The current recommended protocol of miracidia hatching test is been listed in the National Criteria for Diagnosis of Domestic Animal Schistosomiasis formulated in 2002 (GB/T 18640–2002).[7] Although a definitive diagnosis is only dependent on etiological diagnosis, insufficient of direct parasitological techniques is low sensitivity, especially when the prevalence and degree of the infection in most endemic areas are decreasing, and is labor-intensive and time-consuming.

Serological diagnosis

Serologic diagnosis is based on the detection of schistosome-specific circulating antibodies and antigens, or their immune complex. The investigation and application of serologic diagnosis techniques for domestic animal schistosomiasis have had a history of more than five decades, and have undergone a great deal of development with the advances of biotechnology and immunology. Also, several antibody detecting techniques for domestic animal schistosomiasis, including COPT, IHA, ELISA and Strip test, among others, as well as a circulating antigens-detecting technique, McAB-Dot-ELISA, have been developed. Some of them, such as IHA and the Strip test have been widely applied in endemic areas for the screening of chemotherapy individuals.

The protocol for IHA has been listed in the National Criteria for Diagnosis of Domestic Animal Schistosomiasis formulated in 2002 (GB/T 18640–2002).[7] Besides COPT, which uses intact *S. japonicum* eggs as a detecting antigen, the others all apply the schistosome eggs or adult worm soluble extracts as detecting reagents. The application of serologic diagnosis techniques significantly increases the sensitivity of the detection. However, the problem is that cross-reacting results are often encountered in most of the assays, which may be caused by the use of crude antigens that contain a lot of antigens potentially being shared with other species of parasites, such as *Fasciola hepatica*. In addition, the currently available serological assays cannot distinguish active infection from previous infection or reinfection. This results in difficulties in determining the rate of occurrence, identifying infected individuals for selective chemotherapy, and assessing the effectiveness of the chemotherapy and other forms of intervention.

Efforts made for the identification of single defined native or recombinant molecules with potential diagnostic values via immune-proteomics and other large-scale screening techniques have been carried out by parasitologists. Thus, several molecules with higher sensitivity and specificity for bovine, sheep, and goat schistosomiasis diagnosis have been identified, such as LHD-Sj23 (a large hydrophilic domain of 23 kDa membrane protein of *S. japonicum*), SjPGM, etc.[17] For further enhancing the sensitivity of the diagnosis methods that are based on the defined diagnostic antigen studies, several multi-epitope recombinants have been constructed and their potential as diagnosis antigens for domestic animal schistosomiasis have been evaluated. Some of them, such as pGEX-Sj23-SjGCP, have been found with higher sensitivity and specificity over the single molecule of recombinant Sj23 or SjGCP.[18] In general, although the serological diagnosis technique has been included in the schistosomiasis control programme in China, no one of them has been an alternative to parasitological diagnosis until now.

Chemotherapy of domestic animal schistosomiasis

Chemotherapy is generally regarded to be the most important, rapid and cost-effective method to reduce morbidity resulting from schistosome infection. The drugs that have been used for the treatment of domestic animal schistosomiasis include antimony potassium tartrate, metrifonate, hexachloroparaxylol, amoscanate and PZQ. They have all played an important role during different schistosomiasis control periods.

The treatment of schistosome-infected domestic animals not only cures and reduces morbidity among the animals, but more importantly, it has significant effects on the transmission of the disease by preventing further depositing of schistosome eggs into the environment. Currently, PZQ in powder form is the drug that is being widely used. It possesses the benefits of high effectiveness and mild side effects; it generally requires a single-dose administration, has a short treatment term, and can be purchased at a comparatively low cost. Unlike PZQ, the other drugs are no longer in use because they are less effective and/or more toxic. The oral dose of PZQ is 30 mg per kilogram of body weight, with the highest limited weight of 300 kg for yellow cattle, 25 mg per kilogram of body weight with the highest weight limit of 400 kg for water buffalo, 20 mg per kilogram of body weight for goats, and 60 mg per kilogram of body weight for pigs, respectively. However, although praziquantel is safely used in humans, side effects and even death rarely occurred in yellow cattle or dairy cow after praziquantel treatment.[16,19]

One of the drawbacks for the treatment of schistosome with PZQ is that schistosomula have low susceptibility to the drug compared with that of the adult worms. Moreover, parasitologists have found that artesunate and AM are highly effective in the killing of schistosomula, and that both possess an early preventive effect in yellow cattle and water buffalo. However, the cost of these two drugs is high, and also, large-scale application in endemic areas is limited.

Housing of domestic animals

Stable breeding of livestock is strongly recommended and widely performed in the endemic areas by the support of the government. When the livestock, including bovines, goats, sheep, and pigs are housed and fed in a pen, there will be no chance for these animals to contact water containing cercariae and become infected. Thus, the chance of contamination of the feces from schistosome-infected animals to the marshland with snail habitats will reduce.[19] An integrated control strategy aimed at blocking the transmission of *S. japonicum*, mainly through rearing cows in stalls, was implemented in Eryuan County, Yunan Province in 2002. This resulted in the reduction of the rate of *S. japonicum* infection in humans and cows from 9.18% and 6.02% in 2002 to 0.09% and 0.29% in 2005, respectively.

Establishment of safe pastures and safe grazing for livestock

Safe grazing of livestock is encouraged. The selected safe pastures are usually established in grasslands uninhabited by *Oncomelania* snails, in which snails have been eliminated through molluscicides or deep plowing, and they are segregated from those snail habitats by digging isolated ditches or installing fences. All animals must be treated with PZQ 2 – 3 weeks before grazing in the established safe pastures. Monitoring of snail and schistosome-infected animals should be carried out 3 – 4 times per year.[19] It was reported that the prevalence of cattle schistosomiasis was reduced from 26.1% to 2.0%, and both the infected snails and the contamination of cattle dung were efficiently controlled after the establishment and application of safe pastures in He County, Anhui Province.

Banning livestock grazing on marshlands or hillside grasslands with snail habitats

Livestock are not allowed to graze on marshlands or hill grasslands with *Oncomelania* snail populations. Usually livestock are prohibited from grazing from 1 March to 31 October, the season when the livestock become infected easily. In the lake and marshland regions populated with snails, this is found to be effective in protecting animals from schistosome infection, and significantly reduces the contamination of feces from infected animals to the environment.[19,20] In mountainous endemic areas in the Sichuan and Yunnan provinces, every year there is usually a rainy season and a dry season, and the domestic animals are mainly infected during the rainy season. Therefore, restricting the grazing time on hillside land with snail populations is usually carried out during the entirety of the rainy season. Wang *et al.* reported that forbidding grazing from 1 March to 31 October for a total of 2 – 3 years reduced the schistosome infection rates in residents, domestic animals, and snails to 0% in two out of four heavy epidemic towns in the Poyang Lake Region, Jiangxi province.[20]

Quarantine and monitoring of domestic animals from schistosomiasis-endemic areas

With economic development, the circulating of domestic animals among different areas is becoming more and more frequent, and this increases the spreading of schistosomiasis. Thus, the quarantining of domestic animals from schistosomiasis-endemic areas is important and needs to be carried out. Serological techniques such as IHA and the Strip test are usually used for quarantining. Schistosomiasis-positive animals are prohibited for import or export to other endemic areas, and must be eliminated or treated with PZQ immediately.

Development of a schistosomiasis vaccine for domestic animals

Although chemotherapy with PZQ has been performed widely in China, it is still difficult to block the transmission of the disease due to the high rates of reinfection that frequently occur following the chemotherapy of humans and domestic animals. Therefore, the development of an effective vaccine against schistosomiasis is an obviously desirable objective for the control programme.[21] The studies on the development of anti-schistosomiasis vaccines have also received support by the national high technique project and other research programmes in China.

The development studies on the schistosomiasis vaccine undergo a process of examination of different kinds of vaccines including crude whole worm antigens, live attenuated cercaria or schistosomula, and gene engineering vaccines. The efficacy of several kinds of vaccines in protecting bovines, sheep, and pigs from schistosome infection has been evaluated. Partial results of these evaluations are shown in Table 5.4.

In general, although the vaccination of live, attenuated cercaria or schistosomula elicits the highest protection among all the tested vaccines, it is not considered as a practical means of vaccinating humans or domestic animals in the field because of safety and the large number of parasites. Also, purified single molecule worm antigens could induce partial protection against schistosome infection in bovine and sheep, but it is difficult to collect enough worms to prepare the antigens for the vaccination and apply it in the field. There are dozens of *S. japonicum* genes that have been cloned and identified in China, including *S. jGST, S. j Paramyosin, S. j23kD,*

Table 5.4 Evaluation of the protective efficacy against *S. japonicum* infection induced by different kinds of vaccines in domestic animals.

Vaccines/adjuvants	Animals	Protective efficacy (%)		Reporters (reference no.)
		Worm reduction	Egg reduction	
Frozen-thawed schisto-somula/BCG	Sheep	40.36 – 37.26	39.29 – 42.90	Xu *et al.*, (24)
Irradiated attenuated schistosomula	Bovines	65.1 – 75.7	54.9 – 80.9	Hsu and Xu *et al.*, (22)
Native worm GST/FCA	Sheep	24.73 – 35.93	49.29 – 47.9	Xu *et al.*, (24)
Recombinant LHD – Sj23/FCA/FIA	Sheep	66.1	66.4	Xu *et al.*, (23)
Recombinant Sj28GST/ FCA/FIA	bovines	33.5	69.0	Taylor *et al.*, (27)
Recombinant Sj28GST+LHD – Sj23+ SjGCP/206	Water buffalo	55.32 – 73.84	45.62 – 84.34	SVRI, CAAS (unpublished)
Sj23 DNA vaccine/IL-12	Pigs	58.6		Zhu *et al.*,(28)

S. jTPI, S. jFABP, and *S. jIrV-5*, which were recommended as promising vaccine candidates for *S. mansoni* by WHO/TDR. Most of these genes have been expressed in *E. coli,* and some have sub-cloned into eukaryotic expression plasmids to construct DNA vaccines. Sj28GST,[27] Sj23,[23,28] SjGCP, SjParamyosin, and several other *S. japonicum* recombinant proteins or DNA vaccines have been shown to be able to induce partial protection against schistosome infection in domestic animals.

Schistosome-infected domestic animals are the main transmission sources of the disease in China. If an effective vaccine for domestic animal schistosomiasis becomes available, it will greatly promote the control programme by effectively reducing the transmission source to the surrounding environment. Among different developed schistosomiasis vaccines, several have shown promise in protecting hosts from schistosome infection, or significantly reducing the pathological damage caused by the schistosome infection. However, until now, none of the developed vaccines have been available in the control programme.

Other methods for controlling domestic animal schistosomiasis

Several other methods have also been found to be effective in the controlling of domestic animal schistosomiasis or the transmission source from schistosome-infected animals. These included: the replacement of bovine plowing with tractor plowing, replacement of ruminants with poultry, using tap water or well water as drinking water for domestic animals, strengthening the management of animal waste of domestic animals, snail elimination, and health education for the farmers in schistosomiasis transmission areas (section 5.4).

5.3.3   The main experiences for domestic animal schistosomiasis control in China

Both the Chinese central government and local governments in endemic areas place great emphasis on domestic animal schistosomiasis control. The action plan of schistosomiasis control was listed in the outline of the National Programme for Agricultural Development in 1956. Bovine schistosomiasis control is included in the national schistosomiasis control programme. Synchronous chemotherapy of both schistosome-infected bovines and residents is required and carried out in China.[5,7,15]

"Put prevention first" and "active control with comprehensive approaches" is the basic policy for the domestic animal schistosomiasis control. Besides active chemotherapy of the infected animals, several effective integrated prevention approaches are encouraged and widely applied for domestic animal schistosomiasis control in the endemic areas based on local rates of infection and the local socio-economic situation in China. These are: safe grazing of the livestock, using tractor plowing instead of bovine plowing, strengthening the management of animal waste, and snail elimination. Synchronous chemotherapy of both humans and livestock is emphasized so as to control possible infection sources. The schistosomiasis control programme in combination with economic development and basic construction of agriculture and water conservancy projects is promoted to change the environment of snail habitats and minimize the problem in endemic areas.[7,15]

Strengthening the scientific studies for the prevention and control of schistosomiasis. Scientific prevention and control measures or strategies are formulated and carried out in different endemic areas and adapted to the local conditions. The rates of infection in different endemic areas and different seasons vary, and the composition of the main reservoirs in various endemic areas is also different. As a result, several national or provincial domestic animal schistosomiasis monitoring points have been set, and the main reservoir hosts and main transmission seasons in each investigated point are determined based on epidemiological survey results. Finally, the specific comprehensive control approaches targeting each type of endemic area are formulated and carried out. In addition, the effect of each intervention measure is evaluated, and the experiences are then summarized and promoted in other similar types of endemic areas. In turn, the comprehensive application of effective intervention measures greatly facilitates progress in controlling schistosomiasis in China. At the same time, researchers in China do their best to screen effective drugs for chemotherapy and to establish a series of diagnosis techniques for domestic animal schistosomiasis. The application of these products and techniques greatly promotes the control process of the disease in various control periods.[7,15]

5.3.4 New challenges for the control of domestic animal schistosomiasis in China

Great efforts have been made and remarkable success in schistosomiasis control has been achieved over the past six decades, with the schistosomiasis infection rate of bovine, sheep, and other domestic animals being reduced to the lowest level in history by the end of 2015. However, to realize the target of finally eliminating the disease in China is still an arduous task.

An environment with the potential risk for transmission of schistosomiasis still exists in some regions with *Oncomelania* snail habitats in most of the lake and marshland regions. This becomes an important bottleneck in the achievement of significant progress; therefore, the opportunity for the reappearance of a schistosomiasis outbreak may occur in some of these areas.

Lower prevalence of schistosomiasis will last for a longer term in large-scale areas in China. Therefore, transmission surveillance in different types of endemic regions, including transmission interrupted areas or endemic areas, still needs to be strengthened, and rigorous monitoring should be carried out to consolidate the achievements gained.

At present, only residents and bovines are included in the national control programme. For reaching the target of disease elimination, the role of some other important reservoir hosts, such as sheep, dogs, wide animals, in the transmission of schistosomiasis should be determined. That is to say, all of the main reservoir hosts in an area should be involved in the local control programme, and effective control measures should be set and carried out.

Some key techniques for the elimination of schistosomiasis have still not been worked out and need to be developed further. With the gradual decrease in the infection rate and the degree of infection in residents and animal reservoirs, the development of a more sensitive, specific, simple, and quick diagnostic technique, or a technique that could distinguish between active and previous infection of domestic animal schistosomiasis, is urgently needed. If a safe, highly effective schistosomiasis vaccine becomes available for domestic animals in endemic areas, it will greatly advance the disease elimination process. Therefore, the screening of more protective vaccine candidates needs to be stronger.

References

1. Logen OT. A case of dysentery in Hunan province, caused by the trematoda, *Shistosoma japonicum*. Chin Med Mission J, 1905, 19: 243-245.

2. Wang LD. Control Process of Schistosomiasis in China and Expectation. Bejing: People's Health Press, 2006. pp8-15. (in Chinese)

3. Wang XY. Domestic animal schistosomiasis. Shanghai: Shanghai Science and Technology Press, 1959. pp1-4, 36-47. (in Chinese)

4. Shen W. Review and suggestion for domestic animal schistosomiasis control. Chin J Schisto Contr, 1992, 4: 82-84. (in Chinese)

5. Li H, Liu JM, Song JX, et al. Domestic animal schistosomiasis in 2012 in China. Chin J Animal Infect Dis, 2014, 22: 68-71. (in Chinese)

6. Schistosomiasis Control Office, Ministry of Agriculture, P. R. China. Handbook of Animal Schistosomiasis Control. Beijing: Chinese Agricultural Press on Sciences and Technology, 1998. pp39-40. (in Chinese)

7. Li CY, Lin JJ. Fifty Years Process on Agricultural Comprehensive Measures for the Schistosomiasis Control in China. Beijing: Chinese Agricultural Press on Sciences and Technology, 2008. pp14-15, 37-42, 78, 111-114. (in Chinese)

8. He YX, Salafsky B, Ramaswamy K. Host-parasite relationships of *Schistosoma japonicum* in

mammalian hosts. Trend Parasitol, 2001, 17: 320-324.

9. Liu J, Zhu C, Shi Y et al. Surveillance of *Schistosoma japonicum* infection in domestic ruminants in the Dongting Lake region, Hunan Province, China. PLoS One. 2012, 7: e31876.

10. Chen MG, Zhou XN, Hirayama K. Schistosomiasis in Asia. Chiba: FAP Journals. 2005. pp39-46,151-162.

11. Wang TP, Vang Johansen M, Zhang SQ, et al. Transmission of *Schistosoma japonicum* by humans and domestic animals in the Yangtze River Valley, Anhui Province, China. Acta Trop, 2005, 96: 198-204.

12. Li YS, McManus DP2, Lin DD, et al. The *Schistosoma japonicum* self-cure phenomenon in water buffalo: potential impact on the control and elimination of schistosomiasis in China. Int J Parasitol, 2014, 44: 167-71.

13. Guo JG, Li Y, Gray D, et al. A drug-based intervention study on the importance of buffaloes for human *Schistosoma japonicum* infection around Poyang Lake, People's Republic of China. Am J Trop Med Hyg, 2006, 74: 335-41.

14. Gray DJ, Williams GM, Li Y, et al. Transmission dynamics of *Schistosoma japonicum* in the lakes and marshlands of China. PLoS One, 2008, 3: e4058.

15. Xu BW. Agricultural Comprehensive Measures for the Schistosomiasis Control in China, Beijing: Chinese Agricultural Press on Sciences and Technology, 2004. pp 8-21. (in Chinese)

16. Schistosomiasis Control Office of Agricultural Department, China. Handbook for Animal Schistosomiasis Control. Beijing: Chinese Agricultural Press on Sciences and Technology, 1998. pp38-45, 59-76, 78-98, 111-118, 136-145. (in Chinese)

17. Zhang M, Fu Z, Li C, et al. Screening diagnostic candidates for schistosomiasis from tegument proteins of adult *Schistosoma japonicum* using an immunoproteomic approach. PLoS Negl Trop Dis, 2015, 9: e0003454.

18. Jin YM, Lu K, Zhou WF, et al. Comparison of recombinant proteins from *Schistosoma japonicum* for schistosomiasis diagnosis. Clin Vaccine Immunol, 2010, 17: 476-80.

19. Xu BW, Lin JJ. Technical Guidelines of Agricultural Comprehensive Measures for Schistosomiasis Control in China. Beijing: Chinese Agricultural Press on Sciences and Technology, 2007. pp22-37, 51-55, 56-57, 69-73. (in Chinese)

20. Wang XH, Liu W, Yang YB, et al. Field observation on the effect of control and prevention for schistosomiasis by marshland isolation and farming prohibition in Lake District. Chin J Zoonoses, 2010, 26: 609-610. (in Chinese)

21. Bergquist NR. Schistosomiasis vaccine development: Progress and prospects. Mem Inst Oswaldo Cruz, Rio de Janeiro,1998, 93: 95-101.

22. Hsu SY, Xu ST, He YX, et al. Vaccination of bovines against *Schistosoma japonicum* with highly irradiated schistosomula in China. Am J Trop Med Hyg, 1984, 33: 891-8.

23. Xu ST, Shi FH, Shen W, et al. Vaccination of bovines against schistosomiasis japonicum with crypreserved~irradiated and freeze/thaw schistomula. Vet Parasitol, 1993, 47: 37-50.

24. Xu S, Shi F, Shen W, et al. Vaccination of sheep against schistosomiasis japonicum with either glutathione-S-transferase, key hole limpet haemocyanin or the freeze/thaw schistosomula/BCG vaccine. Vet Parasitol, 1995, 58(4): 301-12.

25. Shi F, Zhang Y, Lin J, et al. Field testing of *Schistosoma japonicum* DNA vaccines in cattle in China. Vaccine, 2002, 20: 3629-31.

26. Shi F, Zhang Y, Ye P, et al. Laboratory and field evaluation of *Schistosoma japonicum* DNA vaccines in sheep and water buffalo in China. Vaccine, 2001, 20: 462-7.

27. Taylor MG, Huggins MC, Shi F, et al. Production and testing of *Schistosoma japonicum* candidate antigens in the natural bovine host. Vaccine, 1998, 16(13): 1290-8.

28. Zhu YC, Ren JR, Harn DA, et al. Protective effects of 23kDa membrane protein DNA vaccine of *Schistosoma japonicum* Chinese strain in infected pigs. Chin J Schisto Contr, 2002, 14: 3-7. (in Chinese)

5.4 Comprehensive agricultural measures for schistosomiasis control in China

In China, *Schistosoma japonicum* is mainly endemic in rural areas, and peasants are the main victims of the disease. The transmission of *S. japonicum* is closely related to peasants' working and living conditions. In 1992, based on experiences from the 1950s through to the 1980s, the Chinese Ministry of Agriculture proposed an applied research project in comprehensive agricultural schistosomiasis control. The central objective was to reach an organic combination of controlling schistosomiasis and developing the rural economy through the comprehensive agricultural exploitation of *Oncomelania hupensis* snail habitats, adjustments to the structure of the agricultural industry, and management of sources of infection. From 1991 to 1994, the Chinese Ministry of Agriculture carried out a pilot project in comprehensive agricultural schistosomiasis control in five counties of Hubei Province including Qianjiang, Xiantao, Jianli, Honghu, and Jiangling. The pilot project was successful in snail control, reducing the infection rate in humans and domestic animals and developing the rural economy. Since then, comprehensive agricultural measures for schistosomiasis control have been widely used in China.

5.4.1 Agricultural measures for reducing the number of grazing ruminants

Domestic animals, especially cattle and buffaloes, play an important role in the transmission of schistosomiasis in China. It has been reported that bovine species contribute 80% or more to local transmission in certain areas.[1-3] The objective of reducing the number of ruminants is to control the source of infection from livestock.

Replacing bovine plowing with tractor plowing

The mechanization of agriculture in the endemic regions of schistosomiasis could reduce the local number of bovines and therefore water-contacting opportunities between farm workers and bovines.

Replacing bovine plowing with tractor plowing for schistosomiasis control is an enormous social project. This includes: the determination of application areas, purchasing farm equipment, technical training in the operation and maintenance of machines, creating a supporting financial policy, constructing tractor roads, eliminating farming bovines, etc. Thus, this work must be conducted with unified leadership at all levels of government, with the relevant departments coordinating implementation. For example, agricultural schistosomiasis control sectors are responsible for making plans; the agricultural machinery department is responsible for purchasing and technical training; and the local authorities at the township and village levels are responsible for coordinating the relationships with farmers.

Governments could organize specialized teams or households to serve the farmer. In recent years, mass organizations to replace bovine plowing with tractor plowing have been set up in many endemic counties or townships. These offer services within five areas, namely: unifying the organization of machine-cultivation; deploying machines; offering technical training; offering maintenance; and setting standard charges. These services have greatly promoted agricultural mechanization and the control of bovine sources of infection.

In Laozhou Township, Tongling County, Anhui Province, there were 3,040,650 m^2 of snail distribution areas. In 2006, the infection rates of *S. japonicum* in snails, humans, bovines, and goats were 2.6%, 5.72%, 41.1%, and 50% respectively. In 2007, an integrated control strategy based on the replacement of bovine plowing with tractor plowing was carried out. A total of 917 bovines and 510 goats were eliminated. The infection rates of *S. japonicum* in snails and humans were reduced to 0.03% and 0.05% by the end of 2008.

Replacing ruminants with poultry

Poultry animals are oviparous and cannot be infected with *S. japonicum*. Poultry animals also eat snails and aquatic plants, thereby reducing the number of environmental snails and changing snail habitats.

With the help of programmes on schistosomiasis control, the local County Center for Animal Disease Control and Prevention closely collaborate with other administrative departments of animal husbandry to provide financial and technical assistance for the construction of poultry farms, poultry animal introduction, and poultry disease control. For instance, in Baisha Town, Yuanjiang City, Hunan Province, the total number of buffaloes and *S. japonicum* infection rate in buffaloes were significantly reduced by 65.42% and 60.46%, respectively between 1998 and 2001 through programmes to replace ruminants with poultry.

Prohibiting livestock grazing on marshlands or hillsides with *Oncomelania* snails

Schistosomiasis is a typical endemic disease. Even in epidemic areas, animals can only be infected when grazing in areas where oncomelanid snails are present. Infected animals are the infection source. Hence, forbidding grazing on marshlands or hillsides with oncomelanid snails is a highly effective method of schistosomiasis control.

In most lake and marshland regions, grazing should be prohibited from 1 March to 31 October each year. In years with dry weather, if the water level is beneath the grassland, the grazing ban could formally end on 15 October. If there are higher temperatures and more rain during fall, the end date will be postponed to 30 November. If there is rich forage for housed animals, marshlands with *O. hupensisi* should be closed to grazing for the whole year.

In mountainous endemic regions in Sichuan and Yunnan provinces, there is usually a rainy season and a dry season every year. Domestic animals are mainly infected during the rainy season. The duration of the grazing prohibition on hillsides with *O. hupensis* should be determined according to climatological data and usually last for the entire rainy season.

The following measures could be implemented for this project. Firstly, the local township (or county) authorities would release an announcement and place warning signs along the forbidden areas. The locations, scope, and durations of grazing bans, and/or telephone numbers for reporting and supervision should be displayed on these warning signs. Secondly, in regions with better economic conditions, fences or isolating canals would be used to prevent animals from grazing. The fences should be installed with concrete piles and barbed wire, and must be over 1 m tall. Both the width and depth of isolating canals should be over 2 m. Thirdly, a management commission for forbidding grazing would be established and professional management staff employed to ensure that no grazing occurs.

Wang et al.[4] report that grazing bans enforced between 1 March and 31 October reduced the schistosoma infection rates in residents, domestic animals and snails to 0% in two of four heavy epidemic towns in Poyang Lake region, Jiangxi Province, in a total of 2 – 3 years. Liu et al.[5] report that after fencing the marshland in a village of Yuanjiang City in Dongting Lake region (Hunan Province) for 2 – 5 years, the infection rates of residents, cattle, and snails dropped by 88.89%, 100%, and 100% respectively. The number of cattle decreased by 73.60% and the ecological economic benefits in the marshland increased by 15 – 20%.

5.4.2   Feces management

Based on the life cycle of *S. japonicum*, the keys to the prevalence and transmission of this disease are: eggs entering into water inside feces; the presence of snails in the water; and humans and animals making contact with infectious water containing cercaria. Only *S. japonicum* eggs that are dropped into fresh water in the feces of domestic animals are involved in the transmission of the disease. The aims of this measure are to prevent the entrance of eggs into fresh water and to kill the parasite's eggs through fermentation.

Constructing biogas pools

The feces of domestic animals are widely used to produce biogas throughout the country. The practice is supported as a new energy technique by the Ministry of Agriculture of China. This technique is important for improving the environment, saving energy materials, and preventing zoonotic infectious disease.

The mechanisms by which biogas pools prevent zoonotic parasitic disease are as follows: i) Biogas pools are airtight with an aerobic environment. They contain a large amount of organic acids, ammonium ions and proteases, which are produced during the metabolic fermentation process of feces and can kill the parasite eggs. ii) A biogas pool is also a sedimentation tank in which the eggs of parasites will be deposited and stored for at least half a year.

The design, construction, quality assurance, and use of rural household biogas pools should be carried out with reference to the national technical standards (GB/T4750–2002; GB/T4751–2002; GB/T4752–2002; GB76360–1987; GB7637–1987; GB9958–1988).

Construction of septic tanks for the treatment of animal feces

Rural household septic tanks for animal feces usually have three chambers (or cesspools). If the number of domestic animals is limited, the rural household septic tank could be co-constructed with household lavatories. The parasite eggs will be killed by the organic acids and other chemical materials such as sulfuretted hydrogen, which are produced during the metabolic fermentation process of feces.

Stacking fermentation of the feces

Common practice is to dig a small pool near the animal house and pour the collected feces of domestic animals into this pool. Once it has achieved a certain amount, the feces will be covered with mud or a plastic membrane. After five to 10 days of fermentation, according to the different ambient temperatures (generally five days in summer, seven days in spring and fall, and ten days in winter), the parasite eggs are killed.

5.4.3　Comprehensive agricultural measures for snail control

O. hupensis, the only intermediate host of *S. japonicum*, are amphibious animals. Hatching from snail egg and the development of young snails both occur in water. Mature snails live in wetlands or watery areas. The most favorable environments for snail habitats are humid, with fertile soil and weeds growing. Dry land is not suitable for snail survival and the snails will die when they are submerged in water for around eight months. Therefore, several measures combined with agricultural production can be used to modify the habitat environment and kill the snails. The practice in China shows that these comprehensive agricultural measures could have a significant effect on snail control, increase farmers' incomes and preserve the ecological environment by reducing the polluting effect of chemical molluscicides.

Before carrying out agricultural snail control, local agricultural authorities should have an overall plan and select suitable agricultural measures according to the local natural conditions, snail survey data from health institutes, local development plans for the agricultural economy, and previous successful experiences. The principle of snail control in China includes dividing snail habitats according to the water system, from upper stream to lower stream; proximity to the village; and from simple to complicated environments. During the implementation of agricultural snail control measures, careful attention should be paid to technical requirements and quality control. After implementation, the effectiveness of snail control must be evaluated in detail.

Changing rice paddies to dry fields

Snails will gradually die when rice paddies are changed to dry fields, due to the dramatic change in environment. Changing or rotating rice paddies into dry fields is a suitable measure for snail control in all endemic areas.

The basic methods of changing rice paddies into dry fields include digging a deep ditch to lower the water levels, and raising the fields to keep it out of the water. This measure can be carried out in rice fields located on higher ground, where oncomelanid snails have been present, and there are no influence factors such as clay for planting the dryland crop. After several years, the dry land could be rotated back to rice fields if the snails have been eliminated.

Beyond snail control, there are two benefits of this measure. Firstly, the opportunity for *S. japonicum* to infect farm workers and bovines is reduced because cultivation and planting are done without water. Secondly, this measure could reduce the number of working bovines because the newly dry fields are used to plant fruits.

This measure is involved in the adjustment of planting structures and diversifies the structure of agricultural production. After changing to dry fields, the farmers have the choice of several planting patterns, such as greenhouse vegetables, fruits, medicinal herbs, cotton, and other cash crops. This will increase the income of the farmer, especially after they form a certain market scale under the guidance of the local government. So, farmers in some endemic areas are enthusiastic to carry out this measure.

Rotational planting of rice and other crops

Rotational planting in the same field has two models. One is seasonal rotation in one year, such as the wheat-rice and rapeseed-rice rotation systems. The second model is yearly rotation, such as the rice-cotton rotation system. In this system, the duration of one cycle could be two, four, and six years, with one, two, and three years for rice, and another one, two, and three years for cotton. The duration could be determined according to the planting habit, geo-environment, water conservancy conditions, and market demand. However, six-year cycle rotational planting is the best system for the prevention and control of schistosomiasis.

Rotational planting, as a measure of schistosomiasis control, could be used in endemic regions with an annual rainfall of 700 – 1,600 mm, low underground water levels, and good drainage-irrigation systems.

Cementing ditches

Ditches in many schistosomiasis-endemic regions have become full and these muddy ditches are good for snail breeding. Cementing the muddy ditch could remove the mud and weeds in the ditches and have good long-term results for snail control.

Building ponds for aquatics breeding

Lowlands, wastelands and rice fields with low yields in the endemic regions could be used for building ponds for aquatics breeding and to submerge the snail habitats to kill the snails.

Programmes for this measure must be located in low-lying areas that have snails, as well as convenient transportation and an abundance of good-quality water. If the water is from lake areas, it must meet the requirements of aquaculture, namely: over 4 mg/L dissolved oxygen, pH 7 – 8.5, 5 – 8 degrees of hardness, and no methane or hydrogen sulfide.

Cultivation of high-altitude floodplain

Some high-altitude places could be used for cultivation by planting early-maturing crop such as barley, fava beans, rape, and vegetables after the waters recede in fall. This measure can reduce the density of the snails in flood plain areas but cannot eliminate the snails entirely. It is therefore important to educate farm workers to keep up good physical protection.

Storing water to raise aquatic products

This approach is to build a dam or a dike dividing the lake and its branches, then fill the branches with water in order to breed aquatics. As a result, the snail habitats in the branches are submerged.

5.4.4　Propaganda and education

Agricultural measures of schistosomiasis control can only be smoothly carried out and have good results with the cooperation of local residents. Propaganda and education are critical parts of an integrated strategy and should play an active role in schistosomiasis control.

The objects of propaganda and education in agricultural schistosomiasis control are the local residents in the endemic areas, especially the farmers. The aims are to improve their ability to protect themselves, and their enthusiasm and initiative to cooperate on the carrying out of agricultural approaches to schistosomiasis control. This work should mainly be organized and implemented by the agricultural authorities of schistosomiasis control at the county level, using the cooperation of veterinary stations in villages and towns, meetings, school education, bulletin boards, television, etc. The contents of programmes should include: basic knowledge of *S. japonicum* infection and transmission; national laws and local regulations; the local epidemic situation, including the main high-risk areas; the results and benefit of agricultural interventions, etc.

References

1. Wang TP, Vang Johansen M, Zhang SQ, et al. Transmission of *Schistosoma japonicum* by humans and domestic animals in the Yangtze River Valley, Anhui Province, China. Acta Trop, 2005, 96: 198-204.

2. Gray DJ, Williams GM, Li YS, et al. Transmission dynamics of *Schistosoma japonicum* in the lakes and marshlands of China. PLoS One, 2008, 3: e4058.

3. Li H, Dong GD, Liu JM, et al. Elimination of schistosomiasis japonica from formerly endemic areas in mountainous regions of southern China using a praziquantel regimen. Vet Parasitol, 2015; 208: 254-8.

4. Wang XH, Liu W, Yang YB, et al. Field observation on the effect of control and prevention for schistosomiasis by marshland isolation and farming prohibition in Lake District. Chin J Zoonoses, 2010, 26: 609-10. (in Chinese)

5. Liu ZC, He HB, Wang ZX, et al. Effect of marshland isolation and grazing prohibition on schistosomiasis control in Dongting Lake region. Chin J Schisto Contro, 2010, 22: 459-62. (in Chinese)

5.5   Schistosomiasis prevention through afforestation

Controlling snails through afforestation is one of the most effective methods of schistosomiasis prevention in China. Professor Peng Zhenhua first proposed the new idea of schistosomiasis prevention through afforestation in the 1980s. Schistosomiasis prevention through afforestation is based on the ecological-economic principle. Utilizing technical integration, an afforestation project aims to control snail populations in order to prevent the spread of schistosomiasis.[1] This occurs by means of the plants' allelopathy directly killing the snails and by afforestation destroying the snails' living habitat and preventing people from making contact with schistosome-contaminated water (Figure 5.12). It not only has chronic effects of schistosomiasis control, but also has the benefits of protecting the environment and improving the ecology, promoting local economic incomes, and preventing contact between local people and schistosomiasis-contaminated water. Thanks to a lot of research and experimentation, great progress has been made in schistosomiasis prevention through afforestation in China over the past 30 years. China has made great efforts to find the best mechanisms and techniques for snail control through afforestation. The national project of afforestation for schistosomiasis prevention was carried out along the middle-lower Yangtze River, and the mountainous and hilly epidemic regions. Schistosomiasis prevention through afforestation has greatly improved many people's health in several provinces in China.

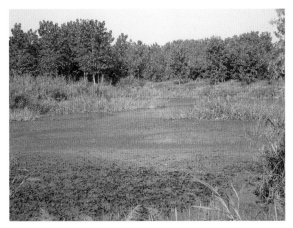

Figure 5.12   Afforestation on weed banks for schistosomiasis prevention.

5.5.1   Why does afforestation prevent schistosomiasis?

As we know, snails are the only intermediate host of the schistosoma japonicum. Controlling and eliminating snails has been always the most common method of schistosomiasis prevention. Schistosomiasis prevention through afforestation is also based on the principle controlling the number of snails. Due to the plants' allelopathy that directly kills the snails and destroys the snails living habitat, afforestation can effectively decrease the snails' density and the occurrence rates of living snails.[2]

It is reported that there are 113 allelopathic plants, which have a positive effect of killing snails. These include trees, shrubs, and herbaceous plants, such as *Astragalus sinensis, Belamcanda chinensis, Euphorbia helioscopia, Gleditsia sinensis, Melia azedarach, Sabia japonica, Sapindus mukorossi, Croton tiglium*, and *Rhododendron sinensis* (Table 5.5). Most of them are medicinal plants. These plants can be categorized into 20 families, as shown in Table 5.6.

Table 5.5   Allelopathic plants species and their families.

	Name of plant species
Trees	*Pterocarya stenoptera, Sapium sebiferum, Melia azedarach, Toxicodendron verniciluum, Sapindus mukorossi, Camptotheca acuminata, Gleditsia sinensis, Cinnamomum bodinieri, Ginkgo biloba, Morus alba, Alangium platanifolium, Croton tiglium, Liquidambar styraciflua, Eucalyptus spp., Camellia oleifera, Juglans regia, Carya cathayensis Sarg, Ailanthus altissima, Glyptostrobus pensilis*
Shrubs	*Atiina piluiiferam, Datum met, Buddleja lindleyan, Strychnos nux-vomica, Nerium indicum, Jatropha curcas, Zanthoxylum bungeanum.*
Herbs	*Phytolacca acinosa, Pulsatilla chinensis, Aconitum carmichaelii, Calystegia hederacea, Euphorbia pekinensis, Euphorbia helioscopia, Cannabis sativa, Humulus scandens, Reynoutria japonica, Polygonum hydropiper, Polygonum lapathifolium, Astragalus sinicus, Chenopodium ambrosioides, Lobelia chinensis, Xanthium sibiricum, Artemisia capillaris, Perilla frutescens, Veratrum nigrum, Arisaema consanguineum, Pinellia ternata, Equisetum arvense, Agrimonia pilosa, Duchesnea indica, Lycoris radiata, Belamcanda chinensis, Datura stramonium, Leonurus artemisia, Rumex japonicus, Hedychium flavum, Vetiveria zizanioides.*

Table 5.6   20 Families of allelopathic plants that have the effect of directly killing snails.

20 Families of allelopathic plants			
Phytolaccaceae	Thymelaeaceae	Sapindaceae	Papilionaceae
Euphorbiaceae	Ranunculaceae	Anacardiaceae	Araceae
Polygonaceae	Loganiaceae	Juglandaceae	Amaryllidaceae
Rutaceae	Buddlejaceae	Mimosaceae	Compositae
Berberidaceae	Meliaceae	Caesalpiniaceae	Stemonaceae

Allelopathic plants are more effective for killing and controlling snails. However, some allelopathic plants cannot survive with flooding, so are not suitable for many years of afforestation. Can plants with no allelopathic effects control snails? Experts found that snail growth and breeding were extremely correlated with the surrounding ecological characteristics. Based on these experiments, seasonal changes in rainfall, ground water levels, temperature and the community structure of vegetation (as snails' food) cause marked fluctuations in snail densities and transmission rates. Afforestation could largely alter these environmental conditions, and adversely impact the snails' living habitat.

Afforestation has isolated humans from making contacting with schistosome-infested water, by preventing livestock from going into the area, and reducing the contamination of water with dung. Schistosomiasis-prevention forestry has changed people's way of life and further reduced the probability of human infection with schistosomiasis.

> **How schistosomiasis prevention through afforestation changes local farmers' lifestyles**
>
> In the past, farmers often became infected with schistosomiasis because they had frequent contact with schistosome-contaminated water, due to swimming, washing clothes or fishing in rivers, or cultivating rice in paddy fields. As forestry for schistosomiasis prevention was planted, the riverbank environment changed. Thus, farmers seldom work or live near the contaminated water, and the infection rate of schistosomiasis has sharply decreased.

5.5.2　The secrets behind afforestation control of schistosomiasis

Experts have proven that afforestation changes the snails' habitat and reduces the density of snails, or directly kills the snails. But what are the secrets behind afforestation-based snail control? Are the snails' bodies harmed because of the plant's allelopathy, or is it because their environment is destroyed? In long-term experiments, experts found that the snails' physiology, biochemistry, and body structure were deeply influenced by the agroforestry system. Afforestation changes the essential nutritional substances of the snails, such as amino acids, and the protein and glycogen content of snails.[3] It also had a large influence on the activity of the transaminase, the ultra-microstructure of snails.

Differences between impacts of afforestation on female and male snails

Many studies have indicated that female snails are more sensitive to changes in habitat. Afforestation leads to a lack of food for the snails, and reduces their protein and amino acid content, changing the activity of the transaminase. These changes would not only cause the female snails to be poorly nourished, but would also reduce the amount of eggs they lay. Nutrition and breeding were both the primary causes of the decrease in snail density. This means that male snails have a stronger resistance to environmental changes than female snails.

5.5.3 The main afforestation techniques for schistosomiasis prevention

Since the 1980s, many technical afforestation measures have been developed for schistosomiasis prevention. There are some notable differences between the afforestation techniques for schistosomiasis prevention and common afforestation techniques. There are many special techniques of selecting the appropriate afforestation region, tree species, and planting techniques.[4]

Afforestation techniques should be different in different types of endemic areas. The afforestation techniques that are suitable for different types of the endemic areas were shown to be as follows.

Tree species selection

Marshland and lake regions; plains regions with waterway networks

Tree species chosen for afforestation in marshland and lake regions, and plain regions with waterway networks, in the middle-lower Yangtze River should be strongly water-resistant, fast-growing, harmful to the snails, and value-adding. Because winters are dry in this area and flooding often occurs in summer, afforestation techniques for schistosomiasis prevention are more difficult here than elsewhere. Riverbanks can be submerged for 1–3 months. Therefore, afforestation managers should choose large trees that can survive for a long time in waterlogged conditions, and make sure that tree tops are not submerged during the flood season.

Due to their strong water resistance and suitability to the riverbank environment, the survival rate of poplars, hybrid willow trees, and *Taxodium ascendens* were very high on the river banks. In consideration of their effectiveness for controlling snails and the water resistance of the trees, appropriate tree species also include *P. stenoptera*, *S. sebiferum*, and *Alnus cremastogyne*.

In plains regions with waterway networks, afforestation should also be combined with Green Village Project, and suitable tree species should be chosen according to the local hydrological conditions.

Mountainous and hilly regions

Conditions for afforestation in mountainous and hilly areas are more favorable than those in marshland and lake regions, and plains regions with waterway networks. Suitable tree species are more abundant.

It is suggested to plant tree species which are effective at directly killing snails in this region, such as *Gleditsia sinensis*, sumac, *Pistacia chinensis*, ginkgo, camphor, *Schima superba*, camellia, magnolia, *Carya illinoensis*, and geum. These tree species are suitable for growing in fertile soil, and many are food plants with positive medicinal effects.

Choosing appropriate areas for afforestation

It is very important to choose the appropriate area for afforestation. Long-term practice has led to valuable experience in choosing areas for afforestation. The main concerns when choosing an area for afforestation are: the density of living snails, waterlogging time, soil conditions for plant growth, and adverse effects on flood control.

Some studies have assessed the suitability of afforestation areas for schistosomiasis prevention, as shown in Table 5.7.

Table 5.7　Assessment indexes for the suitability of afforestation areas chosen for schistosomiasis prevention.

Index	Best condition	Good condition	Moderate condition	Bad condition
Living snails density	High	High	Moderate	Low
Waterlogging time (d)	< 25	25 – 40	40 – 65	65 – 90
Soil bulk density (g/cm³)	< 1.30	1.30 – 1.40	≥ 1.40	≥ 1.40
Drainage conditions	Good drainage	Good drainage	Normal drainage	Poor drainage
Soil texture	Loamy soils	Sandy loam soils	Sandy loam soils	Sandy loam soils
Soil structure	Crumb structure	Crumb structure	Block structure	Block structure

(Continued)

Index	Best condition	Good condition	Moderate condition	Bad condition
Type of bank	Islet beaches	Lake beaches	River beaches	River beaches
Available K content (mg/100 g)	≥ 15	10 – 15	5 – 10	< 5
Available N content (mg/100 g)	≥ 5.0	4.0 – 5.0	< 4.0	< 4.0
Available P content (mg/100 g)	≥ 1.25	0.75 – 1.25	< 0.75	< 0.75

Digging ditches and drainage; making ridges

When trees are in the young seedling stage, they cannot withstand long-term water-logging. Oxygen deficiency caused by waterlogging damages the roots of the trees, induces root-rot and prevents the growth of the plant. Drainage ditches are convenient for discharging floods (Figure 5.13). Planting trees on ridges can prevent them from becoming waterlogged. It clearly increases the trees' survival rate. Digging ditches and making ridges must be done in the winter of the year before planting.

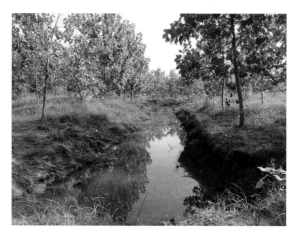

Figure 5.13   Digging ditches in forests for schistosomia-sis prevention.

Suitable seedlings and seeds choice

Marshland and lake regions; plains regions with waterway networks

In these regions, afforestation should be done by planting trees as seedlings. To ensure a high survival rate, it is also very important to choose the right seedlings. In June and July, the riverbanks are always submerged under 3.4 – 4.5 m of floodwater. Transplanting cultivation is a suitable method of afforestation in this area. To ensure the success of afforestation on the banks, the seedlings should generally be 1 m taller than the maximum water level during the flooding season. Seedling selection will have a serious impact on trees' survival rates and their effectiveness for snail control (Table 5.8). Seedlings chosen for afforestation should be large and vigorous. Studies have shown that seedlings of poplars should be taller than 4.5 m. *P. stenoptera*, *S. sebiferum*, *T. ascendens*, and *A. cremastogyne* should be taller than 3.5 m.

Table 5.8   Impacts of seedling selection on trees' growth and effectiveness for snail control.

Seedling chosen	Growing time (a)	Average height (m)	Average diameter (cm)	Survival rate (%)	Snail density (/0.11 m²)
Seedling height: 3.2 m; diameter at breast height: 2.6 cm	3	9.20	7.50	82	3.2
Seedling height: 4.5 m; diameter at breast height: 2.6 cm	3	11.81	9.92	96	1.1

Mountainous and hilly regions

In these regions, governments and farmers can choose afforestation methods with seedlings or vegetative propagation, according to the tree species and the local afforestation area conditions. It is better to select a good seed source or seeds from an improved seed base. Tree seed quality inspection should be done according to the rules for forest tree seed testing (GB /T 2772), set by the State Forestry Administration of China. It is also necessary to choose large well-growing seedlings to plant. Tests of seedling quality, lifting, packaging, transportation, and storage should be done according to the tree seedling quality grading of major species for afforestation (GB/T 6000), set by State Forestry Administration of China.

Land preparation

Land preparation is necessary at the initial stage of afforestation. Generally, the land preparation period should begin at least one year prior to afforestation. The best seasons are fall, winter, or early spring. Land preparation should be combined with the activities of the departments of health, agriculture, water conservancy, land, and others. After land preparation, drainage and ditches should be connected with each other, the land flattened, and there should be no shrubs, weeds or other plants, no rough dirt or waterlogged land in the afforestation areas.

Marshland and lake regions

It is advised to clear away all miscellaneous items from the afforestation lands. Comprehensively, all land should be claimed. For the lower land, it is important to dig ditches and make ridges, which follow the direction of the water flow. The ridge heights must be suitable for the trees' growth. The depth of land prepared should be greater than 5 cm. The depth of earth piled up should be greater than 20 cm.

Plains regions with waterway networks

It is suggested to clear away all miscellaneous items and level the afforestation area. Dredging channels, ditching new drainage and filling in the old drainage are advocated. It is also recommended to pile up soil and conduct slope protection. Land preparation methods can use cavity preparation or strip-like site preparation.

Mountainous and hilly regions

The cavity site preparation method is the most suitable method in mountainous and hilly regions. The cavity preparation depth for high forest and economic forest should be more than 45 cm, while in the shrub forest it should be more than 25 cm. Strip-like site preparation is suitable in areas where the slope is more than 20°C. Strip-like site preparation is along the contour, and the preparation depth is less than 30 cm.

Proper afforestation density design and afforestation patterns

The most specific and important factor is that the afforesting patterns and afforestation density configuration for schistosomiasis prevention must be different from common afforestation practice in the endemic areas. Rational afforestation density is critical to the success or failure of the afforestation project. Afforestation for schistosomiasis prevention should not only have the best effects of controlling snails, but also not prevent flood discharge. Afforestation density should be determined according to local hydrological conditions, tree species, and the different types of schistosomiasis epidemic region.

In marshland and lake regions

During summer, floods frequently occur on the banks of the marshland and lake regions in the middle-low Yangtze River.[5] Experts have made a lot of effort to find the proper afforestation patterns that will not have an adverse effect on flooding discharge in the area. They found that afforestation for schistosomiasis prevention requires special management.

Afforestation pattern in marshland and lake regions

- In flood channels, afforestation for schistosomiasis prevention should be done with broad row spaces and narrow stand spaces between the trees. The row spaces should be more than 8 m, and the stand spaces less than 3 m. The row spaces and stand spaces are defined in the Technical Regulations of Afforestation for Schistosomiasis Prevention by State Forestry Administration of China. For example, row-space and stand-space are 3 m and 8 – 12 m in afforestation for poplars (Figure 5.14). It is important to note that row spaces should be in the same direction as the flood flow. This pattern is convenient for flooding discharge, intercropping, and snail elimination. The afforestation pattern's technical specifications for schistosomiasis prevention with different tree species is shown in Table 5.9.

- In bank areas that do not release floodwaters, the afforestation density can be planned to be higher for the best schistosomiasis prevention effects, or according to the embankment protection target.

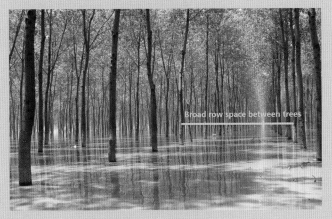

Figure 5.14 Afforestation patterns of poplar trees for schistosomiasis prevention.

Table 5.9   Technical specifications of afforestation patterns for snail control for different tree species.

Tree species	Afforestation pattern (stand space × row space)
Poplar	3 m × (8 m – 12 m)
Hybrid willow, *T. ascendens*, swamp, *Metasequoia glyptostroboides*	2 m × (6 m – 8 m)
P. stenoptera, alder and cypress	3 m × 10 m
S. sebiferum	3 m × 9 m

In plains regions with waterway networks

Afforestation patterns in plains regions with waterway networks

- Broad row spaces and narrow stand spaces should be used for afforestation on the riverbanks. The row space should be designed in accordance with the direction of flooding flow.

- It is suggested that tree species, shrubs, or herbs, which have the effect of directly killing snails, be planted in the side slope of the bank or near the water line.

- Along the canals, afforestation patterns should take account of the water flow direction in the canal, the width of the canal, and be combined with the development of a farmland shelterbelt. To best control snails, it is suggested to plant at least two rows of trees, and one row of shrub grass isolation belt between the tree row spaces.

In mountainous and hilly regions

Afforestation patterns in mountainous and hilly regions

- Cultivation objectives and intercropping conditions will determine a reasonable row spacing and configuration according to the tree species.

- Tree species that can directly kill snails should be planted. A planting zone near the waterline must be configured, with a width of 1 m.

- For ground-cover plant species that have the effect of killing snails, the afforestation density should be 90% after three years of planting. For the plant species whose litter cover has the effect of killing snails, the afforestation density should be 50% after three years of planting.

Afforestation regulations, operation design, and afforestation times

Afforestation regulations and operation design

The afforestation techniques should be according to the "Technical Regulation of Afforestation for Snail Control and Schistosomiasis Prevention on Riverbanks" (LY/T165-005) by State Forestry Administration of China. The operation design is according to the "Design Code for Afforestation Operations" (LY/T 1607). The operation design for forests for schistosomiasis prevention should take into consideration of the epidemic situation of schistosomiasis, including the snail distribution area, the occurrence rate of living snails, the average density of living snails, the snail infection rate, density of infected snails, etc.

Afforestation time

Afforestation should be arranged in the proper time according to the phenological characters for different tree species and local climatic conditions.

Tending and managing forests

Forest management and protection

- Weed control with a hoe should be implemented in forests with no intercropping plants.
- According to the characteristics of the tree species, timely removal of litter, pruning, shaping, fertilizing, irrigation, draining, and thinning can promote the growth of trees.
- Afforestation needs to be combined with pest control and forest fire prevention measures.
- When flooding, heavy snow and other natural disasters occur. Thus, tree restoration work should be completed in good time.

Accompanying measures

- A notice board to ban human and animal entry should be set up for the protection of trees and prevention of schistosomiasis infection.
- Isolation ditches, fences, roads or other isolation measures must be provided to prevent cattle and sheep from entering the forests.

Renewal of trees

Trees that are not growing well or are having little effect on schistosomiasis prevention should be harvested and renewed. Forest managers must carry out renewal and maintenance activities on harvested areas to ensure the sustainability of the forests. All areas harvested are required to be regenerated.

Archive management

According to the archive's nature, the archive can be divided into two types: technical files and management files. According to the archive content, the archive can be divided into the afforestation files and schistosomiasis files.

The archive must be complete, unified, and scientific.

- Complete: it should include all the historical records and database of afforestation for schistosomiasis prevention. No records should be missing from the archive.

- Unified: the format, data and standards in the archive should be uniform, and set by the State Forestry Administration. File archiving takes the small forest land patch as the basic unit.

- Scientific: the administrative government at or above the county should have assigned specific persons to be in charge of archive management. The archive should record the forests' construction in lots of permanent sample plots, in order to observe the changes in tree growth and the snail control conditions.

5.5.4　Typical modes for schistosomiasis prevention through forestry

Constructing a forest ecosystem for schistosomiasis prevention aims to control snails and prevent schistosomiasis. The effect of schistosomiasis prevention is closely related to the standing structure of forest. An excellent forest structure includes correctly selected plant material and the construction of an optimized mode. A variety of forest management modes are suggested to be carried out within the forests. Continuous composite management within the forests can help to enhance the effectiveness of snail control. It also improves land use efficiency and increases economic profits.

- Proper intercropping plants must be planted under the trees. Crops, vegetables and some medicinal plants are suggested to be planted under trees.

Plants with good snail controlling effects are suggested for planting. At least three years of intercropping is advised in regions which are susceptible to landslides and in the forests which were reclaimed from farmland.

- It is advised to promote the raising of chickens, ducks, geese, and fish between the forests. The raising of cattle and sheep in the forests are prohibited, as these livestock are hosts of schistosoma.

Composite management in forests for schistosomiasis prevention mainly includes five modes. The Agroforestry Mode; Forestry and Husbandry Mode; and the Forestry, Fishery, and Husbandry Mode are all suitable for all three kinds of epidemic areas. The Courtyard Forestry Mode and the Special Agroforestry Mode are usually suitable in the mountainous and hilly epidemic areas.

Agroforestry Mode

The Agroforestry Mode is the most common way to increase the short-term economic profits of local farmers. For a long time, the banks along the Yangtze River were not exploited and farmers' incomes were low. In the short term of 1 – 3 years, afforestation could not bring farmers economic income, meaning that local people had no enthusiasm for afforestation. However, intercropping cash crops like soybeans, corn or vegetables under the forest could generate some economic incomes and improve the farmers' annual economic benefits (Figures 5.15). Intercropping can also improve the soil quality and promote the growth of trees.

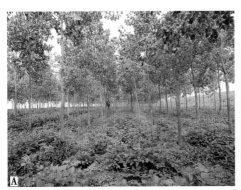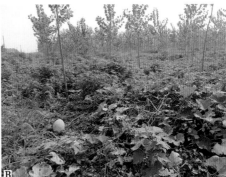

Figure 5.15　The agroforestry mode within forestry for schistosomiasis prevention. A, Planting soybeans in the poplar forest; B, Planting *Cucurbita moschata* in the forest.

How afforestation increases local people's incomes

Intercropping with different crops produces different profits. Planting rice paddies will generate about CNY 1,500 per mu (1 mu = 666.7 m^2). Planting soybeans could generate CNY 200 – 300 more than rice paddies. Planting vegetables could produce more profits. Tree stock also brings good profits for the local farmers: about CNY 6,000 – 8,000 per mu for 10 years of tree growth. In mountainous and hilly regions, farmers planted walnut or grapefruit trees for more economic profits (Figure 5.16). The increased incomes could be more than CNY 10,000 per mu.

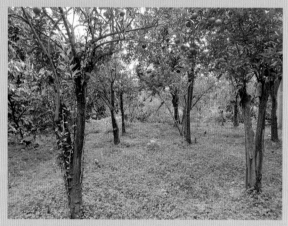

Figure 5.16   Grapefruit plantation in the forest for schistosomiasis prevention.

Forestry and Husbandry Mode

The Forestry and Husbandry Mode is another important mode for schistosomiasis prevention. This mode is always applied in the three types of prevailing regions for schistosomiasis prevention. Breeding poultry, such as ducks, geese, and chickens in the forests can not only increase the income of the farmers, but also increase the land use rate (Figure 5.17). Poultry manure can promote tree growth. However, local farmers are forbidden to raise sheep or cows between the forests because these livestock are susceptible to infection by schistosoma. Forestry and animal husbandry benefit each other and improve the effects of schistosomiasis prevention. Traditional afforestation for schistosomiasis prevention gradually turns into modern intensive and efficient afforestation.

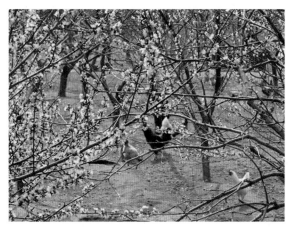

Figure 5.17　Forestry and Husbandry Mode: breeding chickens in the forest.

Forestry, Fishery, and Husbandry Mode

The Forestry, Fishery, and Husbandry Mode is a good mode for schistosomiasis epidemic areas. The water resources on the banks are convenient for developing fisheries. Establishing fisheries in the shallow water, and raising ducks and geese along the banks of the lakes is combined with tractor plowing to eliminate weeds and reeds for afforestation. The Forestry, Fishery, and Husbandry Mode is the most economic method for schistosomiasis prevention on riverbanks.

Courtyard Forestry Mode

The Courtyard Forestry Mode depends on making the best use of courtyard spaces. Families work to extensively develop the courtyards' economic potential, producing bamboo, flowers, fruits, medicine, and vegetables. In mountainous and hilly regions, the Courtyard Forestry Mode can play an important role in improving rural beauty and improving the living environment and economic conditions.

Special Agroforestry Mode

The Special Agroforestry Mode aims to intercrop plants with special roles in the forest for schistosomiasis prevention. It includes the Forestry-Medicinal Plants Intercropping Mode, the Forestry-Edible Fungus Intercropping Mode, and the Forestry-

Resource Insects Compound Mode. Intercropping between the forests is very important for the Special Agroforestry Mode. It has the added effect of maintaining good forest structure and function for schistosomiasis prevention.

5.5.5   Successful experiences of schistosomiasis prevention through afforestation

The prevention of schistosomiasis through forestry is actually a form of bioengineering. The techniques combine multiple subjects and the processes are complex. Governments and local people have obtained many valuable experiences for the long-term practice of schistosomiasis prevention through afforestation. The details of these experiences were summed up as follows.

Combination of economic, social, and ecological effects

Schistosomiasis-prevention forestry has multiple benefits to society, the local economy, and ecology. The primary purpose of the forests is for controlling snails to prevent schistosomiasis. However, afforestation also enhances ecological and economic considerations, such as protecting wetlands, promoting and exploiting riverbanks, effectively decreasing snail density, developing the forestry industry, and so on.

Combination of multiple departments

Schistosomiasis prevention through forestry-ecological engineering is an emerging multidisciplinary technique. Extensive coordination between the works of various related departments would assist the implementation of projects and improve achievements. Schistosomiasis prevention through afforestation is related to schistosomiasis prevention projects by the department of health, and to the departments of forestry, agriculture, water resources, and light industry. Various departments have different tasks. For example, the department of schistosomiasis prevention is in charge of land preparation; the agricultural and forestry departments provide tree seedlings and intercropping seeds; the water conservancy department is responsible for riverbank ownership; and the light industrial department for investment, timber processing and marketing.

Combination of scientific research with practical education

Afforestation for schistosomiasis prevention is a system project and many techniques of afforestation are very complex. In the past 30 years, various failures have occurred in afforestation, such as trees being submerged to death, plants having minimal effectiveness for snail control, and projects producing low economic benefits for local farmers. Scientific research and experiments are necessary to avoid repeating these failures. More scientific research needs to be carried out in the key endemic areas in order to promote afforestation techniques, control snails more effectively, and create more economic profits and ecological benefits. This scientific research would play an important role in choosing tree species with strong water resistance and effectiveness for killing snails; improving the effect of altering the snails' living environment; and promoting afforestation survival rates.

It would be very helpful to train local government workers and farmers in the use of these techniques, and in key points in the afforestation processes. The local governments are suggested to open training courses and immediately communicate the results of new scientific research to the afforestation workers.

5.5.6 Planning schistosomiasis control through forestry-ecological engineering

In order to deal with an emergency situation of schistosomiasis proliferation, beginning in 2004 China started to make plans for the comprehensive management of schistosomiasis control. The government of China drew up the "Comprehensive Management of Key Schistosomiasis Projects Plan 2004 – 2008 and 2009 – 2015". The project aimed to reach the criteria of a transmission control threshold of less than 1% in the lake and marshland provinces and reach a transmission interruption threshold in the hilly provinces of Sichuan and Yunnan provinces by the end of 2015.

At the same time, China began systematic afforestation for schistosomiasis prevention and established the national afforestation project. The "National Planning of Schistosomiasis Control through Forestry Ecological Engineering (2006 – 2015)" was issued in 2006. The field of engineering considered forestry for snail control and schistosomiasis prevention as a new type of forestry (the abbreviation is Schistosomiasis-Prevention Forestry). This plan involved 194 counties in seven provinces across the endemic areas. It suggested the targets of reducing the level of infection in all endemic counties to less than 5% by 2008 and to less than 1% by 2015. It included 102 counties of the lake-beach type and 92 hill-type counties. The plan aimed to build 496.2×10^4 mu area of schistosomiasis prevention forest from 2004 – 2008. The average snail density would drop by 30% by 2008. It would build 534.8×10^4 mu area of schistosomiasis prevention forest from 2009 – 2015, and the average snail density would drop by 50% from 2004. The density of infected snails would also drop by 50%. The project was to ensure a survival rate of afforestation for schistosomiasis of more than 85%; the growth rate of trees needed to reach 1 m per year on riverbanks, and 0.5 m in hilly areas.

In the future, the government will attach more importance to schistosomiasis prevention through afforestation. The State Forestry Administration of China will make new afforestation plans for medium- and long-term schistosomiasis control between 2016 and 2025. This planning will enhance the investment in afforestation in the next 10 years, and ensure the successful implementation of afforestation for snail control. Afforestation will continue to play an important role in schistosomiasis-control projects in the future.

References

1. Peng ZH, Jiang ZH. China's new type of forest—studies on the snails control and schistosomiasis prevention. 1st ed. Beijing: China's Forestry Publishing House, 1997. (in Chinese)

2. Sun QX, Peng ZH. Screening of Biological Materials for Plantations for Snail Control and Schistosomiasis Prevention and Research Progress in Studies on Inhibiting Mechanism. Wetland Science & Management. 2013; 9(3): 8-11. (in Chinese)

3. Zhang XD. The secrets behind vegetation control on snail fever. Chinese Forestry Science and Technology. 2002; 1(1): 85-89. (in Chinese)

4. Liu GH, Peng ZH, Zhang XD. Mechanisms and Techniques of Agroforestry Ecosystem on Snail Control and Schistosomiasis Prevention. Chinese Forestry Science & Technology. 2005;

4(4): 33-36. (in Chinese)

5. Zhou JX, Sun QX, Yang YF. Research on sustainable use of the middle and lower beach land of the Yangtze River. Resources & Environment in the Yangtze Basin, 2010; 19(8): 878-883. (in Chinese)

Chapter 6

National Plan for Schistosomiasis Control and Achievements

**Bo Zhong, Chen Lin, Jing Xu, Kun Yang, Li-juan Zhang,
and Shi-zhu Li**

6.1 Public Health Campaign

6.1.1 Patriotic health movement

The patriotic public health movement, also known as the "public health campaign" which is a mode based on communities participated health movement in China, aims to strengthen health knowledge awareness among the people; to improve the living environment and quality of life; to reduce disease risk factors; to promote the levels of social comprehensive health and public health. Through the launching of governmental policies and cooperation between collectives and individuals, it is possible to achieve the goals of disease prevention and having a better life and health for local people by environmental improvement in the urban and rural, national health education and health promotion, and pest and its transmitted diseases control. Simply to say, the goal of patriotic public health movement is to improve the living environment, to control pests and its transmitted diseases, and to promote health education and conditions in people. It is a health promotion model with Chinese characteristics, it is also the most influential health event in our history and a great innovation in health field in China.

When the People's Republic of China was established in 1949, the health condition was very poor. The plague, malaria and schistosomiasis were rampant, and the spread of vector-borne diseases such as lymphatic filariasis posed a serious threat to the public health. According to historical records, when plague spread through the country, the average annual number of fatalities was more than 20,000. Malaria, filariasis, and schistosomiasis were mainly prevalent in south of the Yellow River in China, threatened tens of millions of the population. In 1952, in order to curb the spread of disease transmission and to consolidate Chinese new government, Chairman Mao Zedong issued a call to "pay attention to health, reduce disease infections, improve health condition, and defense germ warfare". He appealed to implement "hygiene movement" nationwide focused on control of "four pests" (mice, mosquito, flies, and fleas). This was the prelude of "patriotic public health campaign". It led to the establishment of the central and local levels of the Patriotic Health Campaign Committee, which is responsible for the organization, coordination, and implementation of the patriotic public health campaign activities.

Over the past 60 years, the patriotic health movement — which is based on the national politics, organizations, and cultural superiority, and its effective social mobilization—has improved greatly the human cultural quality and health conditions across the entire nation. In different stages of economic development and health needs, this movement developed different strategies to cope with different situations such as carrying out activities to control disease transmissions and the "four pests", to promote hygiene condition and to defense germ warfare in the 1960s and 1970s. As the same time, "Two Managements and Five Improvements" policy was conducted (two managements: water supply management and feces management; five improvements: water well improvement, toilet improvement, domestic animal corral improvement, kitchen stove improvement, and environment improvement). These activities effectively curbed the spread of cholera, plague, malaria, schistosomiasis, and other acute and chronic infectious and parasitic diseases. The first health care revolution was completed in a relatively short time and the health level of Chinese people significantly improved. During the 1980s, monthly civilized manner activity (encouragement of good manners in civilization; politeness, hygiene, order, morality; praise of good performances in spirit, language, behavior, and environment) was implemented in urban and rural areas in China in order to create a social trend of "good health behavior was an honor, bad health behavior was a shame". Since the 1990s, health-related activities such as improvement of water toilets, implementation of health education, elimination of pests, diseases control, conducting the patriotic health campaign in both urban and rural areas, environmental cleaning, etc., have made a great contribution in environmental improvement, disease prevention and control, living standard enhancement and health condition changing. In urban areas, the patriotic health movement has played a key role in environmental sanitation. In rural environments, the patriotic health movement focused on management in water supply and feces. At the very beginning, pilot was established to show how to improve sanitary latrines. Step by step, there have been improvements in water quality, feces treatment combined with energy supply with biogas. All these activities helped people fight against schistosomiasis and provide strong support to control other parasitic diseases and its transmission media.

After continuous efforts, the patriotic public health campaign, with its unique influence and full range of coverage in China, has had a subtle influence on the Chinese people's lifestyle and mode of thinking. It also has made a contribution to control disease and achieve a higher health outcome with a lower cost. Among these efforts, "Two Managements and Five Improvements" has played an important role in the implementation of national health education, health promotion, and other measures for the prevention and control of schistosomiasis in China.

Sanitary toilets

Schistosomiasis is a zoonotic disease. Under suitable conditions, eggs in the feces of patients, and domestic animals with schistosomiasis get into water, hatch into miracidia, and infect snails. The life cycle described above is one of the key epidemic stages of schistosomiasis transmission. It is reported that there is a close relationship between water contamination caused by feces and schistosomiasis. Schistosomiasis is one of the 7 kinds of diseases caused by feces.[1] In 2002, WHO pointed out that schistosomiasis was caused by unsafe water, sanitation and personal hygiene.[2] Therefore, feces management to prevent eggs from entering water is one of the most important measures for schistosomiasis control. In addition to improving livestock management and avoiding environmental pollution caused by livestock feces, another feasible method is to alter toilets or to build biogas digester in schistosomiasis transmission areas, in order to make all toilets meet requirements for the safe treatment of feces. However, government guidance, funding support, people participation, and improved management are essential to ensure the implementation of these technical measures. Since the 1960s, the central government of China has repeatedly given instructions to improve the quality of drinking water and environment sanitation, especially in rural areas, through the patriotic health campaign. Then, the government began to implement improvements in drinking water supply and lavatories in rural areas, in order to prevent the transmission of parasitic diseases, especially schistosomiasis.

Chinese government has improved toilet renovation project through the development of the patriotic health campaign. During the 21st century, the central and local governments have continued to increase investment in toilet renovation project in rural areas. Since 2004, the central Department of Finance has established a transfer payment project for rural latrine improvement by promoting the construction of sanitary toilets. In 2009, rural latrine renovation was incorporated into a major public health service project to deepen medical reform. Through the centralized implementation of latrine renovation over these years, the coverage rate of sanitary toilets in rural areas in China increased significantly from 7.5% in 1993 to 76.1% in 2014. Great improvements were achieved in rural toilets, poor sanitation, and infectious and intestinal parasitic disease control, which were seriously harmful to people's health. In the rural areas in central and western regions of China, basic health conditions were dramatically improved and the occurrence and spread of disease was effectively controlled. The comprehensive benefit evaluation of toilet renovation project in rural areas from 2009 to 2011 showed that the morbidity rate of fecal-oral transmitted diseases decreased significantly, from 37.5/100,000 to 22.2/100,000. Cases of dysentery, typhoid, and hepatitis A also decreased by 35.2%, 25.1%, and 37.3%, respectively. In schistosomiasis-endemic areas, the infection rate of schistosomiasis dropped significantly in villages with toilet renovation projects. This played an important role in achieving the goal of schistosomiasis prevention and control in the Twelfth Five-Year Plan.

The construction of sanitary latrines has become an important measure and means of controlling the sources of schistosomiasis infection. The main types of safe sanitary toilet in use include three-grid feces digesters, double and triple biogas digesters that use gravity sedimentation to prolong the fermentation time of feces in the manure pits. The parasite's eggs can be deposited in an anaerobic environment at the bottom of biogas digesters for a long time. In addition, the urea in human urine is also in the digesters. The ammonia created by the urea can penetrate the shell of eggs and kill the miracidia: the higher the concentration of ammonia, the faster the death of the eggs.

Several data showed that the infection rate of schistosomiasis in the epidemic villages significantly decreased after the implementation of latrine renovation project. Dong Xiaorong[3] evaluated the safe treatment of household waste in rural schistosomiasis endemic areas in Hubei Province. The results showed that the acceptability rate of *Ascaris* eggs occurred in the liquid manure from the discharge holes of the third pool in three-grid type and biogas digesters was 95.6% and 98.6%, respectively. In addition, no live ascaris eggs or *Schistosoma* eggs were detected in the feces. The prevalence of schistosomiasis among people with sanitary household toilets (8.45%) was 43.7% lower than people with non-sanitary toilets (15.02%). Wei Haichun[4] investigated the concentration of parasitic eggs in the feces of household toilets in rural schistosomiasis endemic areas in Hunan, Hubei, Jiangxi, Anhui, Jiangsu, Yunnan, and Sichuan provinces. Seven hundred and eighty sanitary toilets were tested: the average sedimentation rate of parasitic eggs was 75.41%, the average mortality of ascarid eggs was 91.62%, the acceptability rate of ascarid eggs was 69.6% and the acceptability rate of live *Schistosoma* eggs was 99.9%. Jin Lijian[5] surveyed the effectiveness of toilet renovation in schistosomiasis prevalent areas in Sichuan Province. The average number of live *Ascaris* eggs in 100 ml liquid manure at the exits among the 60 samples from three-grid toilets was 0.39, and the survival rate of *Ascaris* was 5.24%. According to the sanitary standard of the non-hazardous treatment of feces (GB7959–87), the mortality rate of *Ascaris* eggs in liquid manure at the exits should be 95–100%. The survival rates of *Ascaris eggs* inside and outside sanitary toilets and non-sanitary toilets were statistically different. This suggested that the three-grid septic tanks had the effect to kill parasite eggs and could reduce the harmfulness of feces, or made it harmless. This result is basically consistent with the reports given by Cao Qin and Tan Xiaodong.[6] These reports showed that sanitary latrines in rural schistosomiasis endemic areas in China had a better effect than those areas without sanitary latrines. The rural sanitation environment was improved by the promotion and construction of sanitary latrines. Thus, the number of parasitic eggs, including schistosomiasis eggs was low, and the infection rate of parasitic diseases including schistosomiasis decreased, resulting in positive health benefits.

In 2014, the State Council released new goals for patriotic public health programme. The contents included: accelerating the pace of lavatory renovation in rural areas, taking actions that suit local circumstances, concentrating on the advancement at village level, and fastening the process of constructing safe sanitary toilets. The goals were to fulfill the construction of safe sanitary toilets in rural households in eastern, central, and western regions by 2020. Then, the epidemic of intestinal infectious diseases and parasitic diseases will be effectively prevented and controlled.

Early-stage problems occurred in the toilet renovation projects were adaption of purifying effects of several types of toilets, lack of understanding among farmers for construction sanitary toilets, shortage of funds for toilet renovation in underdeveloped areas and no counterpart funds from locals. In addition, the technologies for construction of sanitary toilets and the surveillance of safe feces disposal needed to replenish. The State Council proposed to resolve these problems by strengthening follow-up services and management of the lavatories, educating and guiding farmers to use sanitary toilets, and to establish a long-term management mechanism. We should strengthen research into technology suitable for toilet renovation, rationally integrate project resources, effectively mobilize social forces to participate in projects, and form a financing pattern for toilet renovation with multiple inputs.

Biogas production

Biogas is a form of combustible gas generated by the microbial fermentation of human and animal feces, rubbish, weeds, fallen leaves, and other kinds of organic materials under air-isolation conditions. It belongs to the category of secondary and renewable energy. Biogas is a mixture of various gases, generally containing 50 – 70% methane. Other gases present are carbon dioxide and a small amount of nitrogen, hydrogen, hydrogen sulfide, etc. The characteristics of biogas are similar to those of natural gas. At present, rural household biogas digesters in China are mostly circular methane fermenters with hydraulic system underground. The normal volume of biogas digester is 8 – 10 m^3 according to the types of raw materials input. Biogas itself is not toxic to *Schistosoma* eggs. However the effect of removing eggs is achieved by natural death after sedimentation and the temperature produced during fermentation. The specific gravity of the mixture of human feces and urine is 1.010 – 1.020, 1.005 – 1.010 for biogas liquid, and 1.060 for hookworm eggs, 1.140 for ascarid eggs, and 1.20 for *Schistosoma* eggs. In the process of fermentation, the manure gradually is decomposed and liquefied and the viscosity of the liquid manure gradually decreases. The eggs sink to the bottom of the digester because of the higher gravity. The *Schistosoma* eggs and the *Ascaris* eggs will sink to the digester bottom after 2 h and 8 h, respectively, in a digester with 1 meter in depth. Some eggs will be floating in night soil on the top layer of digester, as eggs are contained in feces filled with bubbles. The eggs on the top layer and those at the bottom of the digester account for about 95% of the total eggs in the digester. Eggs suspended in the middle liquid only account for a few percent. Therefore, the middle part should be chosen to design the outlet. The survival of *Schistosoma* eggs is directly influenced by the temperature and humidity of the environment. When the temperature is above 0 ℃, the higher the temperature, the faster the eggs die. In wet feces with a temperature of 28 ℃, only 3.2% of eggs survive after 12 days in wet feces. The temperature in a normal biogas digester is around 35 ℃. The temperature in the digester can reach 42 – 50 ℃ when there is sufficient plant fiber present.

The feces of schistosomiasis patients and infected livestock directly entering water without safe treatment are the key factor for the transmission of schistosomiasis. The construction of biogas digesters in schistosomiasis endemic areas is an important means of stopping the transmission of schistosomiasis. The biogas digesters were constructed in China in the 1980s. In 1983, the National Patriotic Health Committee and the leading group of biogas construction jointly proposed the document of "biogas health requirements" (Trial Edition). These regulations stated that the deposition rate for parasite eggs should be over 95% in liquid manure from biogas digesters. No live *Schistosoma* and hookworm eggs should be tested in biogas liquid. Currently in China, most biogas digests are constructed combining with renovation of human toilets, animal housings and kitchens. This kind of biogas construction in rural areas has exceeded the scope of traditional fuel uses and provides clean and worm environment for farmers. It also creates an efficient courtyard economy, and makes agricultural production safe and harmless. The construction of biogas digesters has played a major role in the prevention of schistosomiasis. Ling *et al.* regularly collected feces samples at the inlets and outlets of biogas digesters in areas with endemic schistosomiasis and the samples were inspected. The results showed that no *Schistosoma* miracidia survived after 15 days in the biogas liquid with temperature 30 – 35℃. No live schistosoma eggs could be detected in the outlet during the 100-day retention period[7]. Chen *et al.* put human feces with live *Schistosoma* eggs directly and the feces wrapped in nylon bags into household biogas digesters to observe the hatching of eggs for 9 weeks. The results showed that the number of hatched miracidia in biogas liquid was zero in 9 weeks. The presence of hatched miracidia in wrapped feces became negative from the fourth week. Usually, feces could be stored in the biogas digesters up to 120 days. Laboratory and field tests both showed that toilets with biogas digesters have a clear fatal impact on Schistosome eggs. This is completely in line with the sanitary requirements for the non-hazardous treatment of feces (GB7959-2012), as reported by Chen *et al.*[8] Cao Qin *et al.* chose four counties in Hubei Province as observation points, according to different geographic locations and different modes of safe fecal treatment. The infection rate of schistosoma, KAP for knowledge and behaviors related with schistosomiasis control were investigated. They found that the sedimentation rate of Schistosome eggs in three-grid and biogas digester was 90% and 90% respectively. The infection rate of residents in villages with renovated toilets was 47% lower than those residents from villages without renovated toilets. After health education interventions in villages with renovated toilets, farmers and residents had acquired more knowledge about schistosomiasis control than people from villages without renovated toilets. Toilet renovation prompted farmers to better understand schistosomiasis control, and had a significant impact on their living habits.

In addition to the effect on disease control, the construction of biogas digesters also has economic and social benefits. Biogas digesters can provide clean energy and reduce the energy expenditure of households; the feed liquid and sediments drained from the biogas device contain abundant nutrients, which can be used as efficient organic fertilizer for farmers. The biogas byproduct can be used to breed fish, plant fruit trees, improve soil, and reduce farmers' fertilizer expenses. Biogas has taken the place of firewood, thereby forest and vegetation resources are protected. The construction of biogas digesters plays an important and significant role in effectively managing human and animal feces, improving environmental sanitation in rural areas, enhancing the health of the masses and promoting the popularization of breeding technology in rural areas.

However, there are some disadvantages in the construction and promotion use of biogas digesters: the construction cost is high, the amount of land occupied is significant, and the comprehensive benefits of biogas digester are not as high as of those farmers who engaged in planting and breeding. In schistosomiasis endemic areas, we suggested that biogas digester should be constructed with livestock breeding and other new countryside construction action in order to have a good management in human and animal feces, to reduce the infection rate of people and livestock.

6.1.2 Health education

Health education is a series of activities and processes that are carried out by means of communication, education and intervention to help individuals and groups change unhealthy behaviors and establish healthy behaviors. Schistosomiasis is not only a biological pathogen-based disease, but also a kind of behavioral disease. People get infection by being in contact with cercariae-contaminated water. In 1984, the WHO proposed that human and livestock chemotherapy combined with health education, supplemented with local or seasonal snail control strategies, play an important role in schistosomiasis control. The experience of schistosomiasis prevention and control in China has been based on carrying out investigations, offering treatments, and investigating the elimination of snails as a means of disease prevention, while at the same time health education was carried out in the epidemic areas. This was effective in voluntarily population screening and receiving treatment for schistosomiasis in local residents and changing unhealthy behavior; and increasing awareness of schistosomiasis prevention.

In most of the endemic areas in China, adult males and females contact infested water for food production and living habit. For example, they contact infested water when planting fields, mowing weeds on the banks of lakes, herding, fishing, doing laundry, and washing vegetables. Children contact the contaminated water for fun, such as swimming, catching fish, playing in water. If there is no alternative or change in the environment, it is almost impossible to change the human behavior of being in contact with infested water. Health education for primary and secondary school students is an obvious way to facilitate their behavioral change in the fight against schistosomiasis. Moreover, primary and secondary school students with low immunity to *S. japonicum* would easily become infected after being exposed to contaminated water. Therefore, students are classified as being targets for health education interventions to combat schistosomiasis in China.

The "national medium- and long-term plan for the prevention and control of schistosomiasis (2004 – 2015)" pointed out that health education, especially for children and adolescents, could effectively improve the awareness and ability of the masses to protect themselves. In 2006, the State Council promulgated the "Regulations on the prevention and control of schistosomiasis". It also clearly stipulated that departments of education in local governments, at or above the county level, should be responsible for providing education on the knowledge, control, and prevention of schistosomiasis in all types and levels of school. Schools of all levels should provide education on the prevention and control of schistosomiasis. The experience of prevention and treatment shows that schistosomiasis health education courses is easiest and most effective way to protect children and adolescents in primary and secondary schools from infections in the endemic areas during the annual schistosomiasis epidemic season. The opening of schistosomiasis health education courses in primary and secondary schools in many major endemic areas also launched a wide range of "four-in-one" activities in a class of schistosomiasis health education. Namely, these activities are: watching a schistosomiasis health education video or listening to a lecture, carrying out a schistosomiasis survey in health-related extracurricular activities, and writing articles related to schistosomiasis health education. Sichuan Province has carried out a wide range of "small hands" activities requiring students to pass on the knowledge they have learned to their families and other members of the community, in order to expand the coverage of health education for the prevention and control of schistosomiasis. This kind of communication is spread by the doctor and the teacher, to one student, one family, three neighbors, and thus to the society. The propagation of knowledge about schistosomiasis prevention and control, especially for developing countries with epidemic schistosomiasis achieved best with little investment but high output. It does not increase the students' academic burden, so it is a value-adding health education intervention. As to the characteristics of their age and interests of teenagers, a variety of health education intervention models has been developed for students in the endemic areas in China. Guang Han *et al.* studied the effect of audiovisual education (videos of schistosomiasis, schistosomiasis control classes, real pictures of schistosomiasis specimens, training skills, etc.) on students in Poyang Lake Primary School. They found that audiovisual education, skill training, protective medicine providing and rewarding are the best ways to be accepted by students. This is a good model of health education for pupils in Poyang Lake schistosomiasis region.[9] Wei Wangyuan planned and produced popular schistosomiasis cartoons and materials for cartoon pictures to appeal to children's preferred graphic form. He craftily integrated the characteristics and environment of the Dongting Lake into a fairy tale in health education to depict contact with contaminated water and the use of knowledge of self-protection methods.[10] This information is widely spread in schools with serious schistosomiasis epidemics, hence, an intervention effect was produced. Usually, acute cases occur every year from July to August, thus, health education intervention to students before summer holidays is essential. The health education courses should be arranged before the holidays, focusing on transmission knowledge and the harm of contacting with infested water. Before school summer holidays start, all students were asked to sign an agreement with "not in contact with infested water" and related information was released to their parents. These measures help to enhance awareness of the disease prevention in summer and effectively control the occurrence of acute schistosomiasis. In primary and secondary schools in endemic schistosomiasis areas, the control guards selection or "no schistosomiasis patients school selection" were conducted in order to establish an incentive mechanism for correct behavior, thus creating a good atmosphere for schistosomiasis prevention and control. In addition, full use of school radio, newspapers, posters, brochures, blackboard lectures, extracurricular activities, essay competitions, knowledge contests, and other methods of achieving universal knowledge of schistosomiasis control is practical way for health education. This helps the students to understand schistosomiasis transmission and increase self-protective capability from getting the disease by being exposed to contaminated water.

For adults, it is unlikely that they will avoid contacting with infested water during crop production. Therefore, an alternative for crop producers is devised to implementing interventions for treatment compliance and protection awareness. Also, contaminated water can be disinfected by implementing of comprehensive management projects, such as water supply projects, which treat water for use safely. Health education is mainly focusing on the labor people and housewives in endemic areas. The main mode of health education for mass communication is launched in special radio and television programmes that spread knowledge quick and wide. This is complemented by the distribution of a variety of communication materials, such as posters, calendars, and practical promotional items, like basins. Among the scattered labor population, information about schistosomiasis is spread via warning signs, placards, mobile radio vehicles, and other means. Small media materials are also distributed as a form of interpersonal communication. On the basis of mass communication, the use of rural health care networks combined with physical examination and medicine treatment, the killing of snails, and personal skills training, are very effective intervention measures for adult residents. Xu *et al.* reported that use the model of "the sense of value for schistosomiasis prevention + protection skill training" is the best intervention for schistosomiasis prevention in adult women. In this model, mechanism of avoiding infested water is interpreted and reinfection by washing clothes in contaminated water decreases. Liu *et al.*[11] carried out a group discussion and a prize activity in housewives. Authors asked doctors to give health education to patients before treatment, encouraged the patients to tell their story to other people. The results showed that these activities created more effective results.[12] Hu *et al.* suggested that the model of "schistosomiasis prevention, chemotherapy compliance education, plus protection skills training" was the best way for health education in male adults. This intervention model significantly improved physical examination and medicine treatment compliance in the target population.[13] In addition, the schistosomiasis control knowledge was spread by different cultural life among people, such as dancing, singing, dramatic performances. These forms of education can attract the attention of common people in the endemic areas, and appeal more people to join the campaign for schistosomiasis control.

With social and economic development, there are more than two million people as surplus labor flows in rural areas moving to urban and some economically developed areas. At least 30 million people from endemic schistosomiasis areas have moved to cities throughout the country. This situation has brought new difficulties to the work of schistosomiasis control in China. Compared to the residential population in the endemic areas, the floating population has a high infection rate, higher mobility, and low awareness of schistosomiasis prevention and control. Imported acute cases have been reported in some transmission interrupted areas in recent years. It is very important to monitor the infections in floating population in many transmission control and transmission interrupted areas. The people living in the Lake District must use the safe public toilets. Feces and waste collection containers are asked to equip on the fishing boats. Fishermen with higher education are selected as volunteers to release knowledge about schistosomiasis prevention and control. They can use their own experiences to tell other peers about the benefits of using waste collection containers and personal legal obligations. After this kind of intervention, the awareness of schistosomiasis prevention and control increased in fishermen, therefore, the infective risks decreased. Migrant workers from endemic areas must be constantly monitored. The short message service (SMS) is used to disseminate information and knowledge about the prevention and control of schistosomiasis.[14] This way, a better effect has achieved in improving treatment compliance rates and knowledge awareness. The level of education of the floating population is generally not very high. Therefore, communication materials for health education should be easy to understand. It is advised to use pictures, music, animations, and so on, to explain some key information. In addition, radio, television, and other mass media can be used as propaganda carriers to release intervention knowledge. All these methods is helpful in improving of awareness about schistosomiasis among the floating population.

References

1.　Mara DD, Feachem RGA. Water and excreta related disease: unitary environmental classification. J Environ Engin, 1999, 4: 335.

2. World Health Organization. Guidelines for the safe use of wastewater and excreta in agriculture and aquaculture: measures for public health protection (executive summary). Geneva: World Health Organization, 2002.

3. Dong X, Kong L, Tang F, et al. Investigation of decontamination of feces in household latrine in some epidemic areas of schistosome in Hubei. J Environ Health, 2009, 8: 711-712

4. Wei H, Kong L, Tian H, et al. Analysis of the status of parasitic ova in latrine night soil in areas of China where schistosomiasis is prevalent. J Pathogen Biol, 2010, 5: 758-761. (in Chinese)

5. Jin L, Zhang C, Yan L, et al. Cross-sectional study of the latrine innovation and analysis of the effect of the excrement disposal in Sichuan Province. Modern Prevent Med, 2009, 3: 427-429,438. (in Chinese)

6. Cao Q, Tan X, Kong Q, et al. Reforming latrine for schistosomiasis control in Hubei. J Pub Health Prev Med, 2006, 6: 28-32. (in Chinese)

7. Ling B, Zuo JZ, Gao JX, et al. Health assessment on safe treatment of night-soil on schistosomiasis endemic areas. J Hygiene Res, 1997, 26: 20-23. (in Chinese).

8. Chen L, Xu FS, Yin HZ, et al. Effect of killing schistosome eggs by family-size biogas tanks. Parasitoses Infect Dis, 2008, 6: 25-27. (in Chinese).

9. Hu GH, Lin DD, Zeng XJ, et al. Health education for primary school students in Poyang Lake district. Chin J Health Edu, 1995, 11: 34-36 (in Chinese).

10. Wei WY, Yuan LP, Jiang QX, et al. Study on health education to reduce the primary water contact behavior. Chin J Schisto Control, 2000, 12: 143-145. (in Chinese)

11. Xu LW, Hu GH, Zhang J, et al. Effectiveness of the spread application of intervention modes on health education for schistosomiasis control among adult women. Chin J Schisto Control, 2002, 14: 283. (in Chinese)

12. Liu QH, Liu BZ, Chen YW, et al. Health education for mid-term evaluation of World Bank Loan Project for schistosomiasis control in Sichuan Province. J Pract Parasit Dis, 1995, 3: 114-116. (in Chinese)

13. Hu GH, Lin DD, Zhang SJ, et al. Study on the intervention model of health education for schistosomiasis. Chin J Schisto Control, 2000, 14: 283. (in Chinese)

14. Chen L, Cao CL, Bao ZP, et al. Study on schistosomiasis control to migrant population by new pattern. Modern Prev Med, 2013, 9: 1754-6. (in Chinese)

6.2 Strategic plan for the elimination of schisto-somiasis in the P.R. China (2016–2025)

6.2.1 Background

Schistosomiasis is one of the major infectious diseases caused by *Schistosoma japonicum* infection, with a history of more than 2,100 years in China.[1] The national survey conducted in the 1950s revealed that schistosomiasis was endemic in 12 provinces/municipalities/autonomous regions along the Yangtze River, including Anhui, Fujian, Guangdong, Guangxi, Hubei, Hunan, Jiangsu, Jiangxi, Shanghai, Sichuan, Yunnan, and Zhejiang. It was estimated that more than 10 million individuals were infected with *S. japonicum* and more than 100 million people were at risk of infection in the 1950s.[2,3] After the founding of the People's Republic of China, schistosomiasis was given high priority by the central government and the Communist Party. Chairman Mao issued the slogan "We must eliminate schistosomiasis" in 1955 and a vigorous national control programme was established since 1956.[1]

The morbidity and mortality rates associated with schistosomiasis have decreased significantly throughout more than 60 years of the implementation of suitable strategies for various settings and stages. The number of estimated schistosomiasis cases decreased from 1.7 million in 1992 to 874,500 in 1998 due to the implementation of the World Bank Loan Project (WBLP) for schistosomiasis control. Five locations, comprising Shanghai, Zhejiang, Fujian, Guangdong, and Guangxi, interrupted schistosomiasis transmission by 1995.[4] However, schistosomiasis has re-emerged in some endemic regions due to environmental changes caused by flood or large water conservancy projects and the termination of the WBLP.

To protect human health and decrease the impact of schistosomiasis on the development of socioeconomics, the state council published a notice to further strengthen schistosomiasis control in 2004 and a regulation for schistosomiasis control was legislated in 2006. Meanwhile, a strategic plan comprising medium- and long-term national goals for schistosomiasis prevention and control (2004 – 2015) was issued. Two control programmes, in which an integrated control strategy was implemented, were conducted in 2004 – 2008 and 2009 – 2015, resulting in the interruption of schistosomiasis japonica transmission in many areas in China and its control in the remaining endemic areas. By the end of 2015, transmission was interrupted in 343 of the 453 endemic counties (no local cases of individuals and livestock occurred in five consecutive years) and 110 reached the criteria of transmission control (prevalence of schistosomiasis < 1% in human beings and livestock). The estimated number of infected humans has decreased from 842,530 in 2004 to 77,190 in 2015. The largest number of cases and infected cattle were concentrated in marshland and lakes regions in Hubei, Hunan, Jiangxi, and Anhui.

Based on worldwide achievements, interest in schistosomiasis control and discussion on the strategies and approaches towards elimination have been raised internationally in the last decade.[5-9] The World Health Assembly (WHA) adopted the resolution WHA65.21 in 2012, calling for increased investment in schistosomiasis control in order to initiate elimination programmes where appropriate.[10] A strategic action plan was also drafted for guiding endemic countries to control and/or eliminate schistosomiasis.[11]

Although achievements have been made in schistosomiasis control, challenges still exist in China. These include: i) infection risk still exists in areas where transmission was under control; ii) difficulty for snail control due to complicated environments and extensive breeding areas; iii) the presence of more than 40 animal reservoirs of schistosomiasis and large numbers of cattle raised in endemic areas; iv) unavailability of sensitive diagnostic methods and effective intervention tools; and v) a weak surveillance and active response system.

To accelerate the progress of schistosomiasis elimination in China, a national schistosomiasis control conference was organized at the state level in Hunan in November 2014. The Prime Minister Keqiang Li underlined the importance of persisting with the implementation of an integrated control strategy to interrupt schistosomiasis transmission. The Vice Premier Yandong Liu attended this meeting and demanded that a new strategic plan for the years of 2016 – 2025 be drafted, and that reliable and operational approaches on how to interrupt transmission and elimination of schistosomiasis nationwide by 2020 and 2025, respectively, be established. In 2015, the National Health and Family Planning Commission (NHFPC) organized for governmental officials from various ministries and professional staff to draft the new strategic plan, aimed at guiding the endemic areas in planning and implementing integrated approaches for the elimination of schistosomiasis.

6.2.2　Vision, goals, and objectives

The vision of China's strategic plan contemplates a nation free of schistosomiasis. To achieve this vision, medium- and long-term goals are set:

Medium-term goals to be achieved by 2020:

- to interrupt the transmission of schistosomiasis in more than 90% of the endemic counties; and

- to eliminate schistosomiasis in 75% of the endemic counties.

Long-term goals to be achieved by 2025:

- to interrupt the transmission of schistosomiasis in all endemic counties; and

- to eliminate schistosomiasis in 90% of the endemic counties.

Here, the transmission interruption and elimination are defined according to the criteria for schistosomiasis control and elimination issued by Chinese government (Table 6.1).

Table 6.1　Criteria for schistosomiasis control and elimination (GB 15976-2015).

The criteria for schistosomiasis control and elimination issued by Chinese government divides the process into four stages including stage of infection control, transmission control, transmission interruption and elimination.

1. Infection control

(1) The prevalence of schistosomiasis in humans is less than 5%

(2) The prevalence of schistosomiasis in livestock is less than 5%

(3) No outbreaks of acute schistosomiasis

2. Transmission control

(1) The prevalence of schistosomiasis in humans is less than 1%

(2) The prevalence of schistosomiasis in livestock is less than 1%

(3) No local acute schistosomiasis cases

(4) No infected snails for two consecutive years

3. Transmission interruption

(1) No local infected humans for five consecutive years

(2) No local infected livestock for five consecutive years

(3) No infected snails for five consecutive years

(4) Established and improved sensitive and effective surveillance systems at the county level

4. Elimination

After reaching transmission interruption, no local infected cases, livestock, and snails for another five consecutive years.

To accomplish this vision and these goals, the following operational objectives must be met:

1) integrated interventions must be scaled up;

2) the mechanism of governmental leadership, inter-sectoral collaboration, and resources mobilization must be enhanced;

3) the capacity building of professional staff and research for schistosomiasis elimination must be strengthened; and

4) monitoring and surveillance to quickly respond to schistosomiasis emergence must be enhanced.

6.2.3　Guiding principles

To ensure the realization of these goals, the policy of "prevention first, scientific control, guiding intervention adapted to local settings, integrated control, collaborative prevention and control" should be persisted with and put into practice. The campaign for schistosomiasis elimination should be integrated with the strategic plans of beautiful villages' or new townships' construction, as well as the regional developing plans of the Yangtze River Economic Zone, and the ecologic-economic zones of Dongting Lake and Poyang Lake.

Governmental leadership and multi-sector collaboration

The transmission of schistosomiasis is complex, involving social, natural, and economic factors. Efforts should be made to enhance the leadership and financial support from various levels of government. Long-term collaborative mechanisms between the civil society and private sector, pharmaceutical firms, non-governmental development organizations, and international cooperation should be established to mobilize internal and external social resources, as well as to intensify integrated schistosomiasis control interventions.

Comprehensive interventions adapted to local settings

To block transmission from infection sources to surroundings, reservoir control should be enhanced while the feces of humans and livestock should be disposed of harmlessly. Snail control should be integrated with projects of other sectors such as land resources, water conservancy, agriculture, or forestry to modify the environments of snail-infested areas.

Empowerment of people and communities

The involvement of populations affected by or at risk of schistosomiasis is important for the success of the interventions. Communities should be empowered and involved in activities to prevent and control schistosomiasis. Effective information, education, and communication should be enhanced in the communities in endemic areas to improve the perceptive knowledge and awareness of residents so that they can avoid contact with potentially contaminated water.

Sensitive and effective surveillance and response

As morbidity and prevalence rates of schistosomiasis have decreased to a low level, surveillance and pre-warning activities with sensitive tools should be strengthened to detect the outbreak of schistosomiasis in the early stages and thus respond timely. Active case finding should be conducted and appropriate therapy should be given once determinate cases are found.

Improved capacity for control and surveillance

To overcome the shortcomings of current techniques, projects for schistosomiasis research should be listed as a part of national key natural and science programmes to explore sensitive and effective tools for schistosomiasis diagnosis, surveillance, drugs, snail control, etc. Training courses and supervisory visits for case detection and management, and implementation of control activities should be organized. Guides or manuals could be complied to provide guidance for governmental officials and/or professional staff when they are drafting or implementing control plans or activities.

6.2.4   Strategy

An integrated strategy, which emphasizes blocking the contamination from reservoirs to the surroundings should be implemented and adapted to local settings and endemic situation.

Areas with ongoing transmission

In areas where schistosomiasis is still endemic, control of reservoirs and environmental modification in snail-infested areas should be enhanced to interrupt transmission. Preventive chemotherapy should be delivered simultaneously to humans and livestock, and their feces should be disposed of harmlessly. To manage animal reservoirs, prohibiting grazing in the grassland where there are snails, replacing buffalo with machines, razing livestock in pens, etc., should be implemented and adapted to local settings. Safe water should be provided and effective health education should be conducted as supplementary methods. To control snails, mollusciciding should be conducted in high-risk environments, while snail breeding areas could be modified to make them unsuitable for snail survival. This could be integrated with projects from departments of land resources, agriculture, water conservancy, forestry, etc.

Areas where schistosomiasis has been eliminated or transmission interrupted

In areas where schistosomiasis has been eliminated or transmission has been interrupted, schistosomiasis surveillance should be enhanced to detect local and/or imported cases, or infected livestock earlier and thus respond in a timely manner. Snail-infested areas should be reduced with integration with the projects from departments of land resources, agriculture, water conservancy, forestry, etc.

Areas with potential risk of schistosomiasis transmission

Non-endemic areas of schistosomiasis affected by great water conservancy projects such as the Three Gorges Dam reservoir and the South-to-North Water Diversion Project, which diverts water from the Yangtze River to the Huai River, etc., surveillance should be strengthened on imported snails and reservoirs.

6.2.5   Intervention package

Interventions from the health sector

Screening and treatment of schistosomiasis cases

To detect and cure schistosomiasis, case screening using sensitive tools should be conducted followed by timely treatment using standardized PZQ dosages. The epidemiological survey of determined cases and management should be strengthened. Screening and chemotherapy should be focused on high-risk populations, including field workers with high frequencies of water contamination, fishers or boat people, etc., with collaboration from the transport and agriculture sectors. Help and treatment also should be given to advanced schistosomiasis cases.

Clearing and management of schistosomiasis foci

After an outbreak of schistosomiasis, a timely epidemiological survey should be conducted. Approaches such as treatment of cases, preventive chemotherapy, decontamination of feces, mollusciciding, or modifications of snail-infested environments, as well as health education should be promptly implemented.

Snail survey and control

To understand the distribution of snails and determine the snail-infested areas and high-risk environments, a snail survey should be conducted in areas suited to snail survival. Interventions through mollusciciding, applying mud, covering black plastic film, etc., should be implemented to compress the snail-breeding areas near to the place of residence to eliminate infection risk.

Construction of harmless latrines

Combined with the patriotic health campaign and new rural construction, rural sanitation projects should be implemented to build latrines in endemic areas. Public toilets to treat feces harmlessly should be constructed in locations or docks where boat people or fishers are concentrated.

Surveillance and early warning of schistosomiasis emergence

To understand changes in endemicity and factors related to schistosomiasis, disease reporting and management should be strengthened. Besides setting up fixed surveillance sites, risk assessment, analysis of data related to schistosomiasis control programme, and early warning should be conducted regularly.

Health education

To disseminate information and knowledge on how to control and prevent schistosomiasis through different ways, the health sector should provide guidance and collaborate with the sectors of education, news publishing, broadcasting, etc. Health education should be focused on high-risk populations such as school-aged children, fishers, or boat people, etc.

Interventions from the agriculture sector

Management of animal reservoirs

To stop infected livestock contaminating the surroundings with schistosome eggs, raising livestock in pens is recommended and should be implemented in endemic areas. Cattle should be dropped out or replaced step by step through the implementation of agricultural mechanization supplemented with the construction of tractor roads. Digesters for feces treatment should be built in combination with the construction of eco-villages or energy development projects. Raising other animals instead of those susceptible to schistosome infection could consolidate the achievements of cattle replacement. Screening, treatment, and enlarging selective chemotherapy should be conducted, while the examination of imported livestock from endemic areas should be strengthened.

Snail control in combination with agricultural activities

Combined with the adjusting the structures of the agricultural industry, changing rice fields to dry land or paddy-upland rotation on farmland where there are snails should be implemented to make them unsuitable for snail survival. Digging fishponds in low-laying swamps to develop aquaculture could eliminate snails by long time of immersion in water.

Surveillance on animal schistosomiasis

Surveillance on animal schistosomiasis should be conducted to understand the changes in schistosomiasis in livestock. Meanwhile, a web-based data reporting and management system should be established to ensure the timeliness and effectiveness of data collection and analysis. Once infected livestock is found, clearing and management of schistosomiasis foci should be conducted in collaboration with the health sector.

Interventions from the water conservancy sector

Comprehensive engineering of rivers and lakes

Lining riversides and canal banks with concrete, increasing the elevation of islands and decreasing the height of beaches, modifying culverts and sluices with adding snails preventing facilities, etc., should be integrated into snail control in endemic areas along rivers or lakes. These could modify the environment where snails habituate and prevent the diffusion of snails along the river system.

Drainage system modification projects

Modification on snail habitats should be conducted in collaboration with slope protection using concrete, modification of culverts and sluices supplemented with barrier blocking, etc., to make snail survival difficult and prevent snails spreading along the canals.

Rural water supply projects

Combined with the national plan for improving the quality and enhancing efficiency of the water supply in rural areas, endemic areas of schistosomiasis should be given priority for water supply programmes to protect humans from contact with schistosome cercaria-contaminated water.

Hydraulic schistosomiasis control projects

According to the endemic status in areas with water management units, safe areas free of schistosomiasis could be constructed through implementing interventions, including water supply, construction of latrines and environmental modification. Capacity building of water management units for schistosomiasis control should be strengthened through surveillance, health education and research activities.

Interventions from the forestry sector

Planting forests in favor of snail control and prevention of schistosomiasis

Ecological forestry safety systems should be established with afforestation as the center. Trees, which are in favor of snail control and schistosomiasis prevention, should be planted in regions where trees are suitable for growing in schistosomiasis-endemic areas. Botanical materials inhibiting snails, compound systems integrated with forestry and agriculture activities, and isolation facilities should be combined to change snail habitats.

Activities to improve the effectiveness of snail control

Measures including digging ditches to elevate ridges in fields, cleaning up cannels, replanting trees, etc., should be implemented to improve the effectiveness of existing forests for snail control in endemic areas.

Ecological environment surveillance

Surveillance and early warning should be strengthened in areas suited to snail survival. Modes to suppress the breeding and proliferation of snails by improving environments should be explored through pilot studies on establishing ecological forests. Snail surveillance should be strengthened and facilities preventing snails spreading should be constructed in combination with projects of wetland conservation and restoration, wildlife and nature reserves, etc.

Interventions from the land resources sector

Land development and consolidation engineering

When implementing land development and consolidation programmes in schistosomiasis-endemic areas, environmental modifications for snail control could be integrated with land consolidation, drainage and irrigation engineering projects, construction of roads on farmland, protection of farmland and environments, or construction of snail-control facilities such as snail precipitation tanks.

Moving villages from high risk areas

Villages that are heavily endemic for schistosomiasis and with complicated environments suitable for snail breeding, which are difficult to eliminate, priority should be given to moving and rebuilding the villages in a safe place.

Interventions from other related sectors

Transport departments should push for the installation of feces collection apparatuses and treat feces harmlessly. Environmental modification for snail control should be integrated with the construction of waterways.

To avoid outbreaks of schistosomiasis, courses to disseminate knowledge on schistosomiasis control and prevention to residents, especially school-aged children, should be organized in a scientific way by the health sector.

Non-profit health education activities for schistosomiasis control and prevention should be organized by news publishing houses or broadcasting sectors to propagate knowledge and related policies for schistosomiasis control and prevention, improve people's self-protection consciousness, and increase people's willingness to get involved in schistosomiasis control activities.

6.2.6   Strategic approaches to guarantee the implementation of the strategic plan

Governmental leadership and coordination among sectors and districts

Leading groups responsible for planning and implementing schistosomiasis elimination plans at various governmental levels should be set up and improved to enhance leadership in schistosomiasis control. The mechanism to communicate and resolve major problems during the stage of schistosomiasis elimination should be established to ensure the implementation of control approaches in practice.

Local governments should organize related sectors to draft local plans for schistosomiasis elimination with the guidance of the national strategic plan and propel the interventions for schistosomiasis elimination according to regulations for schistosomiasis control and prevention. Prohibiting grazing livestock in snail-breeding areas should be enhanced by local governments. Integrated control measures should be implemented based on the strengthened multi-sector collaboration and sharing information mechanism. Guidance on and supervision of schistosomiasis should be strengthened through the organization of a field survey in spring and a conference in the fall at the state level, and by improving the mechanism of reporting progress on schistosomiasis control by related sectors.

Collaborative control and prevention among neighboring areas should be enhanced. According to the endemic characteristics of schistosomiasis, a work plan for schistosomiasis control and prevention among neighboring areas should be drafted and implemented, with well-defined work priorities and concrete interventions according to real situations.

Combined with the requirements of the patriotic health work in the new era, the local governments should involve the population in non-profit activities to improve the production areas and living surroundings. Knowledge of disease prevention and control should be widely disseminated to improve the consciousness and capacity for self-protection.

Financial support

Expenses for schistosomiasis control and prevention activities should be included in the governmental budgets according to the principle of sharing between the central and local governments. Governments at the provincial or city level are responsible for funding the integrated projects, which will be implemented in local areas, and for providing financial support for schistosomiasis control to those counties and towns under jurisdiction. The governments at county and township levels are responsible for arranging enough funds to conduct normal schistosomiasis control and prevention activities.

The central government should intensify its financial support for schistosomiasis control projects of various sectors such as land resources, water conservancy, agriculture, health, and forestry. It should also subsidize funds for local government schistosomiasis control programmes, construction of control stations, screening and treatment for humans and livestock, molluscicide use, staff training, health education, etc. Measures for schistosomiasis control could be incorporated into projects of land resources, water conservancy, agriculture, and forestry sectors, when governments draw up or approve these projects.

Financial department at various levels should strengthen supervision and audits to ensure that the funds are specifically used for schistosomiasis control. Resources from enterprises, private companies, and non-profit organizations should be mobilized for schistosomiasis control.

Technical support

Studies on accelerating schistosomiasis elimination should be conducted based on multi-sector, multi-discipline principles. Research to explore and develop effective tools for reservoir control, disease surveillance and early warning, rapid diagnosis, drugs for schistosomiasis prevention and treatment, and techniques and machines for snail control should be enhanced and emphasized. According to the new criteria for schistosomiasis control and elimination issued in 2015, related guidelines or manuals guiding implementation and assessment of schistosomiasis elimination activities should be drafted as soon as possible. Meanwhile, international cooperation and communication should be strengthened to introduce advanced techniques from abroad and disseminate Chinese experiences and lessons.

Professional workforce support

To ensure the success of schistosomiasis elimination, control stations and the workforce from the national level to the township level should be strengthened, while the schistosomiasis surveillance system should be improved. The structure of professional staff should be adjusted as most staff from basic stations are old, and their knowledge and techniques cannot meet the current demand of schistosomiasis control activities. Education and training courses should be organized to improve their capacity. Platform for schistosomiasis diagnosis should be strengthened to improve their diagnostic techniques. To increase the motivation of professional staff to work on schistosomiasis control, they should be properly remunerated and their salaries should be included in governmental financial budgets. They should also be subsidized appropriately when working in the field.

6.2.7　Monitoring and evaluation

The goals and tasks to eliminate schistosomiasis should be defined and decomposed to related governments and sectors. If the goals are not achieved, the related persons responsible are to be held accountable.

According to standard indicators that include performance and outcome indicators reflecting the endemicity of schistosomiasis, monitoring the implementation of the strategy would be conducted and the periodic assessment on the medium- and long-term goals would be carried out in 2021 and 2026, respectively, organized by the NHFPC. The final goals may be adjusted according to the real situation and the medium-term assessment.

References

1. Wei O. Internal organs of a 2100-year-old female corpse. Lancet, 1973, 2: 1198.

2. Wang HZ, Jia YD, Guo JP, et al. A histroric review or 40 years' control on schistosomiasis in P.R. China. Chin J Schisto Contr, 1989, 1: 1-4. (in Chinese)

3. Xia C, Wang HZ. The endemic status and control of schistosomiasis. Bull Biol, 1989, 9: 26-27.

4. Chen XY, Wang LY, Jiming C, et al. Schistosomiasis control in China: the impact of a 10-year World Bank Loan Project (1992-2001). Bull World Health Organ, 2005, 83: 43-48.

5. Gray DJ, McManus DP, Li Y, et al. Schistosomiasis elimination: lessons from the past guide the future. Lancet Infect Dis, 2010, 10: 733-736.

6. Fenwick A, Savioli L. Schistosomiasis elimination. Lancet Infect Dis, 2011, 11: 346-7.

7. Ross AG, Olveda RM, Acosta L, et al. Road to the elimination of schistosomiasis from Asia: the journey is far from over. Microbes Infect, 2013, 15: 858-865.

8. Tallo VL, Carabin H, Alday PP, et al. Is mass treatment the appropriate schistosomiasis elimi-

nation strategy? Bull World Health Organ, 2008, 86: 765-771.

9. Rollinson D, Knopp S, Levitz S, et al. Time to set the agenda for schistosomiasis elimination. Acta Trop, 2013, 128: 423-440.

10. WHA65.21. Elimination of schistosomiasis. 2012.

11. WHO. Schistosomiasis: progress report 2001-2011 and strategic plan 2012-2020. Geneva: World Health Organization, 2013.

6.3 Monitoring and response systems for schistosomiasis

After nearly 60 years of arduous efforts, there have been remarkable achievements in the prevention and control of schistosomiasis in China. Especially in recent years, with the adjustment of prevention and treatment approaches, as well as the implementation of new control strategy, the outbreak of schistosomiasis has continued to decline in endemic areas, reaching its lowest levels in history. By 2012, in the 12 schistosomiasis-endemic provinces, Shanghai, Zhejiang, Fujian, Guangdong, and Guangxi (municipalities and autonomous regions) achieved the national critera of transmission interrupted. The provinces of Sichuan, Yunnan, and Jiangsu reached the national critera of transmission control. The remaining four provinces—Anhui, Jiangxi, Hubei, and Hunan—reached the national critera of epidemic control. By 2014, in all of the 453 counties (cities and districts), 313 and 135 counties have reached the national critera of transmission interrupted and transmission control, respectively.[1]

With the implementation of the 12th five-year plan and the "Healthy China 2020" programme, China will achieve its stated objectives for 2015 and 2020. At the same time, because China continues to face many challenges, it is necessary to consolidate the achievements of schistosomiasis control. These challenges are manifest in the following factors. First, the repeated infection of humans and animals was more serious in the lake and marshland regions due to the large number of infected livestock, the wide distribution of snail-infested areas, the complex and changing environment of these areas, the highly mobile population, etc.[2] The repeated epidemic outbreaks in the mountainous and hilly regions is due to the complexity of the natural environment, relatively backward social and economic development, the scattered distribution of snails, many types of animals infection source and others.[3] Second, the area of snail distribution is still relatively large, confirmed cases of schistosome infection can still be found in the population every year, and the conditions for transmission have not significantly changed. This is further complicated by reduced funding after compliance, the aging control team personnel structure, the decline in control and prevention awareness, etc.[4-7] Third, imported cases of schistosomiasis have also occurred because of increasing international trade and population migration.[8-11] Fourth, schistosomiasis transmission is influenced by environmental changes due to global warming, flooding and the construction of large-scale water conservancy projects, and behaviors changed because of the market economy system.[12-15]

Especially in recent years, the epidemic status has rebounded in some endemic areas because of ecological and environmental changes, reduced funding after standards have been achieved.[16,17] In order to keep abreast of the factors that influence both infection outbreaks and the spread of schistosomiasis, as well as the dynamics of epidemics and to guide prevention and control work, it is crucial to establish sensitive and effective schistosomiasis monitoring systems in the present situation of low prevalence.

6.3.1 The history and current status of schistosomiasis surveillance systems

The history of schistosomiasis surveillance systems

In general, monitoring is the long-term, continuous, and systematic collecting of information on the dynamic distribution of a disease and its impact factors. It also includes timely reporting and feedback in order to adopt prompt intervention measures and evaluate their effectiveness.[18] Since the founding of the People's Republic of China and the evolution of prevention and control models, the monitoring system of schistosomiasis has gone through three stages: i) disease surveillance; ii) epidemiological surveillance; and iii) public health surveillance.

The schistosomiasis monitoring model used in China includes longitudinal and cross-sectional monitoring, fixed and flow monitoring, active and passive monitoring, etc., all of which have played an important role in promoting the prevention and control of the disease during different periods.[18-21] Over the past decade, with the shift from epidemiological surveillance to public health surveillance, the monitoring of schistosomiasis has gradually improved to a more systematic monitoring network. This network includes: fixed monitoring sites throughout China for surveillance of epidemic and epidemiological factors; potential monitoring sites in areas subject to climate change and with large-scale water conservancy projects; risk monitoring sites that are based on sentinel mice surveillance; and consolidation monitoring sites which focus both on eliminating the remnants of snail populations and monitoring imported infection sources in areas where transmission has been interrupted.[7,22] Except epidemic situations, environmental and social factors related to epidemics should be also monitored, including the economic factors relevant to behavior change and the implementation of control measures. These monitors of factor will provide an important reference for the formulation, evaluation, and adjustment of integrated control strategy.

In general, surveillance can be classified into passive surveillance and active surveillance. In passive surveillance, the surveillance data and information are routinely reported from the primary-level organization to the high-level unit, and the high-level unit passively accepts those data. In China, schistosomiasis is categorized as a Class B notifiable infectious disease, and the statutory reporting of schistosomiasis began in 2004.[23] So far, most reported cases are acute schistosomiasis. In active surveillance, the high-level unit conducts special investigations or the primary-level unit collects information in strict accordance with meeting special needs.

In line with different monitoring purposes, active surveillance of schistosomiasis in China can be divided into three categories: i) repetitive cross-sectional sampling survey, namely national surveys on schistosomiasis endemicity; ii) longitudinal monitoring of fixed sentinel surveillance, namely surveillance on sentinel sites; and iii) risk surveillance, namely consolidated surveillance in areas where schistosomiasis transmission has been interrupted.

The contents of schistosomiasis surveillance systems

The surveillance indicators mainly include schistosomiasis cases, infected domestic animals, intermediat host snails and the related epidemic factors.[24]

Schistosomiasis cases

According to the diagnostic criteria issued in 2006, schistosomiasis cases are classified into the following categories: acute schistosomiasis; chronic schistosomiasis; and advanced schistosomiasis. Acute schistosomiasis is one of the important indexes to measure the severity of the schistosomiasis epidemic situation in a certain area.[25] Therefore, surveillance is focused on acute cases where uncontrolled transmission occurs.

Domestic animals

Livestock are a major reservoir host. The surveillance on domestic animals mainly includes cattle, sheep, pigs, and horses.[26] Cattle are the main surveillance focus, as they play a major role in schistosomiasis transmission, Particulary in marshland and lake regions.[27]

Snail intermediate hosts

Oncomelania hupensis is the only intermediate host involved in the transmission of *Schistosoma japonicum*, playing a key role in schistosomiasis transmission.[28,29] The geographic distribution of the snail is strictly consistent with that of schistosomiasis.[30] Therefore, snail monitoring is an important component of the surveillance system, including snail-ridden areas, density of snail population, and infection rates of snail hosts.

Related epidemic factors

The surveillance on related epidemic factors mainly includes surveillance on water level, rainfall, temperature,[13,31] the occupational activities and lifestyle habits of local residents, and the implementation of schistosomiasis prevention and control measures.[32,33]

The demand of the current schistosomiasis surveillance systems

With the full implementation of the key projects for the comprehensive control and management of schistosomiasis (2009 – 2015), the epidemic status of schistosomiasis has further declined and moved toward elimination based on the consolidation of control achievements. However, the current surveillance systems cannot fully meet the needs of this goal for the following reasons. First, the monitoring tools are outdated. Many studies have shown that the current diagnostic technology as a surveillance tool for infected human and livestock populations has reached the limit of effective detection in the context of low prevalence. The final diagnosis of the disease still relies on pathogenic examination, which has higher missing rates and leads to an underestimated epidemic situation in people and animals.[34-37] During snail monitoring, the traditional method for snail detection has a low sensitivity. The microscopy method is also problematic because of difficulties in identifying the early development of schistosome sporocysts in snails.[28,38] It is therefore difficult to meet the monitoring needs in areas where transmission control and interrupted transmission have been achieved. Second, the professional team is unstable. In recent years, factors such as national health system reform and scarce funding for schistosomiasis control, have resulted in unsustainable teams for schistosomiasis control. The professional losses have been very serious. The age structure of the professionals were unreasonable, added to the aging of the population and fewer training opportunities for further education, it is clear that their knowledge has been slowly updated.[39,40] The laboratories undertaking the main tasks of schistosomiasis monitoring widely lack professional and technical personnel and do not have high levels of diagnosis.[41] Third, the information feedback mechanism is not perfect, the capability of data management and analysis is not strong, and these aspects of monitoring are unable to adapt to epidemic situations in time.[39] During the monitoring process, a sound information feedback mechanism, a reasonable data management and analysis can help detect abnormal phenomena early. However, the existing monitoring systems lack effective information feedback mechanisms and the data cannot provide the guidance for schistosomiasis control. A lot of resources and material are used to collect data. However, they cannot play a significant role, thus delaying the best time to control the epidemic. For example, the snail population has rebounded and infected snails have been found in Midu County, Yunnan Province since 2011. However, local control agencies did not pay sufficient attention to this development and failed to take effective preventive measures in time, which resulted in a serious epidemic after 2012. Fourth, the monitoring indicator system is imperfect. The transmission of schistosomiasis always involves complex ecological environments, social behavior, socio-economic factors and disease management, among other factors. The existing system is still mainly confined to monitoring the occurrence of the disease, which is only a single indicator for active monitoring. With the promotion of schistosomiasis control and elimination, the epidemic situation of schistosomiasis can be reduced to a lower level. However, it is clear that the existing single indicator monitoring system is neither sensitive nor effective enough to detect the presence or potential risk factors of diseases transmission. A comprehensive and considered design is needed to establish and improve scientific, rational, sensitive, and effective monitoring indicators.

6.3.2 Focus on surveillance after schistosomiasis transmission control

The purposes of surveillance after transmission control

With the goal of shifting from schistosomiasis control to elimination, the activities of surveillance, evaluation, and monitoring must also have a corresponding shift. This entails moving from observed disease morbidity and mortality to a focus on finding infection cases and detecting the means of transmission. At the macro level, the purpose of surveillance is to find, investigate, and eliminate sustained transmission so as to ultimately achieve the goal of elimination. At the micro level, the purpose of surveillance is to detect individual cases, confirm and treat these cases, undertake epidemiological and vector investigation, eliminate the epidemic point through chemotherapy, environmental change, and then follow-up individual cases and monitor the wider community to which those individuals belong. In this stage, the surveillance work itself constitutes intervention.[41]

There are still endogenous causes of disease transmission in the transmission control areas. The monitoring system should be focused to find and remove the endogenous human and animal cases, intermediate host snails and the unstable epidemic status, in order to control exogenous sources of infection. Therefore, during the transitional period from disease control to elimination, the surveillance response becomes one of the key measures to eliminate the disease.[42,43]

Perfecting the surveillance system after transmission control

The surveillance system is a complicated systematic project. Minimally, it should be able to identify an epidemic situation. Once transmission control has been achieved, a surveillance system should include a range of other related systems. These are the detection system (passive and active surveillance, sample preparation and testing, pathogen analysis, and disease confirmation), the information processing system (information collection, compilation, analysis, processing, reporting and so on), the warning systems (disease classification index analysis, epidemic information dissemination, epidemic early warning and forecasting and so on) and the epidemic response system (epidemic emergency disposal, evaluation after epidemic control).

If one component part of the surveillance system has a problem, this will affect the sensitivity and effectiveness of the entire surveillance system. Recently, some areas that have reached the transmission control and transmission interrupted stages have witnessed a re-emergence of and rise in the number of schistosomiasis cases. The main reason for this development is that the surveillance system is not perfect and so causes problems. Therefore, it is particularly important to better establish and improve the surveillance system in order to achieve transmission control in these regions. The integrity of the surveillance system is the basic requirement for improving the sensitivity and effectiveness of the system.

Among the revised national criteria for schistosomiasis control and elimination, it was proposed that the endemic county should be established as a basic unit for surveillance. Improving the sensitivity and effectiveness of the schistosomiasis surveillance system should begin at this level. Minimally, the surveillance system at the endemic county level should meet the following basic requirements. First, there is a person who is responsible for surveillance in the county and towns. The responsible person is tasked with the timely discovery and the effective treatment of outbreaks of the disease. Second, there are personnel who have mastered the technology of schistosomiasis detection at the endemic county level. Third, there are information archives for schistosomiasis prevention, control and surveillance at the village level. Fourth, the consolidation measures should be built and implemented. The following aspects should be strengthen to build a sensitive, effective, and robust surveillance system.

To establish the sensitive and efficient surveillance indicators

Surveillance indicators are the most important part of the surveillance system. The target of surveillance should be to establish indicators that are designed to collect relevant data and information. This data and information must then be analyzed to guarantee the effectiveness of the surveillance work and minimize the resources employed in surveillance. According to the principles of sensitivity, timeliness, and operability, a series of indicators should be selected. These indicators should reflect the outbreak and development of the disease—not only the distribution of disease and snails, but also the infection source, genetic information of snails, environment, socio-economic factors and other relevant factors.[44,45]

However, more surveillance indicators are not necessarily better. The conservation of resources and the improvement of efficiency should also be considered. Some surveillance indicators can be acquired from other fields or comprehensive parameters. It is a minimum requirement of a surveillance system to build a basic database based on the surveillance indicators that have been selected.[42]

To explore a comprehensive surveillance and management model

The long-term, effective surveillance of epidemic situations is an important tool for institutions dedicated to disease prevention and control at all levels to master transmission patterns and guide disease control. The effective surveillance and management mode is the basic requirement to ensure the normal operation and quality of the surveillance system. At the stage of epidemic control, surveillance responsibilities belong to a single active surveillance team. This team determines changes in the incidence rate and the key control object of sentinel surveillance in the target community population.

In regions where transmission control and transmission interrupted have been achieved, the infection level of humans and livestock is very low. Given that many factors affect transmission, it would be a huge waste of resources to carry out full and active surveillance. Therefore, the efficiency of the surveillance system should be considered. The measures of increasing passive surveillance, sharing and exchanging surveillance data with other fields, and comprehensive surveillance of other diseases can partly compensate for the deficiencies of active surveillance. There are many measures that can be taken to improve the level of surveillance. These include strengthening health education delivery to high-risk groups and the floating or migration population, improve the awareness among these groups of the value of seeing a medical doctor, and strengthen the knowledge and skills base of medical staff and control personnel who are responsible for addressing the disease.

To develop and utilize advanced techniques and tools

It is very important to develop and use highly sensitive and effective tools to guarantee quality assurance in surveillance of schistosomiasis. These include infection screening and diagnostic tools for humans and animals, surveillance technology for snails and infected snails, mapping the distribution of schistosome infections and high risk areas, emergency response, and so on. Some technologies with high sensitivity and specificity have good prospects, especially those based on nucleic acid detection technologies, for example polymerase chain reaction (PCR) and loop-mediated isothermal amplification (LAMP). However, these technologies require further evaluation because of the costs, the compliance of local residents, and the operability of laboratory testing.

Studies have shown that LAMP infection detection technology can be used to detect snails at the early stage of infection.[46-50] However, sampling design and surveillance efficiency still need verification at the field level. In addition, the techniques of sentinel mice and sentinel snails can be a supplement to conventional surveillance systems.[51-53] The technologies of remote sensing (RS) and geographic information systems (GIS) along with other spatial information technology, can predict and monitor snail habitats, allowing appropriate interventions and control measures to be taken as soon as possible in high-risk areas. Such technologies also greatly improve surveillance efficiency, especially for those areas that lack means for surveillance and/or require prevention interventions.[54-57] With the epidemic status gradually reducing, it is necessary to use advanced technology to carry out applied studies on disease surveillance in order to continuously improve the sensitivity of surveillance tools.

To improve capabilities for detection of and responses to outbreaks

It is very important to have a stable and high-quality monitoring team to improve the effectiveness of schistosomiasis control and consolidate achievements to date. Along with the health system reform, most independent professional schistosomiasis intuitions may merge with the Center for Disease Control and Prevention (CDC) in the area where schistosomiasis transmission is under control and interrupted, and the local government will change the engaged professional and investment funds of schistosomiasis control.[58] Given that there are limited health care resources, there should be at least one professional who has mastered schistosomiasis epidemiological investigation and laboratory testing technology at the local CDC. The schistosomiasis surveillance teams should have access to useful information that can enable them to rapidly respond to potential and actual risks.

6.3.3 Case study of the emergency response for a schistosomiasis outbreak

There was an acute schistosomiasis outbreak in Hukou County, Jiangxi Province in 2013. Eleven people have a history of contact with infested water and eight of these were diagnosed with acute schistosomiasis. In Pingfeng Village, 320 of the total 720 residents living there were tested with a serological method—the indirect hemagglutination assay test (IHA). Among those who were tested, the positive rate of IHA was 3.13%. There were 12 cattle in the village and three were found to be positive, giving an infection rate of 25%. The average density of living snails was 2.1147 per 0.1 square meters. However, no infected snails were found.

According to the requirements of the emergency response scheme for schistosomiasis outbreaks developed by the Ministry of Health, health experts quickly arrived at the outbreak site and held a working conference to guide and deploy the emergency response planning. The group established a lead group and the government provided an adequate budget (an average of one Chinese Yuan per person in the epidemic population).

The steps taken to solve this outbreak were as follows. First, the eight patients who had been diagnosed with acute schistosomiasis were treated in the hospital with praziquantel (PZQ). Second, an epidemiology investigation was carried out among the local residents and animals. PZQ was administered to all local residents who had positive in serological test. All 12 cattle were given extensive chemotherapy. Third, niclosamide was used to kill schistosome larvae and snails in the epidemic location and the surrounding waters. Fourth, health education was delivered to village residents.

6.3.4 Conclusion

Although there have been remarkable achievements in transmission control and interruption of schistosomiasis, there are still many new challenges. After reaching transmission control at the national level, the duty of schistosomiasis control is still a complex, long-term and arduous. Therefore, it is very import to strengthen the existing surveillance system. It is also essential to improve efficiency and responsiveness in order to prevent a rebound of the disease and achieve the goal of schistosomiasis elimination.

References

1. Lei ZL, Zhang LJ, Xu ZM, et al. Endemic status of schistosomiasis in People's Republic of China in 2014. Chin J Schisto Control, 2015, 27: 563-569. (in Chinese)

2. Hao Y, Wu XH, Xia G, et al. Endemic status of schistosomiasis in People's Republic of China in 2005. Chin J Schisto Control, 2005, 18: 401-404. (in Chinese)

3. Chen HG, Xie SY, Zeng XJ, et al. Current endemic situation and control strategy of schisto-somiasis in lake and marsh land regions in China. Chin J Schisto Control, 2011, 23: 5-9. (in Chinese)

4. Hao Y, Wang LY, Zhou XN, et al. Causes and risks of schistosomiasi transmission in Poyang Lake region of Jiangxi Province, China. Chin J Schisto Control, 2009, 21: 345-349. (in Chinese)

5. Wen LY, Cai L, Zhang RL, Zhou XN. Analysis of the imported 37 cases of schistosomiasis in city. Chin J Epidemiol, 2004, 25: 577-579. (in Chinese)

6. Wen LY, Yan XL, Zhang JF, et al. Strategy of solidification and surveillance for schistosomiasis in transmission-interrupted provinces in China. Chin J Schisto Control, 2011, 23: 18-21, 31. (in Chinese)

7. Zhong B, Wu ZS, Chen L, et al. Strengthening the achievements of schistosomiasis control in hilly regions of China. Chin J Schisto Control, 2011, 23: 10-13. (in Chinese)

8. Hua HY, Wang W, Cao GQ, et al. Improving the management of imported schistosomiasis hae-matobia in China: lessons from a case with multiple misdiagnoses. Parasit Vectors, 2013, 6: 1-6.

9. Yi P, Yuan LP, Wang ZH, et al. Retrospective survey of 184 patients infected with Schistosoma haematobium from African countries. Chin J Schisto Control, 2011, 23: 441-442. (in Chinese)

10. Zhou XN, Cai L, Zhang XP, et al. Potential risks for transmission of schistosomiasis caused by mobile population in Shanghai. Chin J Parasitol Parasit Dis, 2007, 25: 180-184. (in Chinese)

11. Zhang YQ, Zhang J, Yang H. Schistosomiasis investigation at 4 villages of Yangjiayuan during a flood in 1999. Chin J Parasitol Parasit Dis, 2002, 20: 59-60. (in Chinese)

12. Yang GJ, Vounatsou P, Zhou XN, et al. A potential impact of climate change and water resource development on the transmission of *Schistosoma japonicum* in China. Parassitologia, 2005, 47: 127-134. (in Chinese)

13. Zhou XN, Yang GJ, Yang K, et al. Potential impact of climate change on schistosomiasis trans-mission in China. Am J Trop Med Hyg, 2008, 78: 188-194.

14. Liang YS, Wang W, Li HJ, et al. The South-to-North Water Diversion Project: effect of the water diversion pattern on transmission of Oncomelania hupensis, the intermediate host of *Schistosoma japonicum* in China. Parasit Vectors, 2012, 5: 52.

15. Huang YX, Hang DR, Gao Y, et al. Study on surveillance and early-warning system of schistosomiasis in first phase of east route of South-to-North Water Diversion Project. III. Indexes of surveillance and early-warning and risk assessment. Chin J Schisto Control, 2011, 23: 32-37. (in Chinese)

16. Collins C, Jing X, Tang S. Schistosomiasis control and the health system in P.R. China. Infectious Diseases of Poverty, 2012, 1: 1-8.

17. Guo J, Zhen J. Advances in the research on the endemicity and control of schistosomiasis in China. Chin J Parasitol Parasit Dis, 1999, 17: 260-263. (in Chinese)

18. Zhou XN, Wang LY, Chen MG, et al. The public health significance and control of schistosomiasis in China--then and now. Acta Trop, 2005, 96: 97-105.

19. Wu XH, Zhang SQ, Wang TP, et al. Schistosomiasis transmission in areas where inhabitants migrated from outside embankment to new settlement. Chin J Parasitol Parasit Dis, 2008, 26: 16-20. (in Chinese)

20. Zhu R, Gray DJ, Thrift AP, et al. A 5-year longitudinal study of schistosomiasis transmission in Shian village, the Anning River Valley, Sichuan Province, the Peoples' Republic of China. Parasit Vectors, 2011, 4: 43.

21. Zhou XN, Wang LY, Chen MG, et al. An economic evaluation of the national schistosomiasis control programme in China from 1992 to 2000. Acta Trop, 2005, 96: 255-265.

22. Zhu R, Lin DD, Wu XH, et al. Retrospective investigation on national endemic situation of schistosomiasis. II. Analysis of changes of endemic situation in transmission-controlled counties. Chin J Schisto Control, 2011, 23: 237-242. (in Chinese)

23. Jin SG, Jiang T, Ma JQ. Brief introduction of Chinese Infectious Disease Detection Report Information System. Chin Digital Med, 2006, 1: 20-22. (in Chinese)

24. Xu J, Yang K, Li SZ, et al. Surveillance system after transmission control of schistosomiasis in P.R. China. Chin J Schisto Control, 2014, 26: 1-5. (in Chinese)

25. Lin DD, Wang SP, Jiang QW, et al. Technical indexes of the criteria for infection control of schistosomiasis in China. Chin J Schisto Control, 2007, 19: 5-8. (in Chinese)

26. Dang H, Zhu R, Guo JG. Report of the result of national surveillance for schistosomiasis in China, 2005. J Trop Dis Parasitol, 2006, 4: 189-193. (in Chinese)

27. Guo JG, Ross AG, Lin DD, et al. A baseline study on the importance of bovines for human *Schistosoma japonicum* infection around Poyang Lake, China. Am J Trop Med Hyg, 2001, 65: 272-278.

28. Zhou XN, Bergquist R, Leonardo L, et al. Schistosomiasis japonica control and research needs. Adv Parasitol, 2010, 72: 145-178.

29. Yang K, Zhou XN, Wu XH, et al. Landscape pattern analysis and Bayesian modeling for predicting *Oncomelania hupensis* distribution in Eryuan County, People's Republic of China. Am J Trop Med Hyg, 2009, 81: 416-423.

30. Li ZJ, Ge J, Dai JR, et al. Biology and control of snail intermediate host of *Schistosoma japonicum* in the People's Republic of China. Adv Parasitol, 2016, 92: 197-236.

31. Wang YJ, Rao YH, Wu XX, et al. A method for screening climate change-sensitive infectious diseases. Int J Environ Res Public Health, 2015, 12: 767-783.

32. Liu L, Yang GJ, Zhu HR, et al. Knowledge of, attitudes towards, and practice relating to schistosomiasis in two subtypes of a mountainous region of the People's Republic of China. Infect Dis Poverty, 2014, 3: 16.

33. Salam RA, Maredia H, Das JK, et al. Community-based interventions for the prevention and control of helmintic neglected tropical diseases. Infect Dis Poverty, 2014, 3: 23.

34. Lin DD, Liu JX, Liu YM, et al. Routine Kato–Katz technique underestimates the prevalence of *Schistosoma japonicum*: a case study in an endemic area of the People's Republic of China. Parasitol Int, 2008, 57: 281-286.

35. Spear R, Seto E, Carlton E, et al. The challenge of effective surveillance in moving from low transmission to elimination of schistosomiasis in China. Int J Parasitol, 2011, 41: 1243-1247.

36. Xu J, Peeling RW, Chen JX, et al. Evaluation of immunoassays for the diagnosis of *Schistosoma japonicum* infection using archived sera. PLoS Negl Trop Dis, 2011, 5: e949.

37. Zhou XN, Xu J, Chen HG, et al. Tools to support policy decisions related to treatment strategies and surveillance of schistosomiasis japonica towards elimination. PLoS Negl Trop Dis, 2011, 5: e1408.

38. Zhou XN, Wayling S, Bergquist R. Concepts in research capabilities strengthening positive experiences of network approaches by TDR in the People's Republic of China and Eastern Asia. Adv Parasitol, 2010, 73: 1-19.

39. Feng T, Xu J, Hang DR, et al. Conditions of schistosomiasis laboratories at county level. Chin J Schisto Control, 2011, 23: 370-376. (in Chinese)

40. Zhu R, Qin ZQ, Feng T, et al. Assessment of effect and quality control for parasitological tests in national schistosomiasis surveillance sites. Chin J Schisto Control, 2013, 25: 11-15. (in Chinese)

41. Yekutiel P. Problems of epidemiology in malaria eradication. Bull World Health Organ, 1960, 22: 669-683.

42. malERA Consultative Group on Monitoring E. A research agenda for malaria eradication: monitoring, evaluation, and surveillance. PLoS Med, 2011, 8: e1000400.

43. Zhou XN, Bergquist R, Tanner M. Elimination of tropical disease through surveillance and response. Infect Dis Poverty, 2013, 2: 1.

44. Abel L, Dessein AJ. Genetic epidemiology of infectious diseases in humans: design of population-based studies. Emerg Infect Dis, 1998, 4: 593.

45. Schrader M, Hauffe T, Zhang Z, et al. Spatially explicit modeling of schistosomiasis risk in Eastern China based on a synthesis of epidemiological, environmental and intermediate host genetic data: Universitätsbibliothek, 2013.

46. Hamburger J, Abbasi I, Kariuki C, et al. Evaluation of loop-mediated isothermal amplification suitable for molecular monitoring of schistosome-infected snails in field laboratories. Am J Trop Med Hyg, 2013, 88: 344-351.

47. Tong QB, Chen R, Zhang Y, et al. A new surveillance and response tool: risk map of infected Oncomelania hupensis detected by Loop-mediated isothermal amplification (LAMP) from pooled samples. Acta Trop, 2015, 141: 170-177.

48. Wang C, Chen L, Yin X, et al. Application of DNA-based diagnostics in detection of schistosomal DNA in early infection and after drug treatment. Parasit Vectors, 2011, 4: 164.

49. Xu J, Guan ZX, Zhao B, et al. DNA detection of Schistosoma japonicum: diagnostic validity of a LAMP assay for low-intensity infection and effects of chemotherapy in humans. PLoS Negl Trop Dis, 2015, 9: e0003668.

50. Xu J, Rong R, Zhang HQ, et al. Sensitive and rapid detection of Schistosoma japonicum DNA by loop-mediated isothermal amplification (LAMP). Int J Parasitol, 2010, 40: 327-331.

51. Sun LP, Liang YS, Wu HH, et al. A Google Earth-based surveillance system for schistosomiasis japonica implemented in the lower reaches of the Yangtze River, China. Parasit Vectors, 2011, 4: 223.

52. Wang J, Yu CX, Yin XR, et al. Monitoring specific antibody responses against the hydrophilic domain of the 23 kDa membrane protein of Schistosoma japonicum for early detection of infection in sentinel mice. Parasit Vectors, 2011, 4: 172.

53. Yang K, Sun LP, Liang YS, et al. *Schistosoma japonicum* risk in Jiangsu province, People's Republic of China: identification of a spatio-temporal risk pattern along the Yangtze River. Geospat Health, 2013, 8: 133-142.

54. Malone JB, Yang GJ, Leonardo L, et al. Implementing a geospatial health data infrastructure for control of Asian schistosomiasis in the People's Republic of China and the Philippines. Adv Parasitol, 2010, 73: 71-100.

55. Yang GJ, Vounatsou P, Tanner M, et al. Remote sensing for predicting potential habitats of Oncomelania hupensis in Hongze, Baima and Gaoyou lakes in Jiangsu Province, China. Geospatial health, 2006, 1: 85-92.

56. Yang K, Wang XH, Yang GJ, et al. An integrated approach to identify distribution of Oncomelania hupensis, the intermediate host of *Schistosoma japonicum*, in a mountainous region in China. Int J Parasitol, 2008, 38: 1007-1016.

57. Zhang ZY, Xu DZ, Zhou XN, et al. Remote sensing and spatial statistical analysis to predict the distribution of *Oncomelania hupensis* in the marshlands of China. Acta Trop, 2005, 96: 205-212.

58. Yu Q, Wan XX, Liu Q, et al. Cost-effectiveness evaluation and investigation of control measure changes in areas of schistosomiasis transmission control in hilly regions of mountain areas I epidemiological investigation and analysis of prevalence factors of schistosomiasis. Chin J Schisto Control, 2012, 24: 250-254, 365. (in Chinese)

6.4 The response mechanism to the epidemic rebound of schistosomiasis

As one of the most serious epidemic diseases in China, schistosomiasis was endemic in 12 provinces, threatening hundreds of millions of people over the course of history. In these endemic provinces, 11,600 thousand patients and 1,200 thousand cattle were infected with the disease reported in 1950s.[1] With political commitment and strong control efforts, in particular, implementation of the medium- and long-term plan (2004 – 2015) for the prevention and control of schistosomiasis has made great progress over the past six decades. The endemic schistosomiasis areas have been significantly reduced and the lowest levels of infection in both humans and livestock in history have been achieved in recent years. However, due to the epidemiology of S. *japonicum infection*, which is governed by biological, ecological, and socio-economic factors—that is, multiple infection sources, snail hosts that are difficult to eliminate, frequent flooding, and human behavior that contributes to the transmission of the disease—the potential risk that transmission in controlled areas can re-emerge has been recognized. In some areas, where transmission had been interrupted or had already been well controlled, progress levelled off. This resulted in growth of snail-infested areas and reports of newly infected cattle and human cases.

6.4.1   The standard for rebound of schistosomiasis epidemics

The rebound of schistosomiasis epidemics mainly refers to the rebound of the disease and the rebound of snails. Indicators to judge the epidemic rebound of schistosomiasis include the following:

- In areas where schistosomiasis transmission has been interrupted, if there are new local infections of people or domestic animals, or there are infected snails, or snail-infested areas reach 2% of their historical levels, the situation is judged as being in an epidemic rebound.
- In areas where schistosomiasis transmission has been controlled, if there are acute schistosomiasis infections among the local population, or the infection rate of residents or domestic animals (as determined by stool examinations) reaches more than 1%, or snail-infested areas reach 10% of their historical levels, the situation is judged as being in an epidemic rebound.

6.4.2   Factors that influence the rebound of schistosomiasis epidemics

There are many factors that could cause the re-emergence of schistosomiasis in areas where transmission has been controlled or interrupted. These include:

Biological factors

Remnant populations of O. hupensis can easily multiply and cause an endemic rebound.

Natural factors

Flood disasters, returning farmland to lake, large-scale water conservancy and the impact of engineering construction projects on ecological environments can create changes leading to the introduction of exogenous snails or the input of infectious source material and cause an epidemic rebound.

Social factors: Reducing funds in the control programme is an important factor. For instance, after the "World Bank Loan Project for Schistosomiasis Control in China" ended in 2001, funding levels for schistosomiasis control decreased and the professional team for schistosomiasis control shrank by a large margin.

6.4.3   The measures to prevent the rebound of schistosomiasis epidemics

In order to prevent the epidemic rebound of schistosomiasis and consolidate the gained achievements for schistosomiasis control, the following measures should be strengthened.

Snail control

Snail control is still a key task in the foreseeable future. In terms of snail control strategies, remnant snail populations should be monitored and eliminated once found, and the import of exogenous snails should be prevented. On the one hand, survey and mollusciciding activities related to remnant snail populations should be strengthened; on the other hand, the surveillance of imported snails should be improved.

Disease control

For disease control of schistosomiasis, endogenous infection sources should be cleaned up. Exogenous infection sources should be prevented and controlled. Surveillance and control systems for migrating populations and for domestic animals must be established and improved.

Professional team

Schistosomiasis control is a prolonged, complicated, and arduous task. It is therefore necessary to maintain a stable professional team in the elimination or post-elimination stage. The professional team for schistosomiasis control cannot be disbanded. Technical capacity should be strengthened for the staff working in the primary health section.

Funding levels

It is necessary to ensure that there are adequate funding levels for ongoing schistosomiasis surveillance and to consolidate achievements to date. The government should include work and activities related to the surveillance and monitoring of schistosomiasis in the overall planning of economic and social development. The government should organize and coordinate the health, agriculture, animal husbandry, water conservancy, forestry, education, and other relevant departments and ministries. In doing so, the government could facilitate and enable these various agencies to cooperate in schistosomiasis surveillance, and also, consolidate and build on achievements to date.

6.4.4 Establishing a sensitive and efficient early warning mechanism for schistosomiasis

Epidemic focus disposal

Treatment of patients

Health administration departments above the county level should organize the deployment of medical teams to epidemic areas immediately so that further treatment can be delivered when a schistosomiasis outbreak occurs. All schistosomiasis patients should be treated promptly.

Preventive chemotherapy for the population at risk

Based on the principle of early detection, early diagnosis, and early treatment, early preventive chemotherapy for people who have a history of exposure to contaminated water should be carried out. Early treatment should occur on a timeline that corresponds to the same period of exposure to contaminated water in order to prevent an outbreak of acute schistosomiasis. The medicine and time for preventive chemotherapy are as follows. Praziquantel (PZQ) treatment should be used after four weeks from the first contact with infested water.[2] Artemether should be used after two weeks from the first contact with contaminated water.[3] Artesunate should be used after one week from the first contact with contaminated water.[4]

Snail control

Niclosamide should be used to kill snails and cercariae in area where schistosomiasis occurs, including surrounding water and snail habitats. For the spraying technique, the dose is 2 g/m^2; for the immersion technique, the dose is 2 mg/L.[2] At the same time, warning signs in susceptible areas should be posted to delineate both safe and unsafe areas. If conditions permit, the surrounding environment should be changed or altered to restructure or eliminate snail habitats and eradicate snails.

Health education

Health education should be carried out using various types of informative materials and pedagogic approaches to develop awareness of schistosomiasis disease prevention and control among local populations. Knowledge-based activities designed to improve self-defense capabilities and encourage active participation in applying this knowledge should be implemented.

Safe water supply

It should be required that residents get their water from designated safe areas. Sanitary treatments should be undertaken before drinking or using water from those sources that may contain schistosome cercariae. The following method should be used in such areas. For each 50 liters of water, 0.5/g of bleach or 1/g of bleaching powders should be added 30 minutes before drinking.

Manure management

The feces of people and animals that are infected with schistosomiasis require special treatment to ensure that schistosome cercariae are killed. The following egg processing method should be used in such cases. For each 50 kg of feces, 250 g of urea should be mixed in to kill the eggs. The mixture should be stored for more than one day before used for fertilization.

Personal protection

Local residents, along with the general public, should be educated to avoid contact with contaminated water. If people must be in contact with infested water, they should apply water-protective lotions (the main component is dibutyl phthalate) and use proper equipment before contact. Field personnel should pay attention to their personal protection.

Epidemiological surveys

In situations where there is an outbreak of schistosomiasis, an investigation is organized by the national health administration and implemented by profossinals from the county-level disease prevention and control (schistosomiasis) center, along with the county-level animal epidemic prevention and supervision agency. The profossinals from the county-level disease prevention and control (schistosomiasis) agency

323

should arrive at the scene of the outbreak within 24 hours after receiving the report of the outbreak in order to investigate the incident.

Case investigation

Individual investigation should be undertaken for all patients with cases of acute schistosomiasis. A follow-up investigation should also be conducted among other people who were in contact with the contaminated water before and after two weeks in the same location where the patient contracted schistosomiasis. Acute schistosomiasis cases survey table should be established according to the "National Schistosomiasis Monitoring Programme (Trial)". The investigators can also report the acute schistosomiasis cases to a higher-level disease prevention and control (schistosomiasis) agency—whichever approach has the fastest means of communication. At the same time, they should also report the incident to the National Institute of Parasitic Diseases, Chinese Center for Disease Control and Prevention.

Investigation on epidemic focus

Epidemic focus and the scope should be confirmed based on the case study, snails and infected snails should be surveyed. If conditions permit, the infectivity of water should be assayed. The state of water contact should be investigated among local residents and livestock around the epidemic points. Also, examination and treatment should be done among the local residents and livestock.

Investigation of environmental and social factors

Relevant factors such as rainfall, temperature, natural disasters, human and animal migrations, as well as the styles of production and living among residents should be investigated.

6.4.5 Case study: the disposal of new snail areas occurring in Xiangyun County, Dali Prefecture, Yunnan Province

A high prevalence of schistosomiasis in Xiangyun County was found in 1973. Schistosomiasis was epidemic in 12 administrative villages in this county. Historically, there were 37.98 million square meters infested with snails and 547 patients with schistosomiasis, including eight advanced schistosomiasis cases. Xiangyun County attained the criteria of transmission interrupted in 1993. The areas infested with snails were reduced 6.5 million square meters.

When implementing the snail survey in October 2013, snails were found in non-endemic areas in Zhoujia Administrative Village. As a result of the survey, many snails were found in the drainage and irrigation ditches on the north side of the highway. The highest snail density reached 124 per frame $(0.1m^2)$. After 5,491 snails were captured and dissected, the results suggested there was one infected snail.

A series of measures were implemented in response to the risk of a rebound of schistosomiasis epidemic. These measures are as follows.

Snail control

Based on the ongoing snail survey and verification, snail control with a molluscicide was carried out in Zhoujia Administrative Village, which had a high density of snails. Snail eradication was carried out three times. At the same time, weeding, channel dredging, and snail control with a molluscicide were also implemented in three other towns where new snails had been detected. In total, the cumulative area of repeated snail control was 348.33 million square meters using 3,180 kg of niclosamide. The areas of weeding and channel dredging produced a total of 1.41 million square meters of organic material.

Schistosomiasis surveyed among people and livestock

In order to obtain information about infection levels in humans and animals, a simultaneous investigation was carried out. Residents and animals from 19 villages or groups in four administrative villages were surveyed. Human feces were collected to examine by the nylon bag incubation method. A total of 3,011 people were screened by B ultrasound and the inspection rate was 88.0%, including 68 people with liver and spleen abnormalities. A total of 3,081 people underwent stool examination and the inspection rate was 90.2%, with four people diagnosed with schistosomiasis. All of these were females, aged 17 – 40 years old; three were in the main labor force of their families (mainly living by agricultural production) and the other one was a student.

The four infected people had no travel history to areas endemic for schistosomiasis. They were infected when undertaking agricultural production, using no protective measures, around the highway. The family members of these four people were also screened by B ultrasound examination, stool examination, and epidemiological investigation. None of them had a schistosomiasis infection. The living environments and toilets of the four families were treated by disinfection in a timely manner. The four patients were treated with PZQ and 11 of the family members were treated by preventive chemotherapy. The animal husbandry department screened 309 animals using a serological test. Ten livestock suspected to be positive for infection were further examined using the nylon bag incubation method. No infected animals were detected.

Health education

In order to raise public awareness of and knowledge about schistosomiasis control, more than 60,000 pamphlets have been distributed to 17 new and former areas endemic for schistosomiasis. The Bureau of Education was coordinated to establish a health education course about schistosomiasis for students from the primary and middle schools in each of the five administrative villages endemic for schistosomiasis. The Radio and Television Bureau was coordinated to broadcast a science programme about schistosomiasis prevention through Xiangyun TV each day. At the same time, medical and health units carried out a full training on schistosomiasis control and prevention for 206 people.

Reference

1.　Chen MG, Feng Z. Schistosomiasis control in China. Parasitol Int, 1999, 48(1): 11-19.

2.　China MoH. Manual for schistosomiasis control. 3rd ed. Shanghai: Shanghai publishing house for science and technology, 2001. (in Chinese)

3.　Xiao SH, You JQ, Yang YQ, et al. Experimental studies on early treatment of schistosomal infection with artemether. Southeast Asian J Trop Med Public Health, 1995, 26: 306-318.

4.　Xiao SH. Development of antischistosomal drugs in China, with particular consideration to praziquantel and the artemisinins. Acta Trop, 2005, 96: 153-167.

6.5　Challenges and requirements relating to schistosomiasis elimination and post-elimination

Schistosomiasis japonica has been endemic in China for more than 2,100 years.

The first national schistosomiasis survey initiated in 1956 revealed that the disease was endemic in 12 locations (provinces, municipalities, and autonomous regions) south of the Yangtze River. More than 10 million individuals were estimated to be infected with *S. japonicum* and more than 100 million people were at risk of infection in 1950s[1,2]. The number of infected bovines was calculated at 1.2 million, while the total area of *O. hupensis* habitat reached 14.5 billion m[2].[3]

With more than six decades of control efforts and the introduction of highly effective antischistosomal drug therapy in the 1980s, the morbidity and prevalence caused by schistosome infection have significantly decreased. The medium- and long-term national control programme initiated in 2004 accelerated the progress of schistosomiasis control in China. By the end of 2015, the whole country controlled the transmission of schistosomiasis while five provinces reached the criteria of transmission interruption (no local cases and infected livestock in five consecutive years).

In November 2014, the national schistosomiasis control conference was organized at the state council level in Hunan Province. Based on the current achievements, a new goal was put forward to eliminate schistosomiasis nationwide following the approaches laid out in two consecutive five-year plans, which continue with an integrated control strategy.[4]

This section aims to analyze the existing challenges to completely eliminating schistosomiasis and preventing its re-emergence in China, in order to provide guidance for policymakers and research scientists.

6.5.1　Challenges to eliminating schistosomiasis and post-elimination

The life cycle of *Schistosoma* involves its intermediate host, definite host, short time of free live in vitro. Natural, social, and economic factors impact schistosomiasis endemicity. The complexity of schistosomiasis transmission and constraints of current control approaches or techniques mean that there are several challenges to eliminating schistosomiasis and preventing its resurgence post-elimination. These are outlined below.

Extensive and complicated snail habitats

S. japonicum is the only species endemic in China and an amphibious, dioecious *O. hupensis* snail serves its intermediate host. The distribution and density of snails can be impacted by temperature, humidity of the soil, and weed growing. Although snail-infested areas have decreased significantly from 14.5 billion m^2 in the 1950s to about three billion m^2 by 1995, there were 3.6 – 3.8 billion m^2 snail-infested areas nationwide over the past decade. In 2013, 96.5% of all snail habitats were located in marshland and lake regions. Among these areas, 94.3% were distributed outside embankments, where they are easily influenced by water level fluctuations.[5] There is a huge challenge to eliminating snails from such extensive areas with complicated ecological characteristics such as unstable water levels or lush vegetation. Furthermore, agricultural activities, flooding, and water conservancy projects may lead to the snails spreading to urban regions or previously uncolonized areas. Between 2002 and 2010, snails were found in areas previously free of snails, measuring 125 million m^2.[2,6]

Management of different sources of infection

Schistosomiasis prevalence in bovines has reduced to a very low level, but the number of livestock including bovines and goats in endemic areas is significant. Other species, especially rodents, which also play important roles as infection source in lake and mountainous regions, make it difficult to completely eliminate schistosomiasis.[7,8] Fishers and boat people are currently at the highest risk of acquiring schistosome infection, but control programmes among such populations are difficult to implement due to their frequent flow. They may also spread schistosomes to other places where intermediate host snails exist. Medical services also need to take into account other forms of schistosomiasis, e.g. in travelers and workers returning from African countries.[9,10]

Unbalanced implementation of the integrated strategy

Despite the significant economic growth that occurred in China since the reform of the economic system in 1978, there are significant differences between urban and rural areas, western and eastern regions, and lake and mountainous regions.[11,12] Many of the proposed integrated measures such as improving safe water supply and sanitation, mechanization of agriculture, building methane tanks, environmental modification, etc., need substantial funding, which is not available in poor areas. Particularly problematic in the Chinese system is that programmes and interventions are centrally planned, but implementation and financing are largely left up to local governments. Prohibiting grazing in snail habitats has also encountered resistance in some regions as it impacts farmers' benefits because such pastures are communal land, and require no or very limited investments for use.[13]

Unavailability of sensitive tools for elimination certification and surveillance

As the prevalence in intermediate and definitive hosts of *S.japonicum* decreases to a very low level, moving towards elimination requires sensitive diagnostic tools. The current diagnostic strategy is screening patients by immunological assays followed by stool examinations only for antibody-positive individuals. This strategy increases compliance of people receiving examination, but risks missing infected individuals due to the relative insensitivity of the Kato-Katz method and/or miracidium hatching technique in identifying light infections. Consequently, the current prevalence of schistosomiasis is probably underestimated and undetected cases continue to serve as infection sources.[14] Snail surveys and dissection are labor-intensive approaches, which require trained technicians. Diagnostic tools and snail examination based on molecular techniques have a higher sensitivity and specificity than traditional approaches, but they are expensive and their performance and applicability need further field assessment.[15-18]

Weak surveillance and active response system

Biological and social factors related to the transmission of schistosomiasis still exist in many areas where active transmission has ceased. Thus, a re-emergence of schistosomiasis can easily happen once infection sources or intermediate hosts are imported. Although systematic surveillance has been conducted since the 1990s and the current surveillance system covers all endemic counties, the tools have not changed fundamentally and shortcomings such as simple monitoring contents, insensitive indicators, obsolete technologies, and insufficient use of collected data become ever more pressing with the decrease in prevalence. In counties that have been at the stage of transmission control or interruption for many years, the diagnostic and epidemiological survey capacity and the ability to respond to outbreaks decreases due to staff turnover, weak infrastructure, and low training levels. From 2011 to 2013, most of the acute cases that were ultimately reported were initially misdiagnosed and new cases were regularly seen in areas where transmission was thought to have ceased.[5,19,20] Surveillance and particularly the ability to actively respond need to be strengthened to ensure early detection and correct handling of schistosomiasis outbreaks, which would thus accelerate progress towards schistosomiasis elimination nationwide.

6.5.2 Achieving elimination and preventing the re-emergence of schistosomiasis post-elimination

To eliminate schistosomiasis in China, a new national plan has been drafted in late 2015. In this plan, the medium-term goals are to interrupt the transmission of schistosomiasis in more than 90% of the endemic counties and to eliminate schistosomiasis in 75% of the endemic counties by 2020. By 2025, schistosomiasis should be eliminated in 90% of the endemic counties. To overcome the challenges in achieving elimination, the following priorities should be considered for schistosomiasis control activities.

Encouraging governmental leadership and intensifying the responsibilities of related departments

The work of schistosomiasis control involves various governmental departments. The government should strengthen its leadership in the field of planning, design, coordination, assurance, monitoring and management, assessment, etc., and involve schistosomiasis control into its socioeconomics developing plan. To ensure that integrated interventions are practiced, the responsibilities of each related departments should be made clear. The enactment and implementation of the regulations of schistosomiasis control and prevention are accelerating the progress of schistosomiasis control in China, as the regulations defined and intensified the responsibility of various governments and departments in schistosomiasis control activities. In the new phase, activities for schistosomiasis control should be designed and implemented according to the law.

Insisting on a comprehensive control strategy and intensifying integrated interventions

Great achievements made during the last decade prove that the comprehensive control strategy is suitable and could meet the current needs of schistosomiasis control in China. The control activities based on integration of the interventions including chemotherapy, snail control, safe water supply, improving sanitation, environmental modification through water conservancy, agriculture, and forestry projects were beneficial to the management of reservoirs and the control of snails. In the process of schistosomiasis elimination in the future, the central government should continue to play a leadership role in the design of a schistosomiasis elimination programme and an integrated control strategy should be implemented continuously in endemic areas. Interventions such as agriculture mechanization, prohibiting pasture in beaches infested with snails, management of fishers and boat people, innoxious disposal of human, livestock feces, etc., should be strengthened. The local governments should better integrate limited resources and enforce comprehensive interventions on the county, township, or valley levels to maximize the overall benefits of projects and interrupt schistosomiasis transmission.

Improving the surveillance and response system to control risk factors

Experience has shown that schistosomiasis would re-emerge if the control activities stop. To prevent the re-emergence of schistosomiasis, the surveillance and response system should be strengthened through the use of scientific and sensitive techniques. A sensitive and effective surveillance system at the county level should include the following basic elements: it should have specially-assigned persons in charge of schistosomiasis surveillance work; it should detect and effectively respond to an outbreak of schistosomiasis; it should have at least one staff member skilled at diagnosing schistosomiasis; it should have a specially-assigned person responsible for file management and archives reflecting the endemicity of schistosomiasis, and control and surveillance activities; and it should implement surveillance and consolidation activities according to the surveillance plan after the transmission of schistosomiasis has been interrupted. Risk assessment and control activities should be conducted in major endemic areas to find the signs of re-emerging schistosomiasis early and manage possible risk factors in a timely manner. In areas where schistosomiasis has been interrupted or eliminated, surveillance should focus on imported cases and snails-infested areas.

Intensifying health education and health promotion

Health education could improve the awareness of residents to get examinations and treatment, and to change their behavior, which in turn can decrease their chances of becoming infected. Currently (when there is a very low prevalence), the willingness of people to receive examinations is decreasing yearly. To overcome this problem and eliminate schistosomiasis, health education should be conducted in endemic areas through various ways such as TV, broadcast, internet, newspapers, etc. To guide the population in developing healthy habits and improving consciousness and self-protection, propaganda and behavioral interventions should focus on high-risk groups such as school-aged children, fishers, boat people, and other mobile populations.

Strengthening scientific research and capacity building to popularization and implementation of new techniques

Breakthrough of key techniques for schistosomiasis control and prevention is needed to eliminate schistosomiasis nationwide. To realize this, scientific research on schistosomiasis, especially applied science, should be strengthened and included in the national research programme. Joint multi-sector and multi-discipline research should be conducted. These should focus on epidemiology and surveillance tools, methods of assessing the effectiveness of interventions, the environment and social ecology, information system and early warning models, as well as basic biology. A batch of new techniques and products appropriate for eliminating schistosomiasis such as rapid diagnostic assays, environmental protecting molluscicides, and sensitive surveillance and monitoring techniques should be developed and implemented. To import and popularize these sorts of techniques from foreign countries, international collaboration and communication should be strengthened. Meanwhile, capacity building of control staff should be intensified to consolidate achievements and prevent the re-emergence of schistosomiasis in endemic areas. The working conditions of the control agencies should be improved and the equipment of laboratories should be updated accordingly. To improve skills of staff for schistosomiasis control and prevention, training courses and rehearsals of schistosomiasis outbreaks should be conducted.

It is believed that multiple-component, integrated control programmes incorporating PZQ treatment with transmission reduction through other control measures, such as use of molluscicides, environmental modification, health education and promotion, as well as improved sanitation, is the best option for schistosomiasis control and elimination. Even if only partly effective, antischistosomal vaccines, incorporated as part of an integrated control strategy, are needed to accelerate efforts to eliminate a disease that has existed for at least two millennia. This integrated approach model has the potential to improve the health of a billion of the world's poorest people, and its effect cannot and should not be underestimated.

References

1. Wang HZ, Jia YD, Guo JP, et al. A histroric review or 40 years' control on schistosomiasis in P.R. China. Chin J Schisto Contr, 1989, 1(3): 1-4. (in Chinese)

2. Xia C, Wang HZ. The endemic status and control of schistosomiasis. Bull Biol, 1989, 9: 26-27.

3. Chen MG. Progress in schistosomiasis control in China. Chin Med J (Engl), 1999, 112: 930-933.

4. Lei ZL, Zhou XN. Eradication of schistosomiasis: a new target and a new task for the national schistosomiasis control program in the People's Republic of China. Chin J Schisto Contr, 2015, 27: 1-4. (in Chinese)

5. Lei ZL, Zheng H, Zhang LJ, et al. Endemic status of schitosomiasis in People's Republic of

China in 2013. Chin J Schisto Contr, 2014, 26: 591-597. (in Chinese)

6. Wang Q, Xu J, Zhang LJ, et al. Analysis of endemic changes of schistosomiasis in China from 2002 to 2010. Chin J Schisto Contr, 2015, 27: 229-34, 250. (in Chinese)

7. Lu DB, Wang TP, Rudge JW, et al. Contrasting reservoirs for *Schistosoma japonicum* between marshland and hilly regions in Anhui, China - a two-year longitudinal parasitological survey. Parasitology, 2010, 137: 99-110.

8. Guo Y, Jiang M, Gu L, et al. Prevalence of *Schistosoma japonicum* in wild rodents in five islands of the west Dongting Lake, China. J Parasitol, 2013, 99: 706-707.

9. Zhu R, Xu J. Epidemic situation of oversea imported schistosomiasis in China and thinking about its prevention and control. Chin J Schisto Contr, 2014, 26: 111-114. (in Chinese)

10. Wang W, Liang YS, Hong QB, Dai JR. African schistosomiasis in mainland China: risk of transmission and countermeasures to tackle the risk. Parasit Vectors, 2013, 6: 249.

11. Bian Y, Sun Q, Zhao Z, Blas E. Market reform: a challenge to public health--the case of schistosomiasis control in China. Int J Health Plann Manage, 2004, 19: S79-S94.

12. Tang S, Meng Q, Chen L, et al. Tackling the challenges to health equity in China. Lancet, 2008, 372: 1493-1501.

13. He HB. Thought of schistosomiasis control strategy with emphasis on controlling sources of infection in lake and marshland endemic regions. Chin J Schisto Contr, 2011, 23: 710-713. (in Chinese)

14. Zhou XN, Xu J, Chen HG, et al. Tools to support policy decisions related to treatment strategies and surveillance of schistosomiasis japonica towards elimination. PLoS Negl Trop Dis, 2011, 5: e1408.

15. Xia CM, Rong R, Lu ZX, et al. *Schistosoma japonicum*: a PCR assay for the early detection and evaluation of treatment in a rabbit model. Exp Parasitol, 2009, 121: 175-179.

16. Xia J, Yuan Y, Xu X, et al. Evaluating the effect of a novel molluscicide in the endemic schistosomiasis japonica area of China. Int J Environ Res Public Health, 2014, 11: 10406-18.

17. Xu J, Rong R, Zhang HQ, et al. Sensitive and rapid detection of *Schistosoma japonicum* DNA by loop-mediated isothermal amplification (LAMP). Int J Parasitol, 2010, 40: 327-331.

18. Tong Q, Chen R, Zhang Y, et al. A new surveillance and response tool: Risk map of infected *Oncomelania hupensis* detected by Loop-mediated isothermalamplification (LAMP) from pooled samples. Acta Trop, 2015, 141: 170-177.

19. Zheng H, Zhang LJ, Zhu R, et al. Schistosomiasis situation in People's Republic of China in 2011. Chin J Schisto Contr, 2012, 24: 621-626. (in Chinese)

20. Li SZ, Zheng H, Gao J, et al. Endemic status of schistosomiasis in People's Republic of China in 2012. Chin J Schisto Contr, 2013, 25(6): 557-563. (in Chinese)

图书在版编目（CIP）数据

中国公共卫生. 热带病防治实践. 血吸虫病 = Tropical
Diseases in China: Schistosomiasis: 英文 / 周晓农主编. —北京：
人民卫生出版社, 2018

ISBN 978-7-117-25999-6

Ⅰ. ①中… Ⅱ. ①周… Ⅲ. ①血吸虫病－防治－中国－
英文 Ⅳ. ①R532.21

中国版本图书馆 CIP 数据核字（2018）第 021049 号

| 人卫智网 | www.ipmph.com | 医学教育、学术、考试、健康，购书智慧智能综合服务平台 |
| 人卫官网 | www.pmph.com | 人卫官方资讯发布平台 |

中国公共卫生：热带病防治实践：血吸虫病（英文）

主　　编：周晓农
出版发行：人民卫生出版社（中继线 010-59780011）
地　　址：北京市朝阳区潘家园南里 19 号
邮　　编：100021
E - mail: pmph @ pmph.com
购书热线：010-59787592　010-59787584　010-65264830
印　　刷：北京盛通印刷股份有限公司
经　　销：新华书店
开　　本：710×1000　1/16　印张：22
字　　数：383 千字
版　　次：2018 年 6 月第 1 版　2018 年 6 月第 1 版第 1 次印刷
标准书号：ISBN 978-7-117-25999-6/R·26000
打击盗版举报电话：010-59787491　E-mail: WQ @ pmph.com
（凡属印装质量问题请与本社市场营销中心联系退换）